# QUICK GUIDE TO
## BENEFITS AND TASTE
# PROFILES OF HERBS

Jodi Walker

LEGAL DISCLAIMER:  The contents of this book are for educational and informational purposes only.  We cannot diagnose health conditions or prescribe medications.  This information is not intended to be a substitute for medical treatment.   Consult your physician or medical care provider before using herbs.  Especially if you have an existing medical condition, take prescription medications, or are pregnant or nursing.

People can react differently to a variety of herbs, including allergic reactions.  The use of herbs may interfere with the effectiveness of other medications.  Some herbs may be confused with harmful substances, and can have adverse or deadly consequences.

Considering the issues mentioned you should consult with your medical professional before using herbs.  Your medical professional can discuss diagnosis and treatment options with you.

SUMMARY:  This book is for educational and reference purposes.  This guide will enable anyone to quickly look up the potential benefits of herbs.  It also has information on taste profiles and if an herb has culinary applications.  The guide is comprised of charts that list the herbs alphabetically, or by categories.  Compiling this information in chart form makes it quicker and easier to find particular details on each herb.

Quick Guide To Benefits And Taste Profiles Of Herbs

# CONTENTS

# SECTION I

Benefits and Details of Herbs

| *Adaptogens* | Enhances resilience to stress and supports overall health. | |
| --- | --- | --- |
| **Herb** | **Scientific Name** | **Benefits** |
| American Ginseng | Panax quinquefolius | Stress resilience, energy, cognition, immunity. |
| American Skullcap | Scutellaria lateriflora | Calmness, relaxation, anxiety. |
| Ashwagandha | Withania somnifera | Stress resilience, energy, immunity. |
| Astragalus | Astragalus membranaceus | Immunity, vitality. |
| Basil | Ocimum basilicum | Stress, immunity. |
| Black Cohosh | Actaea racemosa | Hot flashes, mood swings, sleep disturbances. |
| Cordyceps | Cordyceps sinensis | Energy, endurance, immunity. |
| Eleuthero | Eleutherococcus senticosus | Stamina, resilience. |
| Ginkgo Biloba | Ginkgo Biloba | Cognition, circulation. |
| Gotu Kola | Centella asiatica | Cognition, circulation. |
| Hawthorn | Crataegus app. | Blood pressure, blood flow, heart health. |
| Holy Basil | Ocimum sanctum | Stress, immunity. |
| Indian Gooseberry | Emblica officinalis | Antioxidant, immunity. |
| Jiaogulan | Gynostemma pentaphyllum | Longevity. |
| Kava Kava | Piper methysticum | Relaxation. |
| Korean Ginseng | Panax ginseng | Energy, cognition, immunity. |
| Lemon Balm | Melissa officinalis | Calmness. |
| Licorice Root | Glycyrrhiza glabra | Adrenals. |
| Maca Root | Lepidium meyenii | Energy, hormones. |
| Milk Thistle | Silybum marianum | Liver health. |
| Mucuna Pruriens | Velvet Bean | Mood. |
| Nasturtium | Tropaeolum majus | Helps the body cope with stress. |
| Panax Ginseng | Panax spp. | Energy, cognition, stamina. |
| Passionflower | Passiflora incarnata | Relaxation. |
| Puncture Vine | Tribulus Terrestris | Vitality. |
| Reishi mushrooms | Ganoderma lucidum | Immunity, relaxation. |
| Rhodiola | Rhodiola rosea | Endurance, mood. |
| Saffron | Crocus sativus | Mood. |
| Schisandra | Schisandra chinensis | Endurance, liver. |
| Shilajit | Asphaltum | Vitality. |
| Siberian Ginseng | Eleutherococcus senticosus | Stamina, endurance. |
| Suma | Pfaffia paniculata | Energy. |
| Tulsi | Ocimum sanctum | Stress, immunity. |
| Turmeric | Curcuma longa | Inflammation. |
| Valerian | Valeriana officinalis | Relaxation. |

| *Alterative* | Helps achieve another condition by cleansing the blood & overall detoxification. | |
|---|---|---|
| **Herb** | **Scientific Name** | **Benefits** |
| Alfalfa | Medicago Sativa | Detoxification.  Supports kidney and liver function. |
| Aloe Vera | Aloe barbadensis miller | Healing and repairing skin. |
| Blue Flag | Iris versicolor | Lymphatic cleansing, skin health. |
| Burdock | Arctium lappa | Detoxification.  Supports kidney and liver function. |
| Calendula | Calendula officinalis | Promotes detoxification, skin health. |
| Chaparral | Larea tridentata | Detoxification.  Supports liver function. |
| Cleavers | Galium aparine | Lymphatic cleansing. |
| Comfrey | Symphytum officinale | Tissue repair and healing. |
| Dandelion | Taraxacum officinale | Detoxification.  Supports kidney and liver function. |
| Echinacea | Echinacea purpurea | Immunity. |
| Garlic | Allium sativum | Immunity. |
| Horsetail | Equisetum arvense | Diuretic. |
| Licorice | Glycyrrhiza glabra | Adrenal function.  Endocrine health. |
| Lovage | Levisticum officinale | Supports purification and detoxification. |
| Marshmallow | Althea officinalis | Inflammation in respiratory & digestive systems. |
| Nasturtium | Tropaeolum majus | Cleanses the blood and supports detoxification. |
| Nettles | Urtica dioica | Nutritive. |
| Oregon Grape Root | Mahonia aquifolium | Liver support and function.  Detoxification. |
| Plantain | Plantago spp. | Detoxification. |
| Poke Root | Phytolacca americana | Lymphatic cleansing. |
| Prickly Ash | Zanthoxylum spp. | Stimulate circulation. |
| Purslane | Portulaca oleracea | Cleanses and restores the metabolic processes. |
| Sarsaparilla | Smilax spp. | Detoxification. |
| Uva Ursi | Arctostaphylos uva ursi | Diuretic. |
| Wild Indigo | Baptisia tinctoria | Immunity. |
| Yellow Dock | Rumex crispus | Blood purifying. |

| Amphoteric | Balances bodily functions and have a regulatory effect on various body systems. Many adaptogens have amphoteric or normalizing properties. | |
|---|---|---|
| **Herb** | **Scientific Name** | **Benefits** |
| Ashwagandha | Withania somnifera | Balancing. |
| Ashitaba | Angelica keiskei koidzumi | Adaptogenic. |
| Astragalus | Astragalus membranaceus | Immunity. |
| Cayenne | Capsicum annuum | Stimulating and calming the circulatory system. |
| Chlorella | Chlorella vulgaris | Detoxification. |
| Cordyceps | Cordyceps sinensis | Energizing. |
| Ginseng | Panax spp. | Energizing. |
| Gotu Kola | Centella asiatica | Mental clarity, stress. |
| Holy Basil | Ocimum sanctum | Adaptogenic.  Stress, immunity. |
| Licorice | Glycyrrhiza glabra | Balancing. |
| Maca | Lepidium meyenii | Balancing. |
| Milk Thistle | Silybum marianum | Protects liver from toxins and detoxifies. |
| Nasturtium | Tropaeolum majus | Helps balance and harmonize bodily functions. |
| Purslane | Portulaca oleracea | Balancing. |
| Rhodiola | Rhodiola rosea | Stress, energy, mental clarity. |
| Savory | Satureja | Balancing. |
| Schisandra | Schisandra chinensis | Stimulating.  Focus, stress related fatigue. |
| Spirulina | Arthrospira platensis | Nutrient rich. |
| Turmeric | Curcuma longa | Antioxidant. |

| Analgesic | Decrease pain when taken internally.<br>Some herbs which decrease pain are also antispasmodics or nervines. | |
|---|---|---|
| **Herb** | **Scientific Name** | **Benefits** |
| Arnica | Arnica Montana | Muscle aches, bruises, joint pain. |
| Aspen | Populus grandidentata | Headache, mild pain. |
| Baneberry | Actaea rubra | Mild pain. |
| Birch | Betula pendula | Muscle, joint discomfort. |
| Black Cohosh | Actaea racemosa | Menopausal symptoms. |
| Boswellia | Boswellia serrata | Pain, inflammation, osteoarthritis. |
| Cardamom | Elettaria caramomum | Migraines, headaches. |
| Cayenne | Capsicum annuum | Muscle, joint pain. |
| Chamomile | Matricaria chamomilla | Muscle, inflammation, headache, menstrual cramps. |
| Clematis | Ranunculaceae | Anti-inflammatory, joint pain. |
| Cloves | Syzygium aromaticum | Dental pain, sore throat. |
| Devil's Claw | Harpagophytum procumbens | Inflammation, arthritis, back pain. |
| Feverfew | Tanacetum parthenium | Migraines, headaches. |
| Ginger | Zingiber officinale | Muscle soreness, menstrual cramps. |
| Kava Kava | Piper methysticum | Manage pain from stress and tension. |
| Lavender | Lavandula angustifolia | Headache, muscle tension, mild pain. |
| Marjoram | Origanum marjorana | Provides relief from pains and soothes discomfort. |
| Oregano | Origanum vulgare | Headaches, mild pain. |
| Peppermint | Mentha piperita | Headaches, mild pain. |
| Poplar | Populus tremula | Muscle, joint discomfort. |
| Rosemary | Rosmarinus officinalis | Headaches, mild pain. |
| Sage | Salvia officinalis | Headaches, mild pain. |
| Savory | Satureja | Alleviates pain and discomfort. |
| Skullcap | Scutellaria lateriflora | Tension headaches, pain from stress. |
| Turmeric | Curcuma longa | Pain, inflammation, muscle soreness, osteoarthritis. |
| White Willow Bark | Salix alba | Headaches, mild pain, inflammation. |
| Willow | Salix | Headaches, mild pain, inflammation. |
| Yarrow | Achillea millefolium | Headaches, mild pain, inflammation. |

| **Anodyne** | Alleviate pain, soothe discomfort, or provide relief from various painful conditions. A local anesthesia when applied topically. | |
| --- | --- | --- |
| **Herb** | **Scientific Name** | **Benefits** |
| Arnica | Arnica Montana | Muscle aches, bruises, joint pain. |
| Black Cohosh | Actaea racemosa | Menopausal symptoms. |
| Boswellia | Boswellia serrata | Pain, inflammation, osteoarthritis. |
| Cayenne | Capsicum annuum | Muscle, joint pain. |
| Chamomile | Matricaria chamomilla | Muscle, inflammation, headache, menstrual cramps. |
| Cloves | Syzygium aromaticum | Dental pain, sore throat. |
| Devil's Claw | Harpagophytum procumbens | Inflammation, arthritis, back pain. |
| Kava Kava | Piper methysticum | Manage pain from stress and tension. |
| Lavender | Lavandula angustifolia | Headache, muscle tension, mild pain. |
| Marjoram | Origanum marjorana | Provides relief from pains and soothes discomfort. |
| Savory | Satureja | Alleviates pain and discomfort. |
| Skullcap | Scutellaria lateriflora | Tension headaches, pain from stress. |
| Turmeric | Curcuma longa | Pain, inflammation, muscle soreness, osteoarthritis. |
| White Willow Bark | Salix alba | Headaches, mild pain, inflammation. |
| Yarrow | Achillea millefolium | Headaches, mild pain, inflammation. |

| **Antacids & Anti-ulcers** | Herbs that decrease stomach acid and minimize ulcer formation. | |
|---|---|---|
| **Herb** | **Scientific Name** | **Benefits** |
| Calendula | Calendula officinalis | Anti-inflammatory helps heal ulcers with comfrey. |
| Chamomile | Matricaria chamomilla | Effective for digestive issues brought on by stress. |
| Comfrey | Symphytum officinale | Useful for ulcerations in duodenal ulcers or colitis. |
| Fenugreek seeds | Trigonella foenumgraecum | Supports digestion. |
| Gotu Kola | Centella asiatica | Promotes healing of ulcers. |
| Licorice | Glycyrrhiza glabra | Excellent for ulcers.  Anti-inflammatory, demulcent. |
| Meadowsweet | Filipendula ulmaria | Reduces acidity.  Good for duodenal ulcers. |
| Milk Thistle | Silybum marianum | Aids digestion to alleviate indigestion and bloating. |
| Turmeric | Curcuma longa | Gastrointestinal health. |

| Anthelmintics | Herbs to treat or expel parasitic worms from the body. | |
|---|---|---|
| **Herb** | **Scientific Name** | **Benefits** |
| Black Walnut Hull | Juglans Nigra | Intestinal health and parasite control. |
| Bitter Leaf | Vernonia amygdalina | Digestive health. |
| Boldo | Peumus boldus | Digestive health. |
| Caraway | Carum carvi | Digestive health. |
| Cascarilla | Croton eluteria | Digestive health. |
| Chenopodium Oil | Chenopodium anthelminticum | Gastrointestinal health. |
| Cloves | Syzygium aromaticum | Digestive health. |
| Elecampane | Inula helenium | Gastrointestinal health. |
| Garlic | Allium sativum | Digestive health. |
| Ginger | Zingiber officinale | Digestive health. |
| Hyssop | Hyssopus officinalis | Gastrointestinal health. |
| Male Fern | Dryopteris filix-mas | Digestive health. |
| Neem | Azadirachta | Digestive health. |
| Papaya Seed | Carica Papaya | Digestive health. |
| Pomegranate | Punica granatum | Gastrointestinal health. |
| Pumpkin Seed | Cucurbita pepo | Digestive health. |
| Rue | Ruta graveolens | Digestive health. |
| Savory | Satureja | Expel or eliminate parasitic worms. |
| Sesame Seeds | Sesamum indicum | Digestive health. |
| Tansy | Tanacetum vulgare | Digestive health. |
| Thyme | Thymus Vulgaris | Digestive health. |
| Turmeric | Curcuma longa | Gastrointestinal health. |
| Wormseed | Chenopodium ambrosioides | Digestive health. |
| Wormwood | Artemisia absinthium | Digestive health. |

| Antibiotic | Herbs that can inhibit or kill bacteria, fungi, or other microorganisms. | |
|---|---|---|
| **Herb** | **Scientific Name** | **Benefits** |
| Allspice | Pimenta dioica | Inhibits the growth and spread of bacteria. |
| Andrographis | Andrographis paniculata | Inhibits the growth and spread of bacteria. |
| Anise Seeds | Pimpinella anisum | Inhibits the growth and spread of bacteria. |
| Basil | Ocimum basilicum | Inhibits the growth and spread of bacteria. |
| Barberry | Berberis vulgaris | Inhibits the growth and spread of bacteria. |
| Bay Leaves | Laurus nobilis | Inhibits the growth and spread of bacteria. |
| Bergamot | Monarda fistulosa | Inhibits the growth and spread of bacteria. |
| Black Pepper | Piper nigrum | Inhibits the growth of bacteria. |
| Calendula | Calendula officinalis | Promotes wound healing, soothe skin irritations. |
| Cayenne | Capsicum annuum | Inhibits the growth and spread of bacteria. |
| Chamomile | Matricaria chamomilla | Promotes wound healing, soothe skin irritations. |
| Chaparral | Larea tridentata | Combats bacterial infections. |
| Cinnamon | Cinnamomum verum | Inhibits the growth of bacteria. |
| Cranberry | Vaccinium macrocarpon | Inhibits bacteria adhering to the urinary tract lining. |
| Echinacea | Echinacea purpurea | Boosts immunity to combat bacterial/viral infection. |
| Elecampane | Inula helenium | Combat bacterial infections. |
| Fennel seeds | Foeniculum vulgare | Combat bacterial infections. |
| Garden Sage | Salvia officinalis | Inhibits the growth and spread of bacteria. |
| Garlic | Allium sativum | Combat bacterial infections. |
| Ginger | Zingiber officinale | Inhibit the growth of bacteria. |
| Gentian | Gentiana spp. | Combat bacterial infections. |
| Goldenseal | Hydrastis canadensis | Inhibit bacterial growth. |
| Gumweed | Grindelia integrifolia | Combat bacterial infections, esp. respiratory or skin. |
| Juniper Berries | Juniperus communis | Combat bacterial infection, esp. digestive or urinary. |
| Lovage | Levisticum officinale | Inhibits the growth and spread of bacteria. |
| Marjoram | Origanum marjorana | Mild antibacterial properties |
| Myrrh | Commiphora myrrha | Mild antibacterial properties |
| Nasturtium | Tropaeolum majus | Helps combat certain bacteria. |
| Neem | Azadirachta | Combat bacterial and fungal infections, esp. skin. |
| Olive Leaf | Olea europaea | Inhibits bacterial growth. |
| Onion | Allium cepa | Inhibits bacterial growth. |
| Oregano | Origanum vulgare | Combat bacteria, esp. respiratory or digestive. |
| Oregon Grape | Mahonia aquifolium | Combat bacterial infections. |
| Pau d'Arco | Tabebuia spp. | Combat bacterial and fungal infections. |
| Peppermint | Mentha piperita | Combat bacteria/fungus, esp. respiratory/digestive. |
| Plantain | Plantago spp. | Combat bacterial and fungal infections. |
| Purslane | Portulaca oleracea | Inhibits the growth or kills bacteria. |
| Rosemary | Rosmarinus officinalis | Combat bacterial infections. |
| Rue | Ruta graveolens | Combat bacterial infections. |
| Sage | Salvia officinalis | Inhibit the growth or kill bacteria. |
| Savory | Satureja | Inhibit the growth or kill bacteria. |
| St. John's Wort | Hypericum perforatum | Combat bacterial and viral infections. |
| Sweet Cicely | Myrrhis odorata | Mild antibacterial properties |
| Thyme | Thymus Vulgaris | Combat bacteria/fungus, esp. respiratory/digestive. |
| Turmeric | Curcuma longa | Combat bacterial and fungal infections. |
| Usnea | Usnea spp | Combat bacterial and fungal infections. |
| Uva Ursi | Arctostaphylos uva ursi | Inhibits bacterial growth in the urinary tract. |
| Wormwood | Artemisia absinthium | Combat bacterial and fungal infections. |
| Yarrow | Achillea millefolium | Combat bacterial/fungal infections, esp. in wounds. |

| Anticatarrhal | Useful in reducing or eliminating mucus from the respiratory tract. | |
|---|---|---|
| Herb | Scientific Name | Benefits |
| Cayenne | Capsicum annuum | Reduces mucus and congestion. |
| Chickweed | Stellaria media | Alleviates mucus and congestion. |
| Coltsfoot | Tussilago farfara | Relieves mucus and congestion. |
| Elder | Sambucus nigra | Reduces mucus/congestion, cold/allergy relief. |
| Elecampane | Inula helenium | Relieves mucus and congestion. |
| Eucalyptus | Eucalyptus spp. | Alleviates mucus and congestion, esp. colds. |
| Fenugreek | Trigonella foenum-graecum | Reduces mucus and congestion, esp. colds. |
| Garden Sage | Salvia officinalis | Reduces excess mucus and alleviates congestion. |
| Garlic | Allium sativum | Reduces mucus and congestion, esp. cold & flus. |
| Ginger | Zingiber officinale | Reduces mucus and congestion, esp. cold & flus. |
| Goldenrod | Solidago | Reduces mucus and congestion. |
| Hyssop | Hyssopus officinalis | Reduces mucus and congestion. |
| Irish Moss | Chondrus Crispus | Reduces mucus and congestion, esp. colds. |
| Licorice | Glycyrrhiza glabra | Reduces mucus and congestion, esp. colds. |
| Lovage | Levisticum officinale | Alleviate mucus & congestion in respiratory tract. |
| Marshmallow Root | Althaea officinalis | Reduces mucus and congestion, esp. colds. |
| Marjoram | Origanum marjorana | May aid in the relief of mucus related conditions. |
| Nasturtium | Tropaeolum majus | Alleviates mucus & respiratory congestion. |
| Nettle | Urtica dioica | Reduces mucus and congestion, esp. colds. |
| Oregano | Origanum vulgare | Reduces mucus and congestion, esp. colds. |
| Peppermint | Mentha piperita | Reduces mucus and congestion, esp. colds. |
| Purslane | Portulaca oleracea | Alleviate & prevent the buildup of excess mucus. |
| Sage | Salvia officinalis | Reduces mucus and congestion, esp. colds. |
| Savory | Satureja | Alleviates or prevents excess mucus. |
| Thyme | Thymus vulgaris | Reduces mucus and congestion, esp. colds. |
| Uva ursi | Arctostaphylos uva ursi | Reduces mucus and congestion, esp. colds. |
| Yarrow | Achillea millefolium | Reduces mucus and congestion, esp. colds. |

| Antiemetics | Alleviates nausea and vomiting. | |
|---|---|---|
| **Herb** | **Scientific Name** | **Benefits** |
| Basil | Ocimum basilicum | Digestive discomfort and motion sickness. |
| Black Horehound | Ballota nigra | Motion and morning sickness. |
| Cannabis | Cannabis sativa | Chemotherapy and digestive disorders. |
| Cardamom | Elettaria caramomum | Manages digestive discomfort and motion sickness. |
| Catnip | Nepeta cataria | Relieves digestive discomfort and motion sickness. |
| Chamomille | Matricaria chamomilla | Manages digestive discomfort and motion sickness. |
| Cilantro | Coriandrum sativum | Manages digestive discomfort and motion sickness. |
| Cinnamon | Cinnamomum verum | Relieves digestive discomfort and motion sickness. |
| Cinquefoil | Potentilla spp. | Relieves digestive discomfort and motion sickness. |
| Clove | Syzygium aromaticum | Relieves digestive discomfort and motion sickness. |
| Coriander | Coriandrum sativum | Manages digestive discomfort and motion sickness. |
| Dill | Anethum graveolens | Relieves digestive discomfort and motion sickness. |
| Fennel seeds | Foeniculum vulgare | Manages digestive discomfort and motion sickness. |
| Ginger | Zingiber officinale | Relieves digestive discomfort and motion sickness. |
| Horehound | Marrubium vulgare | Relieves digestive discomfort and motion sickness. |
| Lavender | Lavandula angustifolia | Manages digestive discomfort and motion sickness. |
| Lemon Balm | Melissa officinalis | Relieves digestive discomfort and motion sickness. |
| Lovage | Levisticum officinale | Aids in reducing nausea and vomiting. |
| Marshmallow Root | Althaea officinalis | Relieves digestive discomfort and motion sickness. |
| Meadowsweet | Filipendula ulmaria | Manages digestive discomfort and motion sickness. |
| Mint | Mentha spp. | Relieves digestive discomfort and motion sickness. |
| Nasturtium | Tropaeolum majus | Mitigate nausea & vomiting. Aid digestive comfort. |
| Peppermint | Mentha piperita | Relieves digestive discomfort and motion sickness. |
| Purslane | Portulaca oleracea | Alleviate nausea and vomiting. |
| Savory | Satureja | Alleviate nausea and vomiting. |
| Spearmint | Mentha piperita | Relieves digestive discomfort and motion sickness. |

| Antifungal | Kill or inhibit the growth of fungi or yeasts. | |
|---|---|---|
| **Herb** | **Scientific Name** | **Benefits** |
| Aloe Vera | Aloe barbadensis miller | Topical application inhibits fungal infection growth. |
| Anise Seeds | Pimpinella anisum | Fight fungal infection, promote oral/digestive health. |
| Basil | Ocimum basilicum | Used internally or topically for fungal infections. |
| Bay Leaves | Laurus nobilis | Used internally or topically for fungal infections. |
| Bee Balm | Monarda | Fight fungal infections & promotes skin/nail health. |
| Bergamot | Monarda fistulosa | Used internally or topically for fungal infections. |
| Black Walnut Hull | Juglans Nigra | Treat fungal infections & promotes skin/nail health. |
| Burdock Root | Arctium lappa | Treat fungal infection & promote skin/scalp health. |
| Calendula | Calendula officinalis | Treat fungal skin infections & promote skin healing. |
| Chamomile | Matricaria chamomilla | Soothes and treats fungal skin conditions. |
| Chaparral | Larea tridentata | Treat fungal skin infections & promote skin health. |
| Cinnamon | Cinnamomum verum | Fight fungal infection, promote oral/digestive health. |
| Clove | Syzygium aromaticum | Combats fungal infections, especially in mouth/nails. |
| Echinacea | Echinacea spp. | Fights fungal infections & supports overall health. |
| Fennel seeds | Foeniculum vulgare | Combat fungal infections. |
| Fireweed | Chamaenerion angustifolium | Treats fungal skin infections & supports skin health. |
| Garden Sage | Salvia officinalis | Inhibits the growth of fungi. |
| Garlic | Allium sativum | Combats fungal infections, including skin and nails. |
| Goldenseal | Hydrastis canadensis | Treat fungal infection, esp mucous membranes/skin. |
| Lemon Grass | Cymbopogon citratus | Treat fungal infections & promotes skin/nail health. |
| Myrrh | Commiphora myrrha | Treat fungal infections, especially on skin and nails. |
| Nasturtium | Tropaeolum majus | Inhibits the growth of fungi. |
| Neem | Azadirachta indica | Combat fungal infection, especially on skin and nails. |
| Onion | Allium cepa | Inhibits the growth of fungi. |
| Oregano | Origanum vulgare | Combats fungal infection, promotes overall health. |
| Oregon Grape | Mahonia aquifolium | Treat fungal infection, esp mucous membranes/skin. |
| Pau d'Arco | Tabebuia spp | Treat fungal infections & promotes skin/nail health. |
| Purslane | Portulaca oleracea | Inhibits the growth of fungi. |
| Rosemary | Rosmarinus officinalis | Address fungal skin infections & promote skin health |
| Sage | Salvia officinalis | Treat fungal infection, esp. mucous membranes/skin |
| Savory | Satureja | Inhibits the growth of fungi. |
| Sweet Cicely | Myrrhis odorata | Treat fungal infections, especially on skin and nails. |
| Sweet Root | Acorus calumus | Combat fungal infections & promotes overall health. |
| Tea Tree Oil | Melaleuca alternifolia | Treats fungal infections on the skin and nails. |
| Thyme | Thymus vulgaris | Address fungal skin infections & promote skin health |

| Antihemorrhagic & Hemostatic | Helps control, reduce or stop bleeding. | |
| --- | --- | --- |
| **Herb** | **Scientific Name** | **Benefits** |
| Blackberry | Rubus fruticosus | Aids blood clotting and prevents excessive bleeding. |
| Black Haw | Viburnum prunifolium | Reduce excessive menstrual bleeding. Stop bleeding. |
| Bloodroot | Sanguinaria canadensis | Reduces bleeding, and promotes wound healing. |
| Calendula | Calendula officinalis | Useful for minor cuts and wounds. |
| Cayenne | Capsicum annuum | Reduces bleeding, and promotes wound healing. |
| Comfrey | Symphytum officinale | Reduces bleeding, and promotes wound healing. |
| Cranesbill | Geranium maculatum | Reduces bleeding. |
| Cypress | Cupressus spp. | Reduces bleeding, and promotes wound healing. |
| Germander | Teucrium chamaedrys | Manages bleeding, and minor injuries. |
| Horsemint | Monarda punctata | Manages bleeding, and minor injuries. |
| Horsetail | Equisetum arvense | Aids in cessation of bleeding and wound healing. |
| Lady's Mantle | Alchemilla vulgaris | Reduces bleeding and promotes wound healing. |
| Lamb's Ear | Stachys byzantina | Stops bleeding and promotes wound healing. |
| Mullein | Verbascum thapsus | Manages bleeding and minor injuries. |
| Nasturtium | Tropaeolum majus | Reduces bleeding. |
| Oak Moss | Evernia prunastri | Manages bleeding and wound closure. |
| Plantain | Plantago spp. | Manages bleeding and wound healing. |
| Purslane | Portulaca oleracea | Reduces or prevents bleeding. |
| Raspberry Leaf | Rubus idaeus | Manages hemorrhages and promotes blood clotting. |
| Shepherd's Purse | Capsella bursa-pastoris | Manages bleeding, and minor injuries. |
| Tormentil | Potentilla erecta | Manages bleeding, and minor injuries. |
| Weld | Reseda luteola | Manages bleeding, and minor injuries. |
| White Oak Bark | Quercus alba | Manages bleeding and supports blood clotting. |
| Witch Hazel | Hamamelis virginiana | Manages bleeding and promotes wound healing. |
| Uva ursi | Arctostaphylos uva ursi | Manages bleeding and promotes tissue healing. |
| Yarrow | Achillea millefolium | Manages bleeding and promotes wound closure. |
| Yellow Dock | Rumex crispus | Manages bleeding and anemia. |

| Anti-Inflammatory | Reduces inflammation and alleviate associated symptoms.  May reduce pain. | |
|---|---|---|
| **Herb** | **Scientific Name** | **Benefits** |
| Agrimony | Agrimonia eupatoria | Reduces inflammation. |
| Aloe Vera | Aloe barbadensis miller | Reduces redness and swelling in irritated skin. |
| Arnica | Arnica montana | Reduces pain, bruises, and muscle soreness. |
| Aspen | Populus grandidentata | Reduces pain and inflammation. |
| Bergamot | Monarda fistulosa | Reduces inflammation. |
| Birch | Betula pendula | Reduces inflammation. |
| Black Pepper | Piper nigrum | Reduces inflammation. |
| Boswellia | Boswellia serrata | Manages osteoarthritis & inflammatory bowels. |
| Burdock Root | Arctium lappa | Alleviates inflammatory conditions. |
| Calendula | Calendula officinalis | Reduces skin irritation, redness, & inflammation. |
| Cat's Claw | Uncaria tomentosa | Reduces inflammation and supports immunity. |
| Cayenne | Capsicum annuum | Reduces pain and inflammation. |
| Chamomile | Matricaria chamomilla | Sooths skin irritations and digestive discomforts. |
| Chickweed | Stellaria media | Remedy for skin irritation, eczema, & minor burns. |
| Comfrey | Symphytum officinale | Alleviate pain & inflammation in minor skin injuries. |
| Devil's Claw | Harpagophytum procumbens | Reduces arthritis pain and inflammation. |
| Echinacea | Echinacea spp. | Reduces inflammation and supports immunity. |
| Fennel seeds | Foeniculum vulgare | Reduces inflammation. |
| Frankincense | Boswellia carterii | Alleviates osteoarthritis & inflammatory bowels. |
| Fringe Tree | Chionanthus virginicus | Decrease gallbladder & bile duct inflammation. |
| Garden Sage | Salvia officinalis | Reduces inflammation. |
| Ginger | Zingiber officinale | Alleviate osteoarthritis/gastrointestinal discomfort. |
| Green Tea | Camellia sinensis | Reduces inflammation in the body. |
| Gumweed | Grindellia squarrosa | Soothes respiratory and bronchial inflammation. |
| Hyssop | Hyssopus officinalis | Soothes symptoms of bronchitis or asthma. |
| Licorice | Glycyrrhiza glabra | Reduces inflammation & supports digestive health. |
| Mallow | Malva sylvestris | Reduce respiratory & gastrointestinal inflammation. |
| Marjoram | Origanum marjorana | May help alleviate inflammation. |
| Nasturtium | Tropaeolum majus | Balance immune response & alleviate inflammation. |
| Nettle | Urtica dioica | Alleviates arthritis and allergy symptoms. |
| Onion | Allium cepa | Reduces inflammation. |
| Oregano | Origanum vulgare | Reduces inflammation. |
| Plantain | Plantago spp. | Soothes skin irritations & reduce inflammation. |
| Poplar | Populus tremula | Reduces pain and inflammation. |
| Purslane | Portulaca oleracea | Reduces inflammation. |
| Rosemary | Rosmarinus officinalis | Reduces inflammation. |
| Sage | Salvia officinalis | Reduces inflammation. |

| Anti-Inflammatory | Reduces inflammation and alleviate associated symptoms.  May reduce pain. | |
|---|---|---|
| **Herb** | **Scientific Name** | **Benefits** |
| Savory | Satureja | Reduces inflammation. |
| Skullcap | Scutellaria lateriflora | Reduces inflammation and promote relaxation. |
| St. John's Wort | Hypericum perforatum | Reduces inflammation & depression or nerve pain. |
| Teasel | Dipsacus fullonum | Reduces inflammation. |
| Turmeric | Curcuma longa | Reduces inflammation. |
| White Willow Bark | Salix alba | Reduces headaches, & musculoskeletal discomfort. |
| Willow | Salix | Pain relief and reduces inflammation. |
| Yarrow | Achillea millefolium | Alleviates skin irritations and digestive discomfort. |

| Antilithic | Dissolve stones from the urinary tract or gallbladder. | |
| --- | --- | --- |
| **Gallstone Antilithics** | Helps prevent gallstones or dissolves existing gallstones in the gallbladder. | |
| **Herb** | **Scientific Name** | **Benefits** |
| Artichoke | Cynara scolymus | Prevents the formation of gallstones. |
| Barberry | Berberis vulgaris | Promotes the flow of bile and reduces gallstones. |
| Boldo | Peumus boldus | Stimulates the gallbladder and prevents gallstones. |
| Burdock Root | Arctium lappa | Supports liver function and prevents gallstones. |
| Cascara sagrada | Rhamnus purshiana | Prevents bile accumulation and gallstones. |
| Chicory | Cichorium intybus | Enhances bile production and prevents gallstones. |
| Chicory Root | Cichorium intybus | Stimulates bile production and prevents gallstones. |
| Dandelion Root | Taraxacum officinale | Promotes liver function and prevents gallstones. |
| Ginger | Zingiber officinale | Stimulates bile production and prevents gallstones. |
| Greater Celandine | Chelidonium majus | Enhances bile flow and prevents gallstones. |
| Globe Artichoke | Cynara cardunculus | Supports bile production and reduces gallstones. |
| Lemon | Citrus limon | Dissolves gallstones and reduces gallstones. |
| Milk Thistle | Silybum marianum | Support liver function and prevents gallstones. |
| Nasturtium | Tropaeolum majus | Promotes the flow of bile and dissolves gallstones. |
| Oregon Grape | Mahonia aquifolium | Increases bile production and reduces gallstones. |
| Oregon Grape Root | Mahonia aquifolium | Stimulates the flow of bile and prevents gallstones. |
| Peppermint | Mentha piperita | Facilitates passage of bile and reduces gallstones. |
| Turkish Rhubarb | Rheum palmatum | Prevents bile stasis and gallstone formation. |
| Turmeric | Curcuma longa | Anti-inflammatory properties prevent gallstones. |
| Wild Cherry Bark | Prunus avium | Supports liver function and prevents gallstones. |

| Urinary Antilithics | Prevents urinary stones or helps dissolve existing stones in the urinary tract. | |
| --- | --- | --- |
| **Herb** | **Scientific Name** | **Benefits** |
| Bearberry | Arctostaphylos uva ursi | Prevents the formation of kidney stones. |
| Cleavers | Galium aparine | Dissolves urinary stones & promotes kidney health. |
| Celery Seed | Apium graveolens | Prevents kidney stones and dissolves existing ones. |
| Chanca Piedra | Phyllanthus niruri | Breaks down kidney stones and promotes passage. |
| Corn Silk | Zea Mays | Prevents kidney stones & soothes the urinary tract. |
| Couch grass | Elymus repens | Dissolve urinary stones & support the urinary tract. |
| Dandelion | Taraxacum officinale | Prevent kidney stones & promote their dissolution. |
| Dandelion Root | Taraxacum officinale | Prevents kidney stones and dissolves them. |
| Dill Seed | Anethum graveolens | Prevent kidney stones & promote their dissolution. |
| Garden Sage | Salvia officinalis | Prevents urinary stones from forming. |
| Gravel Root | Eupatorium purpireum | Prevent kidney stones & promote their dissolution. |
| Goldenrod | Solidago spp. | Prevent kidney stones & promote their dissolution. |
| Horsetail | Equisetum arvense | Prevent kidney stones & promote their dissolution. |
| Hydrangea Root | Hydrangea arboescens | Dissolves kidney stones & supports kidney health. |
| Juniper Berry | Juniperus communis | Prevent kidney stones & support their dissolution. |
| Marshmallow Root | Althaea officinalis | Dissolves kidney stones & soothes urinary tract. |
| Nasturtium | Tropaeolum majus | Dissolve urinary stones & support the urinary tract. |
| Parsley Root | Petroselinum crispum | Prevent kidney stones & support their dissolution. |
| Uva Ursi | Arctostaphylos uva ursi | Prevent kidney stones & promote their dissolution. |

| Antiprotozoals | Eliminate protozoans like Giardia or Amoebas from the gut. | |
|---|---|---|
| **Herb** | **Scientific Name** | **Benefits** |
| Barberry | Berberis vulgaris | Has demonstrated antiprotozoal properties. |
| Black Walnut Hull | Juglans Nigra | Kills worms, Giardia, and is anti-fungal. |
| Chaparral | Larea tridentata | Kills bacteria, viruses, parasites, & even cancer cells. |
| Garlic | Allium sativum | Antibiotic, antiviral, antifungal, and kills parasites. |
| Ginger | Zingiber officinale | Effective as an antiprotozoal agent. |
| Goldenseal | Hydrastis canadensis | Effective against Giardia and other protozoans. |
| Licorice | Glycyrrhiza glabra | Antiprotozoal effects against parasites like Giardia. |
| Licorice Root | Glycyrrhiza glabra | Antiprotozoal effects against parasites like Giardia. |
| Milk Thistle | Silybum marianum | Activity against Giardia. |
| Myrrh | Commiphora myrrha | Antibiotic effective against intestinal pathogens. |
| Wormwood | Artemisia spp. | Effective against protozoal infections. |

| Antipyretic & Febrifuges | Lowers fever and reduces body temperatures. | |
| --- | --- | --- |
| **Herb** | **Scientific Name** | **Benefits** |
| Alfalfa | Medicago Sativa | Reduce fevers & alleviates fever related symptoms. |
| Aspen | Populus grandidentata | Reduce fevers & alleviates fever related symptoms. |
| Basil | Ocimum basilicum | Reduce fevers & alleviates fever related symptoms. |
| Bergamot | Monarda fistulosa | Helps break fevers. |
| Bilberry | Vaccinium myrtillus | Reduce fevers & alleviates fever related symptoms. |
| Birch | Betula pendula | Reduce fevers & alleviates fever related symptoms. |
| Boneset | Eupatorium perfoliatum | Reduce fevers & alleviates fever related symptoms. |
| Catnip | Nepeta cataria | Reduce fevers & alleviates fever related symptoms. |
| Chamomile | Matricaria chamomilla | Reduce fevers & alleviates fever related symptoms. |
| Chickweed | Stellaria media | Reduce fevers & alleviates fever related symptoms. |
| Echinacea | Echinacea spp. | Reduce fevers & alleviates fever related symptoms. |
| Elderberry | Sambucus spp. | Reduce fevers & alleviates fever related symptoms. |
| Elderflower | Sambucus nigra | Reduce fevers & alleviates fever related symptoms. |
| Garden Sage | Salvia officinalis | Helps reduce fevers. |
| Ginger | Zingiber officinale | Reduce fevers & alleviates fever related symptoms. |
| Gotu Kola | Centella asiatica | Reduce fevers & alleviates fever related symptoms. |
| Irish Moss | Chondrus Crispus | Reduce fevers & alleviates fever related symptoms. |
| Kelp | Macrocystis pyrifera | Reduce fevers & alleviates fever related symptoms. |
| Lemon Balm | Melissa officinalis | Reduce fevers & alleviates fever related symptoms. |
| Meadowsweet | Filipenula ulmaria | Reduce fevers & alleviates fever related symptoms. |
| Mistletoe | Viscum album | Reduce fevers & alleviates fever related symptoms. |
| Nasturtium | Tropaeolum majus | Regulates body temperature to cool the body. |
| Oregano | Origanum vulgare | Helps reduce fevers. |
| Peppermint | Mentha piperita | Reduce fevers & alleviates fever related symptoms. |
| Poplar | Populus tremula | Reduce fevers & alleviates fever related symptoms. |
| Raspberry Leaf | Rubus idaeus | Reduce fevers & alleviates fever related symptoms. |
| Skullcap | Scutellaria lateriflora | Reduce fevers & alleviates fever related symptoms. |
| Sweet Annie | Artemisia annua | Reduce fevers & alleviates fever related symptoms. |
| Tansy | Tanacetum vulgare | Reduce fevers & alleviates fever related symptoms. |
| Teasel | Dipsacus fullonum | Helps reduce fevers. |
| Thyme | Thymus vulgaris | Reduce fevers & alleviates fever related symptoms. |
| White Willow | Salix alba | Reduce fevers & alleviates fever related symptoms. |
| Willow | Salix | Reduce fevers & alleviates fever related symptoms. |
| Willow Bark | Salix spp. | Reduce fevers & alleviates fever related symptoms. |
| Yarrow | Achillea millefolium | Reduce fevers & alleviates fever related symptoms. |

| Antirheumatic | Alleviates symptoms of rheumatism and arthritis. (I.E. Inflammation & joint pain.) | |
|---|---|---|
| **Herb** | **Scientific Name** | **Benefits** |
| Angelica | Angelica archangelica | Reduces inflammation and relieves joint pain. |
| Arnica | Arnica Montana | Reduces inflammation, relieves muscle & joint pain. |
| Birch | Betula spp. | Reduces inflammation, joint pain and stiffness. |
| Black Current | Ribes nigrum | Reduces joint pain and inflammation. |
| Borage | Borago officinalis | Reduces inflammation, and alleviates joint pain. |
| Boswellia | Boswellia serrata | Reduces inflammation, and alleviates joint pain. |
| Burdock Root | Arctium lappa | Reduces inflammation, & promotes detoxification. |
| Burdock | Arctium lappa | Reduces inflammation, & promotes detoxification. |
| Cat's Claw | Uncaria tomentosa | Reduces inflammation, & eases joint pain. |
| Cayenne | Capsicum annuum | Alleviates inflammation, and joint pain. |
| Chamomile | Matricaria chamomilla | Reduces inflammation, and joint pain. |
| Devil's Claw | Harpagophytum procumbens | Reduces inflammation, and relieves joint pain. |
| Frankincense | Boswellia carterii | Reduces inflammation, and joint pain. |
| Garden Sage | Salvia officinalis | Reduces inflammation, and joint pain. |
| Juniper | Juniperus communis | Reduces inflammation, and soothes joint pain. |
| Licorice | Glycyrrhiza glabra | Reduces inflammation, and offers pain relief. |
| Meadowsweet | Filipenula ulmaria | Reduces inflammation, and joint pain. |
| Nasturtium | Tropaeolum majus | Reduces inflammation & promotes joint health. |
| Nettle | Urtica dioica | Reduced inflammation, and alleviates joint pain. |
| Pineapple Bromelain | Ananas comosus | Reduces inflammation, and improves joint mobility. |
| Rosemary | Rosmarinus officinalis | Reduces inflammation, and eases joint pain. |
| Stinging Nettle | Urtica dioica | Reduces inflammation, and alleviates joint pain. |
| Teasel | Dipsacus fullonum | Reduces inflammation, and joint pain. |
| Turmeric | Curcuma longa | Reduces inflammation, and joint pain. |
| White Willow | Salix alba | Reduces inflammation, and joint pain. |
| Willow Bark | Salix spp. | Reduces inflammation, and joint pain. |
| Wintergreen | Gaultheria procumbens | Alleviates inflammation, and joint pain. |
| Uva Ursi | Arctostaphylos uva ursi | Reduces inflammation, joint pain and discomfort. |

| **Antispasmodic** | Relax and alleviate muscle spasms or cramps. | |
|---|---|---|
| **Herb** | **Scientific Name** | **Benefits** |
| Allspice | Pimenta dioica | Alleviates muscle spasms and cramps. |
| Angelica | Angelica archangelica | Alleviates muscle spasms and cramps. |
| Anise Seeds | Pimpinella anisum | Alleviates muscle spasms and cramps. |
| Baneberry | Actaea rubra | Relieves muscle spasms and cramps |
| Black Cohosh | Actaea racemosa | Eases muscle spasms and cramps. |
| Black haw | Viburnum prunifolium | Relieves muscle spasms and cramps |
| Caraway | Carum carvi | Alleviates muscle spasms and cramps. |
| Catnip | Nepeta cataria | Eases muscle spasms and cramps. |
| Chamomile | Matricaria chamomilla | Soothes and relieves muscle spasms and cramps. |
| Cinnamon | Cinnamomum verum | Soothes and relieves muscle spasms and cramps. |
| Cramp Bark | Viburnum prunifolium | Eases muscle spasms and cramps. |
| Fennel seeds | Foeniculum vulgare | Alleviates muscle spasms and cramps. |
| Garden Sage | Salvia officinalis | Alleviates muscle spasms and cramps. |
| Ginger | Zingiber officinale | Relieves muscle spasms and cramps |
| Hyssop | Hyssopus officinalis | Alleviates muscle spasms and cramps. |
| Lavender | Lavandula angustifolia | Soothes and reduces muscle spasms and cramps. |
| Lemon Balm | Melissa officinalis | Relieves muscle spasms and cramps |
| Lemon Verbana | Aloysia citridora | Relaxes smooth muscle tissue to alleviates spasms. |
| Lobelia | Lobelia inflata | Alleviates muscle spasms and cramps. |
| Marjoram | Origanum marjorana | Aids in relieving muscle spasms. |
| Motherwort | Leonurus cardiaca | Eases muscle spasms and cramps. |
| Nasturtium | Tropaeolum majus | Relaxes muscle to relieve muscle spasms & cramps. |
| Oregano | Origanum vulgare | Eases muscle spasms and cramps. |
| Passionflower | Passiflora incarnata | Reduces muscle spasms and cramps. |
| Peppermint | Mentha piperita | Relieves muscle spasms and cramps |
| Rosemary | Rosmarinus officinalis | Alleviates muscle spasms and cramps. |
| Sage | Salvia officinalis | Alleviates muscle spasms and cramps. |
| Savory | Satureja | Alleviates muscle spasms and cramps. |
| Skullcap | Scutelleria lateriflora | Eases muscle spasms and cramps. |
| St. John's Wort | Hypericum perforatum | Alleviates muscle spasms and cramps. |
| Teasel | Dipsacus fullonum | Eases muscle tension and discomfort. |
| Thyme | Thymus vulgaris | Eases muscle spasms and cramps. |
| Valerian | Valeriana officinalis | Alleviates muscle spasms and cramps. |
| Wild Cherry Bark | Prunus avium | Relieves muscle spasms and cramps |
| Wild Yam | Dioscorea villosa | Eases muscle spasms and cramps. |

| Antiviral | Combats viral infections or boost the immune system's ability to fight viruses. | |
|---|---|---|
| **Herb** | **Scientific Name** | **Benefits** |
| Allspice | Pimenta dioica | Inhibits some viruses. |
| Andrographis | Andrographis paniculata | Boosts viral immunity and inhibits viral replication. |
| Anise Seeds | Pimpinella anisum | Boosts viral immunity and inhibits viral replication. |
| Astragalus | Astragalus membranaceus | Enhance viral immunity & inhibit viral replication. |
| Bay Leaves | Laurus nobilis | Enhance viral immunity & inhibit viral replication. |
| Cat's Claw | Uncaria tomentosa | Stimulates immunity and combats viral infections. |
| Chaparral | Larea tridentata | Boosts viral immunity and inhibits viral replication. |
| Clove | Syzygium aromaticum | Has antiviral properties & inhibits viral replication. |
| Echinacea | Echinacea purpurea | Boosts viral immunity and inhibits viral replication. |
| Elder | Sambucus nigra | Stimulates immunity and combats viral infections. |
| Elderberry | Sambucus spp. | Stimulates immunity and combats viral infections. |
| Fennel seeds | Foeniculum vulgare | Has antiviral properties & inhibits viral replication. |
| Garden Sage | Salvia officinalis | Has antiviral properties & inhibits viral replication. |
| Garlic | Allium sativum | Boosts viral immunity and inhibits viral replication. |
| Ginger | Zingiber officinale | Supports immunity and inhibits viral replications. |
| Goldenseal | Hydrastis canadensis | Has antiviral properties & inhibits viral replication. |
| Japanese Knotweed | Polygonum cuspidatum | Has antiviral properties & inhibits viral replication. |
| Lemon Balm | Melissa officinalis | Has antiviral properties & inhibits viral replication. |
| Licorice | Glycyrrhiza glabra | Has antiviral properties & inhibits viral replication. |
| Lomatium | Lomatium dissectum | Has antiviral properties & inhibits viral replication. |
| Marjoram | Origanum marjorana | Ability to combat viral infections. |
| Mullein | Verbascum thapsus | Manages viral infections of the respiratory system. |
| Nasturtium | Tropaeolum majus | Inhibits the replication of viruses. |
| Olive Leaf | Olea europaea | Has antiviral properties & inhibits viral replication. |
| Onion | Allium cepa | Inhibits viral replication & combats viral infections. |
| Oregano | Origanum vulgare | Inhibits viral replication & combats viral infections. |
| Pau D'Arco | Tabebuia spp. | Has antiviral properties & inhibits viral replication. |
| Peppermint | Mentha piperita | Headaches, mild pain. |
| Rosemary | Rosmarinus officinalis | Combat bacterial infections. |
| Sage | Salvia officinalis | Supports immunity and inhibits viral replications. |
| Savory | Satureja | Combats viruses. |
| Shiitake Mushroom | Lentinula edodes | Enhance viral immunity and inhibit viral replication. |
| St. John's Wort | Hypericum perforatum | Has antiviral properties & inhibits viral replication. |
| Tea Tree Oil | Melaleuca alternifolia | Has antiviral properties & inhibits viral replication. |
| Thyme | Thymus vulgaris | Has antiviral properties & inhibits viral replication. |
| Thuja | Thuja | Has antiviral properties & manages viral infections. |

| Aperient | Mild laxatives that help relieve constipation or promote bowel movements. | |
|---|---|---|
| **Herb** | **Scientific Name** | **Benefits** |
| Alfalfa | Medicago Sativa | Mild laxative that relieves constipation. |
| Aloe Vera | Aloe barbadensis miller | Relief from constipation and digestive discomfort. |
| Buckthorn | Rhamnus frangula | Relieve constipation & promote bowel movements. |
| Cascara sagrada | Rhamnus purshiana | Relieve constipation & promote bowel movements. |
| Cilantro | Coriandrum sativum | Manages digestive discomfort and motion sickness. |
| Coriander | Coriandrum sativum | Supports digestion, alleviates gas and bloating. |
| Dandelion | Taraxacum officinale | Relieve constipation & promote bowel movements. |
| Fennel seeds | Foeniculum vulgare | Reduces digestive discomfort, gas, and bloating. |
| Fenugreek | Trigonella foenum-graecum | Relieve constipation & promote bowel movements. |
| Flax | Linum usitatissimum | Relieve constipation & promote bowel movements. |
| Licorice | Glycyrrhiza glabra | Relieve constipation & promote bowel movements. |
| Marjoram | Origanum marjorana | May help promote mild laxative effects. |
| Marshmallow | Althea officinalis | Relieve constipation & promote bowel movements. |
| Nasturtium | Tropaeolum majus | Promotes mild laxative effects & bowel regularity. |
| Psyllium | Plantago ovata | Relieve constipation & promote bowel movements. |
| Pumpkin | Cucurbita pepo | Relieve constipation & promote bowel movements. |
| Purslane | Portulaca oleracea | Supports digestive health. |
| Rhubarb | Rheum rhabarbarum | Relieve constipation & promote bowel movements. |
| Savory | Satureja | Mild laxative promotes bowel regularity. |
| Senna | Senna alexandrina | Relieve constipation & promote bowel movements. |
| Slippery Elm | Ulmus rubra | Relieve constipation & promote bowel movements. |

| Astringent | A drying or tightening effect on tissues.  Can be sed to tone & contract bodily tissues. | |
|---|---|---|
| **Herb** | **Scientific Name** | **Benefits** |
| Agrimony | Agrimonia eupatoria | Soothes skin irritation, treats minor cuts & bruises. |
| Alum | Aluminum potassium sulfate | Soothes skin & reduces bleeding from minor cuts. |
| Blackberry | Rubus fruticosus | Treats minor wounds & reduces inflammation. |
| Blackberry Leaf | Rubus fruticosus | Tightens tissue & alleviates diarrhea. |
| Cinnamon | Cinnamomum verum | Can contribute to toning and contracting tissues. |
| Cranesbill | Geranium maculatum | Tones tissues, aids wound healing, relieve diarrhea. |
| Garden Sage | Salvia officinalis | Helps tone & constrict tissues, aids wound healing. |
| Geranium | Pelargonium spp. | Manage skin conditions & promote wound healing. |
| Horsetail | Equisetum arvense | Tighten tissue, relieve diarrhea, & control bleeding. |
| Marjoram | Origanum marjorana | Can contribute to toning and contracting tissues. |
| Nasturtium | Tropaeolum majus | Helps tone & constrict tissues, aids wound healing. |
| Oak Bark | Quercus spp. | Treats skin conditions & promotes wound healing. |
| Plantain | Plantago spp. | Promote wound healing, relieves minor skin issues. |
| Purslane | Portulaca oleracea | Tightens and tones tissue. |
| Raspberry Leaf | Rubus idaeus | Tighten tissue, relieve diarrhea, & inflammation. |
| Rose | Rosa spp. | Aids skin conditions and promotes wound healing. |
| Sage | Salvia officinalis | Reduce excessive sweating & aids skin conditions. |
| Savory | Satureja | Tightens & tones tissues, addresses diarrhea. |
| Shepherd's Purse | Capsella bursa-pastoris | Control bleeding to manage minor wounds. |
| Thyme | Thymus Vulgaris | Tightens and tones tissue. |
| Turkey Rhubarb | Rheum palmatum | Promotes bowel regularity to manage constipation. |
| Uva Ursi | Arctostaphylos uva ursi | Tightens tissue to aid urinary tract infections. |
| White Oak | Quercus alba | Tightens tissue and support wound healing. |
| Witch Hazel | Hamamelis virginiana | Soothes skin irritation, treats minor cuts & bruises. |
| Yarrow | Achillea millefolium | Promotes wound healing to manage minor cuts. |

| Bitters | Stimulate digestion and appetite. | |
| --- | --- | --- |
| **Herb** | **Scientific Name** | **Benefits** |
| Agrimony | Agrimonia eupatoria | Improves digestions and prevents indigestion. |
| Angelica | Angelica archangelica | Stimulates the appetite and aids in digestion. |
| Artichoke | Cynara scolymus | Stimulate digestive enzymes/bile to breakdown fat. |
| Barberry | Berberis vulgaris | Aids digestion of fats by stimulating bile production. |
| Bitter Melon | Momordica charantia | Regulate blood sugar & improve insulin sensitivity. |
| Burdock | Arctium lappa | Aids in the elimination of toxins. |
| Centaury | Centaurium erythraea | Stimulates appetite and improves digestion. |
| Chamomile | Matricaria chamomilla | Relieves inflammation, bloating, and gas. |
| Chicory | Cichorium intybus | Promotes the breakdown of food. |
| Dandelion | Taraxacum officinale | Aid fat breakdown to alleviate indigestion/bloating. |
| Garden Sage | Salvia officinalis | Stimulate digestive enzymes to aid digestion. |
| Gentian | Gentiana spp. | Improve digestion and appetite, relieve indigestion. |
| Ginger | Zingiber officinale | Aids digestion, reduces nausea, and discomfort. |
| Goldenseal | Hydrastis canadensis | Supports digestion & relieves digestive discomfort. |
| Horehound | Marrubium vulgare | Aids digestion. |
| Lemon Verbana | Aloysia citridora | Stimulate digestive enzymes to aid digestion. |
| Lovage | Levisticum officinale | Stimulate digestive enzymes to aid digestion. |
| Marjoram | Origanum marjorana | Potentially aids in digestion stimulation. |
| Nasturtium | Tropaeolum majus | Stimulate digestive functions for digestive health. |
| Sage | Salvia officinalis | Promotes digestive secretions to aid in digestion. |
| Savory | Satureja | Promotes digestive secretions to aid in digestion. |
| Wormwood | Artemisia absinthium | Stimulate digestion, appetite, and detoxification. |

| Cardiotonic & Cardioactive | Affects the cardiovascular system: typically, by exerting an influence on heart rate, rhythm, or other cardiac functions. | |
|---|---|---|
| **Herb** | **Scientific Name** | **Benefits** |
| Astragalus | Astragalus membranaceus | Aids the strength & efficiency of heart contractions. |
| Cayenne | Capsicum annuum | Enhance heart contractions & improve circulation. |
| Coleus Forskohlii | Coleus forskohlii | Increases heart contractions. |
| Danshen | Salvia miltiorrhiza | Strengthen heart contractions, improve circulation. |
| Garlic | Allium sativum | Strengthen heart contractions. |
| Ginkgo | Ginkgo biloba | Enhance heart contractions & improve blood flow. |
| Ginger | Zingiber officinale | Aids heart contractions, regulates blood pressure. |
| Hawthorn | Crataegus spp. | Strengthen heart contractions, improve circulation. |
| Lemon Balm | Melissa officinalis | Regulate heart contractions. |
| Lily of the Valley | Convallaria majalis | Strengthens heart contractions.  Can be toxic. |
| Linden | Tilia spp. | Supports heart contractions. |
| Motherwort | Leonurus cardiaca | Enhances heart contractions, reduces palpitations. |
| Olive Leaf | Olea europaea | Support heart contractions, & improve circulation. |
| Savory | Satureja | Regulate heart function and improve circulation. |
| Turmeric | Curcuma longa | Support heart contractions & reduce inflammation. |
| Yarrow | Achillea millefolium | Strengthen heart contractions. |

| Carminative | Relieve or prevent gas and bloating in the digestive tract. | |
| --- | --- | --- |
| **Herb** | **Scientific Name** | **Benefits** |
| Allspice | Pimenta dioica | Aids in digestion by reducing gas and bloating. |
| Anise seeds | Pimpinella anisum | Alleviates gas & bloating in the digestive system. |
| Basil | Ocimum basilicum | Aids in digestion by reducing gas and bloating. |
| Bay Leaves | Laurus nobilis | Aids in digestion by reducing gas and bloating. |
| Black Pepper | Piper nigrum | Reduces gas and bloating.  Promotes digestion. |
| Caraway | Carum carvi | Relieves gas, indigestion, and bloating. |
| Cardamom | Elettaria caramomum | Reduces gas and bloating.  Enhances digestion. |
| Celery Seed | Apium graveolens | Reduces gas and bloating.  Promotes digestion. |
| Chamomile | Matricaria chamomilla | Relieves gas, indigestion, and bloating. |
| Cilantro | Coriandrum sativum | Manages digestive discomfort and motion sickness. |
| Cinnamon | Cinnamomum verum | Alleviates gas, bloating, and digestive discomfort. |
| Cloves | Syzygium aromaticum | Reduces gas and bloating.  Promotes digestion. |
| Coriander | Coriandrum sativum | Relieves gas and bloating.  Enhances digestion. |
| Cumin | Cuminum cyminum | Reduces gas, bloating, and digestive discomfort. |
| Dill | Anethum graveolens | Ease gas, bloating, discomfort, & improve digestion. |
| Fennel seeds | Foeniculum vulgare | Relieves gas and bloating.  Improves digestion. |
| Garden Sage | Salvia officinalis | Reduces gas, bloating, and digestive discomfort. |
| Garlic | Allium sativum | Reduces gas, bloating, and digestive discomfort. |
| Ginger | Zingiber officinale | Reduces gas, bloating, and digestive discomfort. |
| Juniper | Juniperus communis | Relieves gas, bloating, and eases digestive stress. |
| Lavender | Lavandula angustifolia | Reduces gas, bloating, and indigestion. |
| Lemon Balm | Melissa officinalis | Ease gas, bloating, discomfort, & aids digestion. |
| Lovage | Levisticum officinale | Reduces gas and bloating.  Promotes digestion. |
| Marjoram | Origanum marjorana | Relieves digestive discomfort and reduces gas. |
| Parsley | Petroselinum crispum | Reduce gas and bloating.  Improves digestion. |
| Peppermint | Mentha piperita | Relieves gas, bloating, and indigestion discomfort. |
| Rosemary | Rosmarinus officinalis | Combat bacterial infections. |
| Sage | Salvia officinalis | Reduces gas, bloating, and digestive discomfort. |
| Savory | Satureja | Reduces gas, bloating, and digestive discomfort. |
| Thyme | Thymus Vulgaris | Relieve gas, bloating, & gastrointestinal discomfort. |

| Cathartic | Promotes bowel movements and relieves constipation. | |
|---|---|---|
| **Herb** | **Scientific Name** | **Benefits** |
| Alder Buckthorn | Rhamnus frangula | Promotes bowel movements/relieves constipation. |
| Aloe Vera Leaf | Aloe barbadensis miller | Promotes bowel movements/relieves constipation. |
| Barberry | Berberis vulgaris | Promotes bowel movements/relieves constipation. |
| Black hellebore | Helleborus niger | Induces strong bowel movements. |
| Buckthorn | Rhamnus frangula | Promotes bowel movements/relieves constipation. |
| Cascara amarga | Gentiana lutea | Promotes bowel movements/relieves constipation. |
| Cascara Sagrada | Rhamnus purshiana | Promotes bowel movements/relieves constipation. |
| Cassia | Cassia spp. | Promotes bowel movements/relieves constipation. |
| Licorice | Glycyrrhiza glabra | Promotes bowel movements/relieves constipation. |
| Prune | Prunus domestica | Promotes bowel movements/relieves constipation. |
| Rhubarb | Rheum rhabarbarum | Promotes bowel movements/relieves constipation. |
| Savory | Satureja | Mild laxative promoting bowel movements. |
| Senna | Senna alexandrina | Promotes bowel movements/relieves constipation. |
| Yellow Dock | Rumex crispus | Promotes bowel movements/relieves constipation. |

| Cholagogue | Stimulates bile production by the liver and/or bile release from the gallbladder. | |
|---|---|---|
| **Herb** | **Scientific Name** | **Benefits** |
| Artichoke | Cynara scolymus | Aids digestion to alleviate indigestion and bloating. |
| Barberry | Berberis vulgaris | Aids digestion to alleviate indigestion & discomfort. |
| Boldo | Peumus boldus | Aids digestion to alleviate indigestion and bloating. |
| Bupleurum | Bupleurum chinense | Aids digestion to alleviate indigestion & discomfort. |
| Dandelion | Taraxacum officinale | Aids digestion to alleviate indigestion and bloating. |
| Fringe Tree | Chionanthus virginicus | Stimulates bile flow and decongests the liver. |
| Gentian | Gentiana spp. | Aids digestion to alleviate indigestion & discomfort. |
| Greater Celandine | Chelidonium majus | Aids digestion to alleviate indigestion and bloating. |
| Lemon Balm | Melissa officinalis | Aids digestion to alleviate indigestion and bloating. |
| Licorice | Glycyrrhiza glabra | Aids digestion to alleviate indigestion & discomfort. |
| Milk Thistle | Silybum marianum | Aids digestion to alleviate indigestion and bloating. |
| Oregon Grape | Mahonia aquifolium | Aids digestion to alleviate indigestion & discomfort. |
| Rosemary | Rosmarinus officinalis | Aids digestion to alleviate indigestion and bloating. |
| Savory | Satureja | Stimulates bile aids in digestion and liver function. |
| Tinospora Cordifolia | Tinospora cordifolia | Aids digestion to alleviate indigestion & discomfort. |
| Turmeric | Curcuma longa | Aids digestion to alleviate indigestion and bloating. |
| Wild Yam | Dioscorea villosa | Aids digestion to alleviate indigestion and bloating. |
| Yellow Dock | Rumex crispus | Aids digestion to alleviate indigestion & discomfort. |

| Demulcent | Mucilage-rich properties sooth the digestive tract, irritated bronchi and bladders. | |
|---|---|---|
| **Herb** | **Scientific Name** | **Benefits** |
| Aloe Vera | Aloe barbadensis miller | Soothes tissues of skin/digestive tract/throat. |
| Chia Seeds | Salvia hispanica | Soothes the digestive tract & promotes hydration. |
| Cinnamon | Cinnamomum verum | Can contribute to toning and contracting tissues. |
| Comfrey | Symphytum officinale | Soothes skin to aid in wound healing. |
| Coltsfoot | Tussilago farfara | Coats the throat to alleviate coughs & irritation. |
| Corn Silk | Zea Mays | Soothes and coats the urinary tract. |
| Fenugreek | Trigonella foenum-graecum | Soothes the gastrointestinal tract & respiratory. |
| Flax | Linum usitatissimum | Soothes digestive & respiratory linings. |
| Hollyhock | Alcea rosea | Soothes throats, respiratory passages, and coughs. |
| Irish Moss | Chondrus Crispus | Soothes the respiratory and digestive tracts. |
| Licorice | Glycyrrhiza glabra | Coats the throat, stomach, and digestive tract. |
| Mallow | Malva sylvestris | Soothes the throat, digestive & respiratory tracts. |
| Marshmallow | Althea officinalis | Coats the respiratory and digestive systems. |
| Mullein | Verbascum thapsus | Soothes respiratory passages, coughs, and throats. |
| Oats | Avena Sativa | Soothes & protects the gastrointestinal tract. |
| Okra | Abelmoschus esculentus | Soothes & protects the digestive tract. |
| Plantain | Plantago major | Soothes sore throats and respiratory irritation. |
| Purslane | Portulaca oleracea | Soothes and protects irritated muscous membranes. |
| Savory | Satureja | Soothe and protect mucous membranes. |
| Slippery Elm | Ulmus rubra | Soothes throats and digestive tracts. |

| Diaphoretic | Induces perspiration which can help break fevers and help the body eliminate toxins through the skin. | |
|---|---|---|
| **Herb** | **Scientific Name** | **Benefits** |
| Basil | Ocimum basilicum | Regulates body temperature and eliminates toxins. |
| Bay Leaves | Laurus nobilis | Regulates body temperature and eliminates toxins. |
| Bergamot | Monarda fistulosa | Helps break fevers. |
| Black Pepper | Piper nigrum | Induces sweating to reduce fevers. |
| Blessed Thistle | Cnicus benedictus | Aid in detoxification and alleviates fever. |
| Boneset | Eupatorium perfoliatum | Eliminates toxins and relieves cold/flu symptoms. |
| Cayenne | Capsicum annuum | Induces sweating to break fevers & detoxify. |
| Catnip | Nepeta cataria | Eliminates toxins & relieves cold/fever symptoms. |
| Chamomile | Matricaria chamomilla | Induces sweating to reduce fevers. |
| Echinacaea | Echinacea spp. | Promotes sweating to reduce fevers. |
| Elderflower | Sambucus nigra | Stimulates sweating to reduce fevers & detoxify. |
| Fennel seeds | Foeniculum vulgare | Helps break fevers. |
| Garden Sage | Salvia officinalis | Promotes sweating to reduce fevers. |
| Ginger | Zingiber officinale | Induce sweating to reduce fever & eliminate toxins. |
| Hyssop | Hyssopus officinalis | Stimulates sweating to reduce fevers & detoxify. |
| Lovage | Levisticum officinale | Induces sweating to release toxins through the skin. |
| Oregano | Origanum vulgare | Induce sweating to reduce fever & eliminate toxins. |
| Peppermint | Mentha piperita | Promotes sweating to reduce fevers & congestion. |
| Purslane | Portulaca oleracea | Promotes sweating to eliminate toxins via the skin. |
| Rosemary | Rosmarinus officinalis | Induce sweating to reduce fever & detoxify. |
| Sage | Salvia officinalis | Stimulates sweating to reduce fevers & detoxify. |
| Savory | Satureja | Promotes sweating to aid in detoxification. |
| Teasel | Dipsacus fullonum | Promotes sweating and increased perspiration. |
| Thyme | Thymus Vulgaris | Induce sweating to reduce fever & detoxify. |
| Yarrow | Achillea millefolium | Stimulates sweating to reduce fevers & detoxify. |

| Diuretic | Increases urine production.  Promotes the elimination of excess fluids and waste. | |
|---|---|---|
| **Herb** | **Scientific Name** | **Benefits** |
| Agrimony | Agrimonia eupatoria | Removes excess fluid to reduce water retention. |
| Alfalfa | Medicago Sativa | Increase urine production to eliminate excess fluids. |
| Bearberry | Arctostaphylos uva ursi | Aids in eliminating excess fluids and toxins. |
| Black Pepper | Piper nigrum | Removes excess fluid to reduce water retention. |
| Buchu | Agathosma betulina | Relieves bloating and water retention. |
| Burdock | Arctium lappa | Removes excess fluids and waste products. |
| Celery | Apium graveolens | Reduces fluid retention & supports kidney function. |
| Cleavers | Galium aparine | Removes excess fluids & reduces water retention. |
| Corn Silk | Zea Mays | Reduces water retention & supports urinary tract. |
| Couchgrass | Elymus repens | Eliminates excess fluids, & benefits urinary tract. |
| Dandelion | Taraxacum officinale | Removes excess fluids and waste products. |
| Elder | Sambucus nigra | Removes excess fluid to reduce water retention. |
| Fennel seeds | Foeniculum vulgare | Removes excess fluid to reduce water retention. |
| Garden Sage | Salvia officinalis | Increase urine production to eliminate excess fluids. |
| Ginger | Zingiber officinale | Eliminates excess fluids to aid edema and bloating. |
| Goldenrod | Solidago spp. | Reduces fluid and supports urinary tract health. |
| Gravel Root | Eupatorium purpireum | Benefits kidney stones and urinary tract infections. |
| Green Tea | Camellia sinensis | Reduce water retention & aid weight management. |
| Hawthorn | Crataegus spp. | Aids in mild edema and high blood pressure. |
| Hibiscus | Hibiscus sabdariffa | Aids in managing blood pressure and edema. |
| Horsetail | Equisetum arvense | Reduces water retention & benefits urinary tract. |
| Juniper | Juniperus communis | Benefits bloating and urinary tract infections. |
| Lovage | Levisticum officinale | Increase urine production to eliminate excess fluids. |
| Nasturtium | Tropaeolum majus | Increase urine production to aid in fluid balance. |
| Parsley | Petroselinum crispum | Supports kidney function and reduces bloating. |
| Plantain | Plantago spp. | Promotes urine production and fluid balance. |
| Pumpkin | Cucurbita pepo | Promotes urine production and fluid balance. |
| Purslane | Portulaca oleracea | Increases urine production to eliminate excess fluids. |
| Rosemary | Rosmarinus officinalis | Combat bacterial infections. |
| Savory | Satureja | Increases urine production to eliminate excess fluids. |
| Uva Ursi | Arctostaphylos uva ursi | Aids in the removal of excess fluids. |

| Emmenagogue | Stimulates menstrual flow and regulates the menstrual cycle.<br>Don't be take while pregnant. | |
|---|---|---|
| **Herb** | **Scientific Name** | **Benefits** |
| Angelica | Angelica archangelica | Helps regulate menstrual cycle and eases cramps. |
| Bay Leaves | Laurus nobilis | Addresses menstrual irregularities. |
| Black Cohosh | Actaea racemosa | Alleviates menstrual disturbances. |
| Blue Cohosh | Caulophyllum thalictroides | Addresses menstrual irregularities. |
| Calendula | Calendula officinalis | Helps regulate menstrual cycle. |
| Chamomile | Matricaria chamomilla | Aids menstruation, relieves cramps & irregularities. |
| Cinnamom | Cinnamomum verum | Regulates menstruation & reduces pain/discomfort. |
| Cramp Bark | Viburnum prunifolium | Promotes regular cycles & alleviates cramps. |
| Dong Quai | Angelica sinensis | Regulates menstruation and relieves symptoms. |
| Fennel seeds | Foeniculum vulgare | Regulates menstruation and relieves symptoms. |
| Garden Sage | Salvia officinalis | Stimulates menstruation and regulates cycles. |
| Ginger | Zingiber officinale | Stimulate menstruation and reduce discomfort. |
| Motherwort | Leonurus cardiaca | Promotes menstruation, relieves discomfort. |
| Parsley | Petroselinum crispum | Stimulates menstruation and regulates cycles. |
| Pennyroyal | Mentha pulegium | Stimulates menstruation & addresses irregularities. |
| Peppermint | Mentha piperita | Regulates menstruation & eases discomfort. |
| Rue | Ruta graveolens | Stimulates menstruation & addresses irregularities. |
| Sage | Salvia officinalis | Stimulates menstruation & eases discomfort. |
| Savory | Satureja | Stimulates menstruation & addresses irregularities. |
| Tansy | Tanacetum vulgare | Promotes menstruation & addresses irregularities. |
| Yarrow | Achillea millefolium | Regulates menstruation & relieves discomfort. |

| Expectorant | Helps clear mucus from the respiratory tract. | |
| --- | --- | --- |
| **Herb** | **Scientific Name** | **Benefits** |
| Anise seeds | Pimpinella anisum | Helps loosen mucus and ease congestion. |
| Basil | Ocimum basilicum | Helps loosen mucus and ease congestion. |
| Black Pepper | Piper nigrum | Aids in loosening mucus & relieving congestion. |
| Black Seed | Nigella sativa | Aids in loosening mucus & removing congestion. |
| Caraway | Carum carvi | Aids in loosening mucus & removing congestion. |
| Coltsfoot | Tussilago farfara | Helps clear mucus and alleviates congestion. |
| Comfrey | Symphytum officinale | Aids in loosening mucus & relieving congestion. |
| Elder | Sambucus nigra | Helps loosen & expel mucus, relieving congestion. |
| Elecampane | Inula helenium | Helps loosen mucus and alleviates congestion. |
| Eucalyptus | Eucalyptus spp. | Loosens mucus and alleviates congestion. |
| Fennel seeds | Foeniculum vulgare | Regulates menstruation and relieves symptoms. |
| Fenugreek | Trigonella foenum-graecum | Loosens mucus and alleviates congestion. |
| Garlic | Allium sativum | Aids in loosening and expelling mucus. |
| Ginger | Zingiber officinale | Assists in loosening mucus & reducing congestion. |
| Gumweed | Grindelia integrifolia | Help loosen mucus and alleviates congestion. |
| Hyssop | Hyssopus officinalis | Aids loosening of mucus and congestion. |
| Licorice | Glycyrrhiza glabra | Helps loosen mucus and reduces congestion. |
| Lobelia | Lobelia inflata | Assists in loosening mucus & relieving congestion. |
| Lovage | Levisticum officinale | Helps expel mucus from the respiratory tract. |
| Onion | Allium cepa | Helps expel mucus from the respiratory tract. |
| Oregano | Origanum vulgare | Aids in loosening mucus and relieving congestion. |
| Pleurisy Root | Asclepias tuberosa | Assists in loosening mucus & reducing congestion. |
| Savory | Satureja | Expels mucus and facilitates easier breathing. |
| Thyme | Thymus vulgaris | Helps loosen mucus and relieves congestion. |
| Wild Cherry Bark | Prunus avium | Assists in loosening mucus & reducing congestion. |
| Yerba Santa | Eriodictyon californicum | Helps loosen mucus and reduces congestion. |

| Galactogogue | Increase the production of breast milk in lactating individuals. | |
|---|---|---|
| **Herb** | **Scientific Name** | **Benefits** |
| Alfalfa | Medicago sativa | Helps to increase breast milk production. |
| Anise Seeds | Pimpinella anisum | Helps to stimulate/increase breast milk production. |
| Blessed Thistle | Cnicus benedictus | Aids in boosting milk supply. |
| Borage | Borago officinalis | Assists in increasing milk production. |
| Caraway | Carum carvi | Helps stimulate/enhance breast milk production. |
| Chaste Tree | Vitex agnus-castus | Aids in regulating hormones and milk production. |
| Cumin | Cuminum cyminum | Help boost breast milk production. |
| Dill | Anethum graveolens | Aids in increasing milk supply. |
| Fennel seeds | Foeniculum vulgare | Helps stimulate/enhance breast milk production. |
| Fenugreek | Trigonella foenum-graecum | Boosts milk supply. |
| Goat's Rue | Galega officinalis | Aids in increasing breast milk. |
| Nettle | Urtica dioica | Supports increase in breast milk production. |
| Savory | Satureja | Supports milk production. |
| Shatavari | Asparagus racemosus | Enhance milk production. |
| Vervain | Verbena officinalis | Aids in increasing breast milk supply. |

| Hematinic | Support the production of red blood cells.  They often have iron or folic acid. | |
|---|---|---|
| **Herb** | **Scientific Name** | **Benefits** |
| Albizia | Albizia julibrissin | Promotes the production of red blood cells. |
| Alfalfa | Medicago sativa | Helps combat anemia. |
| Ashwagandha | Withania somnifera | Improves iron utilization and helps combat anemia. |
| Astragalus | Astragalus membranaceus | Promotes the production of red blood cells. |
| Bilberry | Vaccinium myrtillus | Strengthens blood vessels, improves circulation. |
| Burdock | Arctium lappa | Helps combat anemia. |
| Chickpeas | Cicer arietinum | Helps prevent and treat anemia. |
| Chickweed | Stellaria media | Enhances red blood cell production. |
| Chicory | Cichorium intybus | Supports the production of red blood cells. |
| Dandelion | Taraxacum officinale | Helps combat anemia. |
| Dong quai | Angelica sinensis | Improves iron absorption & helps combat anemia. |
| Echinacea | Echinacea purpurea | Supports immunity, aids better blood health. |
| Fenugreek | Trigonella foenum-graecum | Aids in the prevention and treatment of anemia. |
| Nettle | Urtica dioica | Promotes the production of red blood cells. |
| Parsley | Petroselinum crispum | Enhances the absorption of iron. |
| Rehmannia | Rehmannia glutinosa | Aids in the management of anemia. |
| Savory | Satureja | Supports and enhances blood health. |
| Stinging Nettle | Urtica dioica | Iron increases red blood cell production. |
| Yellow Dock | Rumex crispus | Support red cell production to alleviate anemia. |

| Hepatic | Support and protect the liver.  Liver detoxification and regeneration of liver tissue. | |
|---|---|---|
| **Herb** | **Scientific Name** | **Benefits** |
| Artichoke | Cynara scolymus | Aids bile production, digestion, and detoxification. |
| Astragalus | Astragalus membranaceus | Enhances antioxidant defenses, protects the liver. |
| Barberry | Berberis vulgaris | Promotes bile secretion and aids digestion. |
| Boldo | Peumus boldus | Aids bile production, digestion, and detoxification. |
| Bupleurum | Bupleurum chinense | Promotes detoxification and reduces inflammation. |
| Burdock | Arctium lappa | Aids detoxification and antioxidant activity. |
| Cleavers | Galium aparine | Assists detoxification and reduces inflammation. |
| Dandelion | Taraxacum officinale | Increases bile production & supports detoxification. |
| Garden Sage | Salvia officinalis | Supports liver health and function. |
| Gentian | Gentiana spp. | Promotes bile production & stimulates digestion. |
| Ginger | Zingiber officinale | Reduces inflammation and aid detoxification. |
| Greater Celandine | Chelidonium majus | Supports bile production and detoxification. |
| Horseradish | Armoracia rusticana | Stimulates enzymes and promotes detoxification. |
| Licorice | Glycyrrhiza glabra | Reduces inflammation & protects against damage. |
| Lovage | Levisticum officinale | Supports liver function & promotes detoxification. |
| Milk Thistle | Silybum marianum | Promotes detoxification & protects against damage. |
| Oregon Grape | Mahonia aquifolium | Promotes bile production & aids detoxification. |
| Savory | Satureja | Supports liver health and function. |
| Schisandra | Schisandra chinensis | Enhances antioxidant defenses, protects the liver. |
| Turmeric | Curcuma longa | Reduces inflammation & protects against damage. |
| Wild Yam | Dioscorea villosa | Aids in detoxification & supports hormone balance. |
| Wormwood | Artemisia absinthium | Aids bile production, digestion, and detoxification. |
| Yellow Dock | Rumex crispus | Aids digestion and supports detoxification. |

| Hypnotic | Induce sleep, alleviate insomnia, or promote relaxation. | |
|---|---|---|
| **Herb** | **Scientific Name** | **Benefits** |
| Ashwagandha | Withania somnifera | Aids relaxation, reduces stress, & improves sleep. |
| Blue Vervain | Verbena hastata | Aids relaxation and helps with sleep. |
| California Poppy | Eschscholzia californica | Promote relaxation and improve sleep quality. |
| Catnip | Nepeta cataria | Aids relaxation, reduces stress, & improves sleep. |
| Chamomile | Matricaria chamomilla | Aids relaxation, reduces stress, & improves sleep. |
| Hops | Humulus lupulus | Alleviate anxiety and improve sleep patterns. |
| Jamaican Dogwood | Piscidia piscipula | Induce relaxation and improve sleep quality. |
| Kava Kava | Piper methysticum | Induce relaxation and improve sleep quality. |
| Kratom | Mityagyna speciosa | Promote relaxation and help with sleep. |
| Lavender | Lavandula spp. | Reduce anxiety, aid relaxation, improve sleep. |
| Lemon Balm | Melissa officinalis | Promote relaxation and improve sleep quality. |
| Linden | Tilia spp. | Reduce anxiety and stress, improve sleep quality. |
| Motherwort | Leonurus cardiaca | Reduce anxiety and improve sleep quality. |
| Passionflower | Passiflora incarnata | Reduce anxiety, promote relaxation, improve sleep. |
| Skullcap | Scutellaria lateriflora | Reduces anxiety and improves sleep quality. |
| Valerian | Valeriana officinalis | Promotes relaxation and improves sleep quality. |
| Vervain | Verbena officinalis | Reduces anxiety and improves sleep quality. |

| Hypotensive | Decrease blood pressure. | |
| --- | --- | --- |
| **Herb** | **Scientific Name** | **Benefits** |
| Arjuna | Terminalia arjuna | Widens blood vessels & reduces stress on the heart. |
| Astragalus | Astragalus membranaceus | Dilates blood vessels and reduces blood pressure. |
| Cat's Claw | Uncaria tomentosa | Relaxes blood vessels and reduces inflammation. |
| Cayenne | Capsicum annuum | Dilates blood vessels and reduces blood pressure. |
| Celery | Apium graveolens | Relaxes blood vessels and lowers blood pressure. |
| Cinnamon | Cinnamomum verum | Improve blood vessels and lower blood pressure. |
| Cramp Bark | Viburnum prunifolium | Relaxes smooth muscles in blood vessels. |
| French Lavender | Lavandula dentata | Reduces stress & anxiety, lowering blood pressure. |
| Garden Sage | Salvia officinalis | Lowers blood pressure. |
| Garlic | Allium sativum | Relaxes smooth muscles in blood vessels. |
| Ginger | Zingiber officinale | Relaxes blood vessels and lowers blood pressure. |
| Hawthorn | Crataegus spp. | Dilates blood vessels and reduces blood pressure. |
| Lemon Balm | Melissa officinalis | Reduces stress & anxiety, lowering blood pressure. |
| Linden | Tilia spp. | Relaxes blood vessels and lowers blood pressure. |
| Mistletoe | Viscum album | Regulates blood pressure. |
| Motherwort | Leonurus cardiaca | Reduces stress & anxiety, lowering blood pressure. |
| Onion | Allium cepa | Relaxes blood vessels and lowers blood pressure. |
| Olive | Olea europaea | Improves cardiovascular health. |
| Olive Leaf | Olea europaea | Relaxes smooth muscles in blood vessels. |
| Parsley | Petroselinum crispum | Regulates blood pressure, by countering sodium. |
| Passionflower | Passiflora incarnata | Reduces stress & anxiety, lowering blood pressure. |
| Siberian Ginseng | Eleutherococcus senticosus | Improve circulation, reduce stress & blood pressure. |
| Skullcap | Scutellaria lateriflora | Reduces anxiety and lowers blood pressure. |
| Valerian | Valeriana officinalis | Reduces stress and lowers blood pressure. |
| Yarrow | Achillea millefolium | Dilates blood vessels & improves blood circulation. |

| Nervine Tonics | Calms the mind and improves overall nervous system function. | |
|---|---|---|
| **Herb** | **Scientific Name** | **Benefits** |
| Ashwagandha | Withania somnifera | Reduces stress and anxiety. |
| Basil | Ocimum basilicum | Reduces stress and anxiety. |
| Blue Vervain | Verbena hastata | Calms nervous system, relieves stress and anxiety. |
| California Poppy | Eschscholzia californica | Relief from nervous tension and mild anxiety. |
| Caraway | Carum carvi | Aids in loosening mucus & removing congestion. |
| Catnip | Nepeta cataria | Reduces anxiety and restlessness. |
| Chamomile | Matricaria chamomilla | Alleviates stress and anxiety symptoms. |
| Garden Sage | Salvia officinalis | Supports the nervous system & promotes relaxation. |
| Gotu Kola | Centella asiatica | Improves cognitive functions, and reduces anxiety. |
| Holy Basil | Ocimum sanctum | Reduce stress and anxiety. |
| Kava Kava | Piper methysticum | Relief from anxiety and nervous tension. |
| Lavender | Lavandula spp. | Reduce stress and anxiety. |
| Lemon Balm | Melissa officinalis | Reduces anxiety and restlessness. |
| Linden | Tilia spp. | Reduce stress and anxiety. |
| Marjoram | Origanum marjorana | Calming effects on the nervous system. |
| Oat Straw | Avena sativa | Reduces anxiety and promotes relaxation. |
| Panax ginseng | Panax spp. | Improves stress response and cognitive function. |
| Passionflower | Passiflora incarnata | Reduces anxiety and restlessness. |
| Sage | Salvia officinalis | Supports the nervous system & promotes relaxation. |
| Siberian Ginseng | Eleutherococcus senticosus | Reduces stress and fatigue. |
| Skullcap | Scutellaria lateriflora | Reduces symptoms of anxiety and tension. |
| St. John's Wort | Hypericum perforatum | Reduces symptoms of mild depression and anxiety. |
| Valerian | Valeriana officinalis | Reduces symptoms of anxiety and insomnia. |
| Wood Betony | Stachys officinalis | Relieves symptoms of stress and tension. |

| **Nervine Relaxants** | Reduce stress, anxiety, & tension.  Promoting relaxation and a sense of calm. | |
|---|---|---|
| **Herb** | **Scientific Name** | **Benefits** |
| Ashwagandha | Withania somnifera | Reduces stress & anxiety, promotes a sense of calm. |
| Black Cohosh | Actaea racemosa | Manages stress & tension, alleviates anxiety. |
| Blue Vervain | Verbena hastata | Manages stress & tension, alleviates anxiety. |
| California Poppy | Eschscholzia californica | Alleviate symptoms of anxiety & insomnia. |
| Catnip | Nepeta cataria | Eases nervousness, alleviates stress and anxiety. |
| Chamomile | Matricaria chamomilla | Soothes nerves, remedy for stress and sleep issues. |
| Cramp Bark | Viburnum prunifolium | Relieves muscle tension to reduce physical stress. |
| Garden Sage | Salvia officinalis | Supports the nervous system & promotes relaxation. |
| Holy Basil | Ocimum sanctum | Reduces stress & anxiety, promotes a sense of calm. |
| Hops | Humulus lupulus | Alleviates anxiety, eases stress and improves sleep. |
| Hyssop | Hyssopus officinalis | Calms nerves, reduces stress, anxiety, and tension. |
| Kava Kava | Piper methysticum | Reduces anxiety, remedy for stress and tension. |
| Lavender | Lavandula angustifolia | Eases anxiety, aids in stress relief and better sleep. |
| Lemon Balm | Melissa officinalis | Reduce nervousness, manages stress and anxiety. |
| Lemon Verbana | Aloysia citridora | Calms the nervous system to promote relaxation. |
| Linden | Tilia spp. | Reduces nervousness and stress, anxiety relief. |
| Lobelia | Lobelia inflata | Relieves muscle tension/spasms, to relax. |
| Marjoram | Origanum marjorana | Helps to soothe and calm the nervous system. |
| Motherwort | Leonurus cardiaca | Reduce anxiety and calm nerves, anxiety relief. |
| Passionflower | Passiflora incarnata | Ease anxiety, manage stress & improve sleep. |
| Passionvine | Passiflora spp. | Alleviate anxiety, stress relief. |
| Red Clover | Trifolium pratense | Calms nerves and reduces stress for relaxation. |
| Rhodiola | Rhodiola rosea | Enhance stress resilience and reduce fatigue. |
| Sage | Salvia officinalis | Supports the nervous system & promotes relaxation. |
| Skullcap | Scutellaria lateriflora | Reduce anxiety, manages stress and tension. |
| St. John's Wort | Hypericum perforatum | Ease symptoms of mild depression and anxiety. |
| Valerian | Valeriana officinalis | Induce relaxation, reduce anxiety, improve sleep. |
| Vervain | Verbena officinalis | Reduce tension, aiding in stress management. |
| Wood Betony | Stachys officinalis | Calm nerves and reduce stress for tension relief. |

| Nervine Stimulants | Stimulates the nervous system. Increases alertness, mental clarity, & energy levels. | |
|---|---|---|
| **Herb** | **Scientific Name** | **Benefits** |
| American Ginseng | Panax quinquefolius | Promotes relaxation and mental clarity. |
| Angelica | Angelica archangelica | Aids in stress reduction and emotional balance. |
| Ashwagandha | Withania somnifera | Reduce stress & anxiety, promotes resilience. |
| Black Pepper | Piper nigrum | Enhance nerve function & mental alertness/clarity. |
| Cardamom | Elettaria caramomum | Promotes mental alertness and relaxation. |
| Cayenne | Capsicum annuum | Enhance nerve function, mental clarity and focus. |
| Cinnamon | Cinnamomum verum | Enhance cognitive function and alertness. |
| Cloves | Syzygium aromaticum | Promote mental clarity and emotional balance. |
| Damiana | Turnera diffusa | Reduce stress and improve mood. |
| Elecampane | Inula helenium | Enhance mental alertness and well-being. |
| Garlic | Allium sativum | Improve cognitive function and mental clarity. |
| Ginger | Zingiber officinale | Enhances mental alertness and focus. |
| Ginkgo Biloba | Ginkgo biloba | Enhances cognitive function and memory. |
| Ginseng | Panax ginseng | Aid stress reduction and mental clarity. |
| Gotu Kola | Centella asiatica | Enhances mental focus and cognitive function. |
| Gravel Root | Eupatorium purpireum | Aid in relaxation & strengthen the nervous system. |
| Guarana | Paullinia cupana | Caffeine boosts alertness & mental clarity. |
| Horseradish | Armoracia rusticana | Increased mental alertness and focus. |
| Juniper | Juniperus communis | Promotes mental clarity and emotional balance. |
| Kola Nut | Cola spp. | Boosting alertness and mental focus. |
| Rhodiola | Rhodiola rosea | Reduce stress, enhance mental alertness. |
| Rosemary | Rosmarinus officinalis | Promotes mental clarity and concentration. |
| Siberian Ginseng | Eleutherococcus senticosus | Reduce stress and improve mental alertness. |
| Yarrow | Achillea millefolium | Calms and strengthen the nervous system. |
| Yerba Mate | Ilex paraguariensis | Caffeine enhances mental alertness and focus. |

| Oxytocic | Stimulate uterine contractions and facilitate or induce labor. | |
|---|---|---|
| | Only use under the supervision of a health professional. | |
| **Herb** | **Scientific Name** | **Benefits** |
| Angelica | Angelica archangelica | Aids in labor and postpartum recovery. |
| Black Cohosh | Actaea racemosa | Aids in labor and menstrual regulation. |
| Blue Cohosh | Caulophyllum thalictroides | Aids in labor. |
| Cotton Root Bark | Gossypium spp. | Induce labor. |
| Cramp Bark | Viburnum prunifolium | Ease labor and manage menstrual cramps. |
| Ginger | Zingiber officinale | Promotes uterine contractions. |
| Juniper Berries | Juniperus communis | Aids in childbirth. |
| Marjoram | Origanum marjorana | Aid in uterine contractions during childbirth. |
| Pennyroyal | Mentha pulegium | Induce labor. |
| Raspberry Leaf | Rubus idaeus | Aids in labor. |
| Rue | Ruta graveolens | Aids in labor. |
| Shepherd's Purse | Capsella bursa-pastoris | Helps control postpartum bleeding. |
| Squaw Vine | Mitchella repens | Aids in labor. |

| **Rubefacient** | Increases blood circulation to the skin when used topically. Warms & reddens skin. | |
|---|---|---|
| **Herb** | **Scientific Name** | **Benefits** |
| Allspice | Pimenta dioica | Promotes skin blood circulation. |
| Arnica | Arnica Montana | Potentially reduces pain and inflammation. |
| Black Mustard | Brassica nigra | Aiding in relieving pain and inflammation. |
| Black Pepper | Piper nigrum | Helps alleviate muscle and joint discomfort. |
| Camphor | Cinnamomum camphora | Helps alleviate muscle and minor discomfort. |
| Cayenne | Capsicum annuum | Eases pain & inflammation in muscles and joints. |
| Eucalyptus | Eucalyptus spp. | Helps relieve muscle and joint discomfort. |
| Garden Sage | Salvia officinalis | Increases blood circulation. |
| Garlic | Allium sativum | Eases pain & inflammation in muscles and joints. |
| Ginger | Zingiber officinale | Alleviate muscle and joint discomfort. |
| Horseradish | Armoracia rusticana | Eases pain & inflammation in muscles and joints. |
| Marjoram | Origanum marjorana | Promotes skin blood circulation. |
| Onion | Allium cepa | Promotes skin blood circulation. |
| Peppermint | Mentha piperita | Aid in relieving muscle aches and tension. |
| Rosemary | Rosmarinus officinalis | Provides relief from muscle and joint pain. |

| Sialogogue | Stimulate saliva flow and improve digestion of starches. | |
| --- | --- | --- |
| **Herb** | **Scientific Name** | **Benefits** |
| Anise seeds | Pimpinella anisum | Aids in digestion and alleviates dry mouth. |
| Black Pepper | Piper nigrum | Aids in digestion. |
| Cayenne | Capsicum annuum | Aids in digestion and relieves dry mouth. |
| Cardamom | Elettaria caramomum | Aids in digestion and improves oral health. |
| Cinnamon | Cinnamomum verum | Aids in digestion and alleviates dry mouth. |
| Echinacea | Echinacea purpurea | Benefits oral health and relieves dry mouth. |
| Fennel Seeds | Foeniculum vulgare | Aids in digestion and freshens breath. |
| Ginger | Zingiber officinale | Aids in digestion and alleviates dry mouth. |
| Licorice | Glycyrrhiza glabra | Sooths dry mouth and supports oral health. |
| Lovage | Levisticum officinale | Stimulates saliva production & aids in digestion. |
| Marjoram | Origanum marjorana | Stimulates saliva production. |
| Peppermint | Mentha piperita | Aids in digestion and alleviates dry mouth. |
| Sage | Salvia officinalis | Helpful for dry mouth and supports oral health. |
| Yerba Santa | Eriodictyon californicum | Alleviates dry mouth and promotes oral comfort. |

| Vasodilator | Relax & widen the blood vessels, to increase blood flow & lower blood pressure. | |
|---|---|---|
| **Herb** | **Scientific Name** | **Benefits** |
| Allspice | Pimenta dioica | Helps widen blood vessels. |
| Astragalus | Astragalus membranaceus | Widens blood vessels and improves blood flow. |
| Butcher's Broom | Ruscus aculeatus | Assists in relaxing and widening blood vessels. |
| Cacao | Theobroma cacao | Facilitates the expansion of blood vessels. |
| Cayenne | Capsicum annuum | Promotes the widening of blood vessels. |
| Cinnamon | Cinnamomum verum | Helps to relax and widen blood vessels. |
| Garlic | Allium sativum | Helps to relax blood vessels. |
| Ginger | Zingiber officinale | Helps widen blood vessels. |
| Ginkgo | Ginkgo biloba | Increases blood flow by dilating blood vessels. |
| Ginseng | Panaz ginseng | Expands blood vessels. |
| Hawthorn | Crataegus spp. | Relaxes and widens blood vessels. |
| Horse Chestnut | Aesculus hippocastanum | Helps relax blood vessels. |
| Linden | Tilia spp. | Helps relax and widen blood vessels. |
| Marjoram | Origanum marjorana | Dilates blood vessels & enhances blood flow. |
| Mistletoe | Viscum album | Helps relax blood vessels. |
| Onion | Allium cepa | Helps relax blood vessels. |
| Rosemary | Rosmarinus officinalis | Aids in relaxing and widening of blood vessels. |
| Prickly Ash | Zanthoxylum americanum | Helps to relax blood vessels. |
| Turmeric | Curcuma longa | Helps to relax blood vessels & enhance blood flow. |
| Yarrow | Achillea millefolium | Helps to relax and widen blood vessels. |

| Vulnerary | Promote the healing of wounds, cuts, injuries, broken bones, and ulcers. Apply topically. | |
| --- | --- | --- |
| **Herb** | **Scientific Name** | **Benefits** |
| Aloe Vera | Aloe barbadensis miller | Promotes wound healing. |
| Arnica | Arnica Montana | Reduces pain, swelling, and bruises. |
| Calendula | Calendula officinalis | Heals skin irritations, cuts, and minor burns. |
| Cayenne | Capsicum annuum | Enhances circulation, reduces pain to aid healing. |
| Chamomile | Matricaria chamomilla | Reduce skin irritation, heal minor wounds & rashes. |
| Comfrey | Symphytum officinale | Heals bruises, sprains, and minor skin injuries. |
| Echinacea | Echinacea purpurea | Supports wound healing. |
| Elderflower | Sambucus spp. | Treats minor burns and skin irritations. |
| Garden Sage | Salvia officinalis | Aids in wound healing and tissue repair. |
| Garlic | Allium sativum | Promotes wound healing. |
| Goldenseal | Hydrastis canadensis | Aids wound healing. |
| Gotu Kola | Centella asiatica | Promotes the healing of wounds, cuts, & burns. |
| Gumweed | Grindelia integrifolia | Aids healing for minor wounds and skin irritations. |
| Lavender | Lavandula spp. | Aids healing for minor burns, cuts, & skin irritations. |
| Marjoram | Origanum marjorana | Aid the healing of wounds & promotes tissue repair. |
| Myrrh | Commiphora myrrha | Useful for wound healing and minor skin irritations. |
| Nasturtium | Tropaeolum majus | Aids in wound healing and tissue repair. |
| Onion | Allium cepa | Helps relax blood vessels. |
| Plantain | Plantago spp. | Aids wound healing, insect bites, & skin irritations. |
| Purslane | Portulaca oleracea | Aids wound healing and promotes tissue repair. |
| Sage | Salvia officinalis | Aids in wound healing and tissue repair. |
| St. John's Wort | Hypericum perforatum | Skin regeneration for minor wounds, burns, etc. |
| Sweet Cicely | Myrrhis odorata | Useful for wound healing and minor skin irritations. |
| Thyme | Thymus vulgaris | Supports healing of minor wound & skin irritations. |
| Witch Hazel | Hamamelis virginiana | Aids healing of minor cuts, bruises, skin irritations. |
| Yarrow | Achillea millefolium | Promotes healing of wounds and skin irritations. |

# SECTION II

## Herb Charts Organized by Classifications

| Herbs By Classifications | Adaptogens | Alterative | Amphoteric | Analgesic | Anodyne | Antacid & Anti-ulcer | Anthelmintics | Antibiotic | Anticatarrhal | Antiemetics | Antifungal | Antihemorrhagic | Anti-Inflammatory | Antilithics-Gallstone | Antilithics-Urinary | Antiprotozoal | Antipyretic | Antirheumatic | Antispasmodic | Antiviral | Aperient | Astringent | Bitters | Cardiotonic | Carminative | Cathartic | Cholagogue | Demulcent | Diaphoretic | Diuretic | Emmenagogue | Expectorant | Galactogogue | Hematinic | Hepatic | Hypnotic | Hypotensive | Nervine Tonics | Nervine Relaxants | Nervine Stimulants | Oxytocic | Rubefacient | Sialogogue | Vasodilator | Vulnerary |
|---|---|---|---|---|---|---|---|---|---|---|---|---|---|---|---|---|---|---|---|---|---|---|---|---|---|---|---|---|---|---|---|---|---|---|---|---|---|---|---|---|---|---|---|---|---|
| *Adaptogens* | | | | | | | | | | | | | | | | | | | | | | | | | | | | | | | | | | | | | | | | | | | | | |
| American Ginseng | X | | | | | | | | | | | | | | | | | | | | | | | | | | | | | | | | | | | | | | | X | | | | | |
| American Skullcap | X | | | | | | | | | | | | | | | | | | | | | | | | | | | | | | | | | | | | | | | | | | | | |
| Ashwagandha | X | | X | | | | | | | | | | | | | | | | | | | | | | | | | | | | | | | X | | X | | X | X | X | | | | | |
| Astragalus | X | | X | | | | | | | | | | | | | | | | | X | | | | X | | | | | | | | | | X | X | | X | | | | | | | X | |
| Basil | X | | | | | | | X | X | X | | | | | | | X | | | | | | | | X | | | | X | | | X | | | | | | X | | | | | | | |
| Black Cohosh | X | | X | X | X | | | | | | | | | | | | | | X | | | | | | | | | | | | X | | | | | | | | X | | X | | | | |
| Cordyceps | X | | X | | | | | | | | | | | | | | | | | | | | | | | | | | | | | | | | | | | | | | | | | | |
| Eleuthero | X | | | | | | | | | | | | | | | | | | | | | | | | | | | | | | | | | | | | | | | | | | | | |
| Ginkgo | X | | | | | | | | | | | | | | | | | | | | | | | X | | | | | | | | | | | | | | | | X | | | | X | |
| Ginkgo Biloba | X | | | | | | | | | | | | | | | | | | | | | | | X | | | | | | | | | | | | | | | | X | | | | X | |
| Gotu Kola | X | | X | | | X | | | | | | | | | | | X | | | | | | | | | | | | | | | | | | | X | | | | X | | | | | X |
| Hawthorn | X | | | | | | | | | | | | | | | | | | | | | | | X | | | | | | X | | | | | | | X | | | | | | | X | |
| Holy Basil | X | | X | | | | | | | | | | | | | | | | | | | | | | | | | | | | | | | | | | | X | X | | | | | | |
| Indian Gooseberry | X | | | | | | | | | | | | | | | | | | | | | | | | | | | | | | | | | | | | | | | | | | | | |
| Jiaogulan | X | | | | | | | | | | | | | | | | | | | | | | | | | | | | | | | | | | | | | | | | | | | | |
| Kava Kava | X | | | X | X | | | | | | | | | | | | | | | | | | | | | | | | | | | | | | | | | X | X | X | | | | | |
| Korean Ginseng | X | | | | | | | | | | | | | | | | | | | | | | | | | | | | | | | | | | | | | | | | | | | | |
| Lemon Balm | X | | | | | | | | X | | | | | | | | X | X | X | | | | | X | X | | | | | | | | | | | | | X | X | X | | | | | |
| Licorice | X | X | X | | | X | | | X | | | | X | | | X | X | X | | X | X | | | | | X | X | X | | | | X | | | X | | | | | | | | X | | |
| Licorice Root | X | X | X | | | X | | | X | | | | X | | | X | X | X | | X | X | | | | | X | X | X | | | | X | | | X | | | | | | | | X | | |
| Maca | X | | X | | | | | | | | | | | | | | | | | | | | | | | | | | | | | | | | | | | | | | | | | | |
| Maca Root | X | | X | | | | | | | | | | | | | | | | | | | | | | | | | | | | | | | | | | | | | | | | | | |
| Milk Thistle | X | | | | | | | | | | | | X | X | | | | | | | | | | | | | X | | | | | | | | X | | | | | | | | | | |
| Mucuna Pruriens | X | | | | | | | | | | | | | | | | | | | | | | | | | | | | | | | | | | | | | | | | | | | | |
| Nasturtium | X | X | X | | | | | X | X | X | X | X | X | X | X | X | X | X | X | X | X | | | | | | | | | | | X | | | | | | | | | | | | | X |
| Panax ginseng | X | | | | | | | | | | | | | | | | | | | | | | | | | | | | | | | | | | | | | X | | | | | | | |
| Passionflower | X | | | | | | | | | | | | | | | | | | X | | | | | | | | | | | | | | | | | X | X | X | X | | | | | | |
| Puncture Vine | X | | | | | | | | | | | | | | | | | | | | | | | | | | | | | | | | | | | | | | | | | | | | |
| Reishi mushrooms | X | | | | | | | | | | | | | | | | | | | | | | | | | | | | | | | | | | | | | | | | | | | | |
| Rhodiola | X | | X | | | | | | | | | | | | | | | | | | | | | | | | | | | | | | | | | | | | X | X | | | | | |
| Saffron | X | | | | | | | | | | | | | | | | | | | | | | | | | | | | | | | | | | | | | | | | | | | | |
| Schisandra | X | | X | | | | | | | | | | | | | | | | | | | | | | | | | | | | | | | | X | | | | | | | | | | |
| Shilajit | X | | | | | | | | | | | | | | | | | | | | | | | | | | | | | | | | | | | | | | | | | | | | |
| Siberian Ginseng | X | | | | | | | | | | | | | | | | | | | | | | | | | | | | | | | | | | | | | X | X | X | | | | | |
| Suma | X | | | | | | | | | | | | | | | | | | | | | | | | | | | | | | | | | | | | | | | | | | | | |
| Tulsi | X | | X | | | | | | | | | | | | | | | | | | | | | | | | | | | | | | | | | | | X | X | | | | | | |
| Turmeric | X | | X | X | X | X | X | X | | | | | X | X | | X | | | | | | | | X | | | X | | | | | | | | X | | | | | | | | | X | |
| Valerian | X | | | | | | | | | | | | | | | | | | X | | | | | | | | | | | | | | | | | X | X | X | X | | | | | | |

The table below is printed sideways on the page: the classification names form the row labels (read down the left edge) and the herb names form the column headers (read along the bottom). The corner cell reads "Herbs By Classifications" / *Alterative*.

**Herbs By Classifications — Herbs 1–11**

| Herbs By Classifications | Alfalfa | Aloe Vera | Blue Flag | Burdock | Calendula | Chaparral | Cleavers | Comfrey | Dandelion | Dandelion Root | Echinacea |
|---|---|---|---|---|---|---|---|---|---|---|---|
| Vulnerary | | X | | | X | | | X | | X | X |
| Vasodilator | | | | | | | | | | | |
| Sialogogue | | | | | | | | | | | X |
| Rubefacient | | | | | | | | | | | |
| Oxytocic | | | | | | | | | | | |
| Nervine Stimulants | | | | | | | | | | | |
| Nervine Relaxants | | | | | | | | | | | |
| Nervine Tonics | | | | | | | | | | | |
| Hypotensive | | | | | | | | | | | |
| Hypnotic | | | | | | | | | | | |
| Hepatic | | | | X | | | | X | X | X | |
| Hematinic | X | | | X | | | | | X | X | X |
| Galactogogue | X | | | | | | | | | | |
| Expectorant | | | | | | | | X | | | |
| Emmenagogue | | | | | | X | | | | | |
| Diuretic | X | | | X | | | X | | X | X | |
| Diaphoretic | | | | | | | | | | | X |
| Demulcent | | X | | | | | | X | | | |
| Cholagogue | | | | | | | | | X | X | |
| Cathartic | | | | | | | | | | | |
| Carminative | | | | | | | | | | | |
| Cardiotonic | | | | | | | | | | | |
| Bitters | | | | X | | | | | X | X | |
| Astringent | | | | | | | | | | | |
| Aperient | X | X | | | | | | | X | X | |
| Antiviral | | | | | | X | | | | | X |
| Antispasmodic | | | | | | | | | | | |
| Antirheumatic | | | | X | | | | | | X | X |
| Antipyretic | X | | | | | | | | | | X |
| Antiprotozoal | | | | | | X | | | | | X |
| Antilithics-Urinary | | | | | | | X | | X | X | |
| Antilithics-Gallstone | | | | | | | | | X | X | |
| Anti-inflammatory | | X | | | X | | | X | | | X |
| Antihemorrhagic | | | | X | | | | X | | | |
| Antifungal | | X | | | X | X | | | | | X |
| Antiemetics | | | | | | | | | X | X | X |
| Anticatarrhal | | | | | | | X | | X | X | X |
| Antibiotic | | | | X | X | | | | | X | X |
| Anthelmintics | | | | | | | | | | | X |
| Antacid & Anti-ulcer | | | | | X | | | X | | X | X |
| Anodyne | | | | | | | | | | | |
| Analgesic | | | | | | | | | | | |
| Amphoteric | | | | | | | | | | | |
| Alterative | X | X | X | X | X | X | X | X | X | X | X |
| Adaptogens | | | | | | | | | | | |

**Herbs By Classifications — Herbs 12–22**

| Herbs By Classifications | Garlic | Horsetail | Licorice | Licorice Root | Lovage | Mallow | Marshmallow | Marshmallow Root | Nasturtium | Nettle | Oregon Grape |
|---|---|---|---|---|---|---|---|---|---|---|---|
| Vulnerary | | | X | | | X | X | X | X | | X |
| Vasodilator | X | | | | | | | | | | |
| Sialogogue | | | X | X | X | | | | | | |
| Rubefacient | X | | | | | | | | | | |
| Oxytocic | | | | | | | | | | | |
| Nervine Stimulants | X | | | | | | | | | | |
| Nervine Relaxants | | | | | | | | | | | |
| Nervine Tonics | | | | | | | | | | | |
| Hypotensive | X | | | | | | | | | | |
| Hypnotic | | | | | | | | | | | |
| Hepatic | | | X | X | X | | | | | | X |
| Hematinic | | | | | | | | | | X | |
| Galactogogue | | | | | | | | | | X | |
| Expectorant | X | | X | X | X | | | | | | |
| Emmenagogue | | | | | | | | | | | |
| Diuretic | | X | | | X | | | | X | X | |
| Diaphoretic | X | | | | | | | | | | |
| Demulcent | | | X | X | X | X | X | X | | | |
| Cholagogue | | | X | X | | | | | | | X |
| Cathartic | | | X | X | | | | | | | |
| Carminative | X | | | | X | | | | | | |
| Cardiotonic | X | | | | | | | | | | |
| Bitters | | | | | X | | | | | X | |
| Astringent | | X | | | | | | | | X | |
| Aperient | | | X | X | | X | X | X | X | | |
| Antiviral | X | | X | X | | | | | X | | |
| Antispasmodic | | | | | X | | | | | | |
| Antirheumatic | | | | | | | | | X | X | |
| Antipyretic | | | | | | | | | X | | |
| Antiprotozoal | | | X | X | | | | | | | |
| Antilithics-Urinary | | X | | | | X | X | X | X | | |
| Antilithics-Gallstone | | | | | | | | | X | | X |
| Anti-inflammatory | | | X | X | | X | X | X | X | X | |
| Antihemorrhagic | | X | | | | | | | X | X | |
| Antifungal | | | | X | | | | | X | | X |
| Antiemetics | X | | | | | | | | | | |
| Anticatarrhal | X | X | | | X | X | X | X | X | X | |
| Antibiotic | | | X | | | | | | | | X |
| Anthelmintics | | | | | | | | | | | |
| Antacid & Anti-ulcer | | | | | | | | | | | |
| Anodyne | | | | | | | | | | | |
| Analgesic | | | | | | | | | | | |
| Amphoteric | | | X | X | | | | | X | | |
| Alterative | X | X | X | X | X | X | X | X | X | X | X |
| Adaptogens | | | X | X | | | | | X | | |

**Herbs By Classifications — Herbs 23–33**

| Herbs By Classifications | Oregon Grape Root | Plantain | Poke Root | Prickly Ash | Purselane | Red Clover | Sarsaparilla | Stinging Nettle | Uva Ursi | Wild Indigo | Yellow Dock |
|---|---|---|---|---|---|---|---|---|---|---|---|
| Vulnerary | | | | | X | | | | | | |
| Vasodilator | | | | X | | | | | | | |
| Sialogogue | | | | | | | | | | | |
| Rubefacient | | | | | | | | | | | |
| Oxytocic | | | | | | | | | | | |
| Nervine Stimulants | | | | | | | | | | | |
| Nervine Relaxants | | | | | | | | X | | | |
| Nervine Tonics | | | | | | | | | | | |
| Hypotensive | | | | | | | | | | | |
| Hypnotic | | | | | | | | | | | |
| Hepatic | X | | | | | | | | | | X |
| Hematinic | | | | | | | | X | | | X |
| Galactogogue | | | | | | | | X | | | |
| Expectorant | | | | | | | | | | | |
| Emmenagogue | | | | | | | | | | | |
| Diuretic | | X | | | X | | | | X | X | |
| Diaphoretic | | | | X | X | | | | | | |
| Demulcent | | X | | | X | | | | | | |
| Cholagogue | X | | | | | | | | | | |
| Cathartic | | | | | | | | | | X | X |
| Carminative | | | | | | | | | | | |
| Cardiotonic | | | | | | | | | | | |
| Bitters | | | | | | | | | | | |
| Astringent | | X | | | X | | | | X | X | |
| Aperient | | | | | X | | | | | | |
| Antiviral | | | | | | | | | | | |
| Antispasmodic | | | | | | | | | | | |
| Antirheumatic | | | | | | | | | X | X | |
| Antipyretic | | | | | X | | | | | | |
| Antiprotozoal | | | | | | | | | | | |
| Antilithics-Urinary | | | | | | | | | X | | |
| Antilithics-Gallstone | X | | | | | | | | | | |
| Anti-inflammatory | | X | | | X | | X | | | | |
| Antihemorrhagic | | X | | | X | | | | X | X | X |
| Antifungal | X | | | | X | | | | | | |
| Antiemetics | | | | | X | | | | | | |
| Anticatarrhal | | | | | X | | | | X | X | |
| Antibiotic | X | | | | X | | | | X | | |
| Anthelmintics | | | | | | | | | | | |
| Antacid & Anti-ulcer | | | | | | | | | | | |
| Anodyne | | | | | | | | | | | |
| Analgesic | | | | | | | | | | | |
| Amphoteric | | | | | X | | | | | | |
| Alterative | X | X | X | X | X | X | X | X | X | X | X |
| Adaptogens | | | | | X | | | | | | |

| Herbs By Classifications | Adaptogens | Alterative | Amphoteric | Analgesic | Anodyne | Antacid & Anti-ulcer | Anthelmintics | Antibiotic | Anticatarrhal | Antiemetics | Antifungal | Antihemorrhagic | Anti-Inflammatory | Antilithics-Gallstone | Antilithics-Urinary | Antiprotozoal | Antipyretic | Antirheumatic | Antispasmodic | Antiviral | Aperient | Astringent | Bitters | Cardiotonic | Carminative | Cathartic | Cholagogue | Demulcent | Diaphoretic | Diuretic | Emmenagogue | Expectorant | Galactogogue | Hematinic | Hepatic | Hypnotic | Hypotensive | Nervine Tonics | Nervine Relaxants | Nervine Stimulants | Oxytocic | Rubefacient | Sialogogue | Vasodilator | Vulnerary |
|---|---|---|---|---|---|---|---|---|---|---|---|---|---|---|---|---|---|---|---|---|---|---|---|---|---|---|---|---|---|---|---|---|---|---|---|---|---|---|---|---|---|---|---|---|---|
| *Amphoteric* |  |  |  |  |  |  |  |  |  |  |  |  |  |  |  |  |  |  |  |  |  |  |  |  |  |  |  |  |  |  |  |  |  |  |  |  |  |  |  |  |  |  |  |  |  |
| Ashitaba |  |  | X |  |  |  |  |  |  |  |  |  |  |  |  |  |  |  |  |  |  |  |  |  |  |  |  |  |  |  |  |  |  |  |  |  |  |  |  |  |  |  |  |  |  |
| Ashwagandha | X |  | X |  |  |  |  |  |  |  |  |  |  |  |  |  |  |  |  |  |  |  |  |  |  |  |  |  |  |  |  |  |  | X |  | X |  | X | X | X |  |  |  |  |  |
| Astragalus | X |  | X |  |  |  |  |  |  |  |  |  |  |  |  |  |  |  |  | X |  |  |  | X |  |  |  |  |  |  |  |  |  | X | X |  | X |  |  |  |  |  |  | X |  |
| Cayenne |  |  | X | X | X |  |  | X | X |  |  | X | X |  |  |  |  | X |  |  |  |  |  | X |  |  |  |  | X |  |  |  |  |  |  |  | X |  |  | X |  | X | X | X | X |
| Chlorella |  |  | X |  |  |  |  |  |  |  |  |  |  |  |  |  |  |  |  |  |  |  |  |  |  |  |  |  |  |  |  |  |  |  |  |  |  |  |  |  |  |  |  |  |  |
| Cordyceps | X |  | X |  |  |  |  |  |  |  |  |  |  |  |  |  |  |  |  |  |  |  |  |  |  |  |  |  |  |  |  |  |  |  |  |  |  |  |  |  |  |  |  |  |  |
| Ginseng |  |  | X |  |  |  |  |  |  |  |  |  |  |  |  |  |  |  |  |  |  |  |  |  |  |  |  |  |  |  |  |  |  |  |  |  |  |  |  | X |  |  |  | X |  |
| Gotu Kola | X |  | X |  |  | X |  |  |  |  |  |  |  |  |  |  | X |  |  |  |  |  |  |  |  |  |  |  |  |  |  |  |  |  |  |  |  | X |  | X |  |  |  |  | X |
| Holy Basil | X |  | X |  |  |  |  |  |  |  |  |  |  |  |  |  |  |  |  |  |  |  |  |  |  |  |  |  |  |  |  |  |  |  |  |  |  | X | X |  |  |  |  |  |  |
| Licorice | X | X | X |  |  | X |  |  | X |  |  |  | X |  |  | X |  | X |  | X | X |  |  |  |  | X | X | X |  |  |  | X |  |  | X |  |  |  |  |  |  |  | X |  |  |
| Licorice Root | X | X | X |  |  | X |  |  | X |  |  |  | X |  |  | X |  | X |  | X | X |  |  |  |  | X | X | X |  |  |  | X |  |  | X |  |  |  |  |  |  |  | X |  |  |
| Maca | X |  | X |  |  |  |  |  |  |  |  |  |  |  |  |  |  |  |  |  |  |  |  |  |  |  |  |  |  |  |  |  |  |  |  |  |  |  |  |  |  |  |  |  |  |
| Maca Root | X |  | X |  |  |  |  |  |  |  |  |  |  |  |  |  |  |  |  |  |  |  |  |  |  |  |  |  |  |  |  |  |  |  |  |  |  |  |  |  |  |  |  |  |  |
| Nasturtium | X | X | X |  |  |  |  | X | X | X | X | X | X | X | X | X | X | X | X | X | X | X |  |  |  |  |  |  | X |  |  |  |  |  |  |  |  |  |  |  |  |  |  |  | X |
| Purselane |  | X | X |  |  |  |  | X | X | X | X | X | X |  |  |  |  |  |  |  | X | X |  |  |  | X | X | X |  |  |  |  |  |  |  |  |  |  |  |  |  |  |  |  | X |
| Reishi mushrooms | X |  | X |  |  |  |  |  |  |  |  |  |  |  |  |  |  |  |  |  |  |  |  |  |  |  |  |  |  |  |  |  |  |  |  |  |  |  |  |  |  |  |  |  |  |
| Rhodiola | X |  | X |  |  |  |  |  |  |  |  |  |  |  |  |  |  |  |  |  |  |  |  |  |  |  |  |  |  |  |  |  |  |  |  |  |  |  | X | X |  |  |  |  |  |
| Savory |  |  | X | X | X |  |  | X | X | X | X |  | X |  |  |  |  | X | X | X | X | X | X | X | X | X | X | X | X | X | X | X | X | X | X |  |  |  |  |  |  |  |  |  |  |
| Schisandra | X |  | X |  |  |  |  |  |  |  |  |  |  |  |  |  |  |  |  |  |  |  |  |  |  |  |  |  |  |  |  |  |  |  | X |  |  |  |  |  |  |  |  |  |  |
| Spirulina |  |  | X |  |  |  |  |  |  |  |  |  |  |  |  |  |  |  |  |  |  |  |  |  |  |  |  |  |  |  |  |  |  |  |  |  |  |  |  |  |  |  |  |  |  |
| Tulsi | X |  | X |  |  |  |  |  |  |  |  |  |  |  |  |  |  |  |  |  |  |  |  |  |  |  |  |  |  |  |  |  |  |  |  |  |  | X | X |  |  |  |  |  |  |
| Turmeric | X |  | X | X | X | X | X | X |  |  |  |  | X | X |  |  |  | X |  |  |  |  |  | X |  |  | X |  |  |  |  |  |  |  | X |  |  |  |  |  |  |  |  | X |  |

| Herbs By Classifications | Adaptogens | Alterative | Amphoteric | Analgesic | Anodyne | Antacid & Anti-ulcer | Anthelmintics | Antibiotic | Anticatarrhal | Antiemetics | Antifungal | Antihemorrhagic | Anti-Inflammatory | Antilithics-Gallstone | Antilithics-Urinary | Antiprotozoal | Antipyretic | Antirheumatic | Antispasmodic | Antiviral | Aperient | Astringent | Bitters | Cardiotonic | Carminative | Cathartic | Cholagogue | Demulcent | Diaphoretic | Diuretic | Emmenagogue | Expectorant | Galactogogue | Hematinic | Hepatic | Hypnotic | Hypotensive | Nervine Tonics | Nervine Relaxants | Nervine Stimulants | Oxytocic | Rubefacient | Sialogogue | Vasodilator | Vulnerary |
|---|---|---|---|---|---|---|---|---|---|---|---|---|---|---|---|---|---|---|---|---|---|---|---|---|---|---|---|---|---|---|---|---|---|---|---|---|---|---|---|---|---|---|---|---|---|
| *Analgesic* | | | | | | | | | | | | | | | | | | | | | | | | | | | | | | | | | | | | | | | | | | | | | |
| Arnica | | | | X | X | | | | | | | | X | | | | | X | | | | | | | | | | | | | | | | | | | | | | | | X | | | X |
| Aspen | | | | X | | | | | | | | | X | | | | X | | | | | | | | | | | | | | | | | | | | | | | | | | | | |
| Baneberry | | | | X | | | | | | | | | | | | | | | X | | | | | | | | | | | | | | | | | | | | | | | | | | |
| Birch | | | | X | | | | | | | | | X | | | | X | X | | | | | | | | | | | | | | | | | | | | | | | | | | | |
| Black Cohosh | X | | | X | X | | | | | | | | | | | | | X | | | | | | | | | X | | | | | | | | | | | | X | | | | X | | |
| Boswellia | | | | X | X | | | | | | | | X | | | | | X | | | | | | | | | | | | | | | | | | | | | | | | | | | |
| Cardamom | | | | X | | | | | | X | | | | | | | | | | | | | | | X | | | | | | | | | | | | | | | | X | | X | | |
| Cayenne | | | X | X | X | | | X | X | | | X | X | | | | | X | | | | | | X | | | | | X | | | | | | | | X | | | | | X | X | X | X |
| Chamomile | | | | X | X | X | | X | | X | X | | X | | | | X | X | X | | | | X | | X | | | | X | | X | | | | | X | | | X | X | | | | | X |
| Clematis | | | | X | | | | | | | | | | | | | | | | | | | | | | | | | | | | | | | | | | | | | | | | | |
| Cloves | | | | X | X | | X | | | X | X | | | | | | | | | X | | | | | X | | | | | | | | | | | | | | | | | | X | | |
| Devil's Claw | | | | X | X | | | | | | | | X | | | | | X | | | | | | | | | | | | | | | | | | | | | | | | | | | |
| Feverfew | | | | X | | | | | | | | | | | | | | | | | | | | | | | | | | | | | | | | | | | | | | | | | |
| Frankincense | | | | X | X | | | | | | | | X | | | | | X | | | | | | | | | | | | | | | | | | | | | | | | | | | |
| Ginger | | | | X | | | X | X | X | X | | | X | X | | X | X | X | X | X | | | | X | X | X | | | X | X | X | | | | X | | X | X | X | X | | | | X | |
| Kava Kava | X | | | X | X | | | | | | | | | | | | | | | | | | | | | | | | | | | | | | | | | X | X | X | | | | | |
| Lavender | | | | X | X | | | | | X | | | | | | | | | X | | | | | | X | | | | | | | | | | | X | | X | X | X | | | | | X |
| Marjoram | | | | X | X | | | X | X | | | | X | | | | | | X | X | X | X | X | | X | | | | | | | | | | | | | X | X | | X | X | X | X | X |
| Oregano | | | | X | | | | X | X | | X | | X | | | | X | X | | | | | | | | | X | | | | | X | | | | | | | | | | | | | |
| Peppermint | | | | X | | | | X | X | X | | | X | | | | X | X | | | | | | | X | | | | X | | X | | | | | | | | | | | | | X | X |
| Poplar | | | | X | | | | | | | | | X | | | | X | | | | | | | | | | | | | | | | | | | | | | | | | | | | |
| Savory | | | X | X | X | | | X | X | X | X | | X | | | | | X | X | X | X | X | X | X | X | X | X | X | X | X | X | X | | | X | | X | | | X | X | X | | X | |
| Sage | | | | X | | | | X | X | | | | X | | | | | X | X | | | X | X | | X | | | | X | | X | | | | | | | X | X | | | | | X | X |
| Skullcap | | | | X | X | | | | | | | | X | | | | X | | X | | | | | | | | | | | | | | | | | X | X | X | X | | | | | | |
| Turmeric | X | | X | X | X | X | X | X | | | | | X | X | | | | X | | | | | | X | | | X | | | | | | | | X | | | | | | | | | X | |
| White Willow | | | | X | X | | | | | | | | X | | | | X | X | | | | | | | | | | | | | | | | | | | | | | | | | | | |
| White Willow Bark | | | | X | X | | | | | | | | X | | | | X | X | | | | | | | | | | | | | | | | | | | | | | | | | | | |
| Willow | | | | X | X | | | | | | | | X | | | | X | X | | | | | | | | | | | | | | | | | | | | | | | | | | | |
| Willow Bark | | | | X | X | | | | | | | | X | | | | X | X | | | | | | | | | | | | | | | | | | | | | | | | | | | |
| Yarrow | | | | X | | | | X | X | | | X | X | | | | X | | X | | | X | | | X | | | | X | | | | | | | | X | | | | | | | X | X |

| Herbs By Classifications | Adaptogens | Alterative | Amphoteric | Analgesic | Anodyne | Antacid & Anti-ulcer | Anthelmintics | Antibiotic | Anticatarrhal | Antiemetics | Antifungal | Antihemorrhagic | Anti-Inflammatory | Antilithics-Gallstone | Antilithics-Urinary | Antiprotozoal | Antipyretic | Antirheumatic | Antispasmodic | Antiviral | Aperient | Astringent | Bitters | Cardiotonic | Carminative | Cathartic | Cholagogue | Demulcent | Diaphoretic | Diuretic | Emmenagogue | Expectorant | Galactogogue | Hematinic | Hepatic | Hypnotic | Hypotensive | Nervine Tonics | Nervine Relaxants | Nervine Stimulants | Oxytocic | Rubefacient | Sialogogue | Vasodilator | Vulnerary |
|---|---|---|---|---|---|---|---|---|---|---|---|---|---|---|---|---|---|---|---|---|---|---|---|---|---|---|---|---|---|---|---|---|---|---|---|---|---|---|---|---|---|---|---|---|---|
| **Anodyne** |  |  |  |  |  |  |  |  |  |  |  |  |  |  |  |  |  |  |  |  |  |  |  |  |  |  |  |  |  |  |  |  |  |  |  |  |  |  |  |  |  |  |  |  |  |
| Arnica |  |  |  | X | X |  |  |  |  |  |  |  | X |  |  |  |  | X |  |  |  |  |  |  |  |  |  |  |  |  |  |  |  |  |  |  |  |  |  |  |  | X |  |  | X |
| Black Cohosh | X |  |  | X | X |  |  |  |  |  |  |  |  |  |  |  |  |  | X |  |  |  |  |  |  |  |  |  |  |  | X |  |  |  |  |  |  |  | X |  | X |  |  |  |  |
| Boswellia |  |  |  | X | X |  |  |  |  |  |  |  | X |  |  |  |  | X |  |  |  |  |  |  |  |  |  |  |  |  |  |  |  |  |  |  |  |  |  |  |  |  |  |  |  |
| Cayenne |  |  | X | X | X |  |  | X | X |  | X |  | X |  |  |  |  | X |  |  |  |  |  | X |  |  |  |  | X |  |  |  |  |  |  |  | X |  |  | X |  | X | X | X | X |
| Chamomile |  |  |  | X | X | X |  | X |  | X | X |  | X |  |  |  | X | X | X |  |  |  | X |  | X |  |  |  | X |  | X |  |  |  |  | X |  | X | X |  |  |  |  |  | X |
| Cloves |  |  |  | X | X |  | X |  |  | X | X |  |  |  |  |  |  |  |  | X |  |  |  |  | X |  |  |  |  |  |  |  |  |  |  |  |  |  |  | X |  |  |  |  |  |
| Devil's Claw |  |  |  | X | X |  |  |  |  |  |  |  | X |  |  |  |  | X |  |  |  |  |  |  |  |  |  |  |  |  |  |  |  |  |  |  |  |  |  |  |  |  |  |  |  |
| Frankincense |  |  |  | X | X |  |  |  |  |  |  |  | X |  |  |  |  | X |  |  |  |  |  |  |  |  |  |  |  |  |  |  |  |  |  |  |  |  |  |  |  |  |  |  |  |
| Kava Kava | X |  |  | X | X |  |  |  |  |  |  |  |  |  |  |  |  |  |  |  |  |  |  |  |  |  |  |  |  |  |  |  |  |  |  | X |  | X | X |  |  |  |  |  |  |
| Lavendar |  |  |  | X | X |  |  |  |  | X |  |  |  |  |  |  |  |  | X |  |  |  |  |  | X |  |  |  |  |  |  |  |  |  |  | X | X | X | X |  |  |  |  |  | X |
| Marjoram |  |  |  | X | X |  |  | X | X |  |  |  | X |  |  |  |  |  | X | X | X | X | X |  | X |  |  |  |  |  |  |  |  |  |  |  |  | X | X |  | X | X | X | X | X |
| Savory |  |  | X | X | X |  |  | X | X | X | X | X | X |  |  |  |  |  | X | X | X | X | X | X | X | X | X | X | X | X | X | X | X | X | X |  |  |  |  |  |  |  |  |  |  |
| Skullcap |  |  |  | X | X |  |  |  |  |  |  |  | X |  |  |  | X |  | X |  |  |  |  |  |  |  |  |  |  |  |  |  |  |  |  | X | X | X | X |  |  |  |  |  |  |
| Turmeric | X |  | X | X | X | X | X | X |  |  |  |  | X | X |  |  |  | X |  |  |  |  |  | X |  |  | X |  |  |  |  |  |  |  | X |  |  |  |  |  |  |  |  | X |  |
| White Willow |  |  |  | X | X |  |  |  |  |  |  |  | X |  |  |  | X | X |  |  |  |  |  |  |  |  |  |  |  |  |  |  |  |  |  |  |  |  |  |  |  |  |  |  |  |
| White Willow Bark |  |  |  | X | X |  |  |  |  |  |  |  | X |  |  |  | X | X |  |  |  |  |  |  |  |  |  |  |  |  |  |  |  |  |  |  |  |  |  |  |  |  |  |  |  |
| Willow |  |  |  | X | X |  |  |  |  |  |  |  | X |  |  |  | X | X |  |  |  |  |  |  |  |  |  |  |  |  |  |  |  |  |  |  |  |  |  |  |  |  |  |  |  |
| Willow Bark |  |  |  | X | X |  |  |  |  |  |  |  | X |  |  |  | X | X |  |  |  |  |  |  |  |  |  |  |  |  |  |  |  |  |  |  |  |  |  |  |  |  |  |  |  |
| Yarrow |  |  |  | X | X |  |  | X | X |  |  | X | X |  |  |  | X |  |  |  |  | X |  | X |  |  |  |  | X |  |  |  |  |  |  |  | X |  |  | X |  |  |  | X | X |

| Herbs By Classifications | Adaptogens | Alterative | Amphoteric | Analgesic | Anodyne | Antacid & Anti-ulcer | Anthelmintics | Antibiotic | Anticatarrhal | Antiemetics | Antifungal | Antihemorrhagic | Anti-Inflammatory | Antilithics-Gallstone | Antilithics-Urinary | Antiprotozoal | Antipyretic | Antirheumatic | Antispasmodic | Antiviral | Aperient | Astringent | Bitters | Cardiotonic | Carminative | Cathartic | Cholagogue | Demulcent | Diaphoretic | Diuretic | Emmenagogue | Expectorant | Galactogogue | Hematinic | Hepatic | Hypnotic | Hypotensive | Nervine Tonics | Nervine Relaxants | Nervine Stimulants | Oxytocic | Rubefacient | Sialogogue | Vasodilator | Vulnerary |
|---|---|---|---|---|---|---|---|---|---|---|---|---|---|---|---|---|---|---|---|---|---|---|---|---|---|---|---|---|---|---|---|---|---|---|---|---|---|---|---|---|---|---|---|---|---|
| **Antacid & Anti-ulcer** | | | | | | | | | | | | | | | | | | | | | | | | | | | | | | | | | | | | | | | | | | | | | |
| Bilberry | | | | | | X | | | | | | | | | | | X | | | | | | | | | | | | | | | | | X | | | | | | | | | | | |
| Calendula | | X | | | | X | | X | | | X | X | X | | | | | | | | | | | | | | | | | | X | | | | | | | | | | | | | | X |
| Chamomile | | | | X | X | X | | X | | X | X | | X | | | | X | X | X | | | | X | | X | | | | X | | X | | | | | X | | X | X | | | | | | X |
| Comfrey | | X | | | | X | | | | | | X | X | | | | | | | | | | | | | | | X | | | | X | | | | | | | | | | | | | X |
| Fenugreek seeds | | | | | | X | | | X | | | | | | | | | | | | | | | | | | | X | | | | X | X | X | | | | | | | | | | | |
| Gotu Kola | X | | X | | | X | | | | | | | | | | | X | | | | | | | | | | | | | | | | | | | | | X | | X | | | | | X |
| Licorice | X | X | X | | | X | | | X | | | | X | | | X | | X | | X | X | | | | | X | X | X | | | | X | | | X | | | | | | | | X | | |
| Licorice Root | X | X | X | | | X | | | X | | | | X | | | X | | X | | X | X | | | | | X | X | X | | | | X | | | X | | | | | | | | X | | |
| Meadowsweet | | | | | | X | | | | X | | | | | | | X | X | X | | X | X | | | | | | | | | | | | | | | | | | | | | | | |
| Milk Thistle | X | | | | | X | | | | | | | | X | | X | | | | | | | | | | | X | | | | | | | | X | | | | | | | | | | |
| Turmeric | X | | X | X | X | X | X | X | | | | | X | X | | | | X | | | | | | X | | | X | | | | | | | | X | | | | | | | | | X | |

| Herbs By Classifications | Adaptogens | Alterative | Amphoteric | Analgesic | Anodyne | Antacid & Anti-ulcer | Anthelmintics | Antibiotic | Anticatarrhal | Antiemetics | Antifungal | Antihemorrhagic | Anti-Inflammatory | Antilithics-Gallstone | Antilithics-Urinary | Antiprotozoal | Antipyretic | Antirheumatic | Antispasmodic | Antiviral | Aperient | Astringent | Bitters | Cardiotonic | Carminative | Cathartic | Cholagogue | Demulcent | Diaphoretic | Diuretic | Emmenagogue | Expectorant | Galactogogue | Hematinic | Hepatic | Hypnotic | Hypotensive | Nervine Tonics | Nervine Relaxants | Nervine Stimulants | Oxytocic | Rubefacient | Sialogogue | Vasodilator | Vulnerary |
|---|---|---|---|---|---|---|---|---|---|---|---|---|---|---|---|---|---|---|---|---|---|---|---|---|---|---|---|---|---|---|---|---|---|---|---|---|---|---|---|---|---|---|---|---|---|
| **Anthelmintics** | | | | | | | | | | | | | | | | | | | | | | | | | | | | | | | | | | | | | | | | | | | | | |
| Bitter Leaf | | | | | | | X | | | | | | | | | | | | | | | | | | | | | | | | | | | | | | | | | | | | | | |
| Black Walnut Hull | | | | | | | X | | | | X | | | | | X | | | | | | | | | | | | | | | | | | | | | | | | | | | | | |
| Boldo | | | | | | | X | | | | | | | X | | | | | | | | | | | | | X | | | | | | | | X | | | | | | | | | | |
| Caraway | | | | | | | X | | | | | | | | | | | | | | | | | | X | | | | | | | | X | | | | | X | | | | | | | |
| Cascarilla | | | | | | | X | | | | | | | | | | | | | | | | | | | | | | | | | | | | | | | | | | | | | | |
| Chenopodium Oil | | | | | | | X | | | | | | | | | | | | | | | | | | | | | | | | | | | | | | | | | | | | | | |
| Cloves | | | | X | X | | X | | X | X | | | | | | | | | | X | | | | | X | | | | | | | | | | | | | | | X | | | | | |
| Elecampane | | | | | | | X | X | X | | | | | | | | | | | | | | | | | | | | | | | X | | | | | | | | X | | | | | |
| Garlic | | X | | | | | X | X | X | | X | | X | | | | | | | X | | | | X | X | | | | | | | X | | | | | X | | | X | | X | | X | X |
| Ginger | | | | X | | | X | X | X | X | | | X | | | | | X | X | | | | X | X | X | | | | X | X | | X | | | | | X | | | X | X | X | | X | |
| Hyssop | | | | | | | X | | X | | | | X | | | | | | | | | | | | | | | | X | | | X | | | | | | | X | | | | | | |
| Male Fern | | | | | | | X | | | | | | | | | | | | | | | | | | | | | | | | | | | | | | | | | | | | | | |
| Neem | | | | | | | X | X | | | X | | | | | | | | | | | | | | | | | | | | | | | | | | | | | | | | | | |
| Papaya Seed | | | | | | | X | | | | | | | | | | | | | | | | | | | | | | | | | | | | | | | | | | | | | | |
| Pomegranate | | | | | | | X | | | | | | | | | | | | | | | | | | | | | | | | | | | | | | | | | | | | | | |
| Pumpkin Seed | | | | | | | X | | | | | | | | | | | | | | | | | | | | | | | | | | | | | | | | | | | | | | |
| Rue | | | | | | | X | X | | | | | | | | | | | | | | | | | | | | | | | X | | | | | | | | | | X | | | | |
| Savory | | | X | X | X | | X | X | X | X | X | | X | | | | | | X | X | X | X | X | X | X | X | X | X | X | X | X | X | X | X | X | | | | | | | | | | |
| Sesame Seeds | | | | | | | X | | | | | | | | | | | | | | | | | | | | | | | | | | | | | | | | | | | | | | |
| Tansy | | | | | | | X | | | | | | | | | | X | | | | | | | | | | | | | | X | | | | | | | | | | | | | | |
| Thyme | | | | X | X | | X | X | | | X | | | | | | X | | X | X | | | | X | X | | | | X | | | X | | | | | | | | | | | | | X |
| Turmeric | X | | X | X | X | X | X | X | | | | | X | X | | | | X | | | | | | X | | | X | | | | | | | | X | | | | | | | | | X | |
| Wormseed | | | | | | | X | | | | | | | | | | | | | | | | | | | | | | | | | | | | | | | | | | | | | | |
| Wormwood | | | | | | | X | X | | | | | | | | X | | | | | | | X | | | | | | | | | | | | X | | | | | | | | | | |

**Herbs By Classifications**

**Antibiotic**

| Herbs By Classifications | Adaptogens | Alterative | Amphoteric | Analgesic | Anodyne | Antacid & Anti-ulcer | Anthelmintics | Antibiotic | Anticatarrhal | Antiemetics | Antifungal | Antihemorrhagic | Anti-Inflammatory | Antilithics-Gallstone | Antilithics-Urinary | Antiprotozoal | Antipyretic | Antirheumatic | Antispasmodic | Antiviral | Aperient | Astringent |
|---|---|---|---|---|---|---|---|---|---|---|---|---|---|---|---|---|---|---|---|---|---|---|
| Allspice |  |  |  |  |  |  |  | X |  |  |  |  |  |  |  |  |  | X | X |  |  |  |
| Andrographis |  |  |  |  |  |  |  | X |  |  |  |  |  |  |  |  |  |  |  | X |  |  |
| Anise seeds |  |  |  | X |  |  |  | X |  |  | X |  |  |  |  |  |  |  |  | X |  |  |
| Barberry |  |  |  |  |  |  |  | X |  |  |  |  |  | X |  | X |  |  |  |  |  |  |
| Basil | X |  |  |  |  |  |  | X |  | X | X |  |  |  |  |  | X |  |  |  |  |  |
| Bay Leaves |  |  |  |  |  |  |  | X |  |  | X |  |  |  |  |  |  | X |  |  |  |  |
| Black Pepper |  |  |  |  |  |  |  | X |  |  |  |  | X |  |  | X |  |  |  |  |  |  |
| Bergamot |  |  |  |  |  |  |  | X |  | X | X |  |  |  |  | X |  |  |  |  |  |  |
| Cayenne |  |  | X | X | X |  |  | X | X |  |  | X | X |  |  |  | X |  |  |  |  |  |
| Chamomile |  |  |  | X | X | X |  | X |  | X | X |  | X |  |  | X | X | X |  |  |  |  |
| Chaparral |  | X |  |  |  |  |  | X |  |  | X |  |  |  |  | X |  |  |  |  |  |  |
| Cinnamon |  |  |  |  |  |  |  | X |  | X | X |  |  |  |  |  |  |  | X |  |  |  |
| Cranberry |  |  |  |  |  |  |  | X |  |  |  |  |  |  |  |  |  |  |  |  |  |  |
| Echinacea |  | X |  |  |  |  |  | X |  | X |  |  | X |  |  | X |  | X |  |  |  |  |
| Elecampane |  |  |  |  |  | X | X | X |  |  |  |  |  |  |  |  |  |  |  |  |  |  |
| Fennel Seeds |  |  |  |  |  |  |  | X |  | X | X |  | X |  |  |  |  |  |  |  |  |  |
| Garden Sage |  |  |  |  |  |  |  | X | X |  | X |  | X |  | X |  | X | X | X | X | X | X |
| Garlic |  | X |  |  |  | X | X | X |  | X |  |  | X |  |  | X |  |  |  |  |  |  |
| Gentian |  |  |  |  |  |  |  | X |  |  |  |  |  |  |  |  |  |  |  |  |  |  |
| Ginger |  |  |  | X |  |  |  | X | X | X | X |  | X | X |  | X | X | X | X | X |  |  |
| Goldenseal |  |  |  |  |  |  |  | X |  |  | X |  |  |  |  | X |  |  |  |  |  |  |
| Gumweed |  |  |  |  |  |  |  | X |  |  |  |  | X |  |  |  |  |  |  |  |  |  |
| Juniper |  |  |  |  |  |  |  | X |  |  |  |  |  |  | X |  | X |  |  |  |  |  |
| Juniper Berries |  |  |  |  |  |  |  | X |  |  |  |  |  |  | X |  | X |  |  |  |  |  |
| Lovage |  | X |  |  |  |  |  | X | X | X |  |  |  |  |  |  |  |  |  |  |  |  |
| Marjoram |  |  |  | X | X |  |  | X | X |  |  |  | X |  |  |  | X | X | X | X | X |  |
| Myrrh |  |  |  |  |  |  |  | X |  |  |  |  | X |  |  | X |  |  |  |  |  |  |
| Nasturtium | X | X | X |  |  |  |  | X | X | X | X | X | X | X | X | X |  | X | X | X | X |  |
| Neem |  |  |  |  |  |  | X | X |  |  | X |  |  |  |  |  |  |  |  |  |  |  |
| Olive Leaf |  |  |  |  |  |  |  | X |  |  |  |  |  |  |  |  |  |  |  |  |  |  |
| Onion |  |  |  |  |  |  |  | X |  |  | X |  | X |  |  |  |  |  |  |  |  |  |
| Oregano |  |  | X |  |  |  |  | X | X |  | X |  | X |  |  | X |  | X |  |  |  |  |
| Oregon Grape |  | X |  |  |  |  |  | X |  |  | X |  | X |  |  |  |  |  |  |  |  |  |
| Oregon Grape Root |  | X |  |  |  |  |  | X |  |  | X |  | X |  |  |  |  |  |  |  |  |  |
| Pau D'Arco |  |  |  |  |  |  |  | X |  |  | X |  |  |  |  |  |  |  |  |  |  |  |
| Peppermint |  |  |  | X |  |  |  | X | X | X |  |  | X |  |  |  | X | X | X |  |  |  |
| Plantain |  | X |  |  |  |  |  | X |  |  |  |  |  | X | X |  |  |  |  |  |  |  |
| Purslane |  | X | X |  |  |  |  | X | X | X | X | X | X |  |  |  |  |  |  |  | X | X |
| Rosemary |  | X |  |  |  |  |  | X |  |  | X |  | X |  |  |  | X | X | X |  |  |  |
| Rue |  |  |  |  |  |  | X | X |  |  |  |  |  |  |  |  |  |  |  |  |  |  |
| Sage |  |  |  | X |  |  |  | X | X |  | X |  | X |  |  |  | X | X |  |  |  |  |
| Savory |  |  | X | X | X |  |  | X | X | X | X | X | X |  |  |  |  |  |  |  |  | X |
| St. John's Wort |  |  |  |  |  |  |  | X |  |  |  |  | X |  |  |  |  |  |  |  |  |  |
| Sweet Cicely |  |  |  |  |  |  |  | X |  | X |  |  |  |  |  |  |  |  |  |  |  |  |
| Thyme |  |  |  |  |  |  | X | X |  |  | X |  |  |  |  |  | X | X | X |  |  |  |
| Turmeric | X |  | X | X | X | X | X | X |  |  |  |  | X |  |  |  |  |  |  |  |  |  |
| Usnea |  |  |  |  |  |  |  | X |  |  |  |  |  |  |  |  |  |  |  |  |  |  |
| Uva Ursi |  | X |  |  |  |  |  | X | X |  | X |  |  |  | X |  |  | X |  |  |  | X |
| Wormwood |  |  |  |  |  |  | X | X |  |  |  |  |  | X |  |  |  |  |  |  |  |  |
| Yarrow |  |  |  | X | X |  |  | X | X |  |  | X | X |  |  |  | X |  |  |  |  | X |

| Herbs By Classifications | Bitters | Cardiotonic | Carminative | Cathartic | Cholagogue | Demulcent | Diaphoretic | Diuretic | Emmenagogue | Expectorant | Galactogogue | Hematinic | Hepatic | Hypnotic | Hypotensive | Nervine Tonics | Nervine Relaxants | Nervine Stimulants | Oxytocic | Rubefacient | Sialogogue | Vasodilator | Vulnerary |
|---|---|---|---|---|---|---|---|---|---|---|---|---|---|---|---|---|---|---|---|---|---|---|---|
| Allspice |  |  | X |  |  |  |  |  |  |  |  |  |  |  |  |  |  |  |  | X |  | X |  |
| Andrographis |  |  |  |  |  |  |  |  |  |  |  |  |  |  |  |  |  |  |  |  |  |  |  |
| Anise seeds |  |  | X |  |  |  |  |  |  | X | X |  |  |  |  |  |  |  |  |  | X |  |  |
| Barberry | X |  |  | X | X |  |  |  |  |  |  |  | X |  |  |  |  |  |  |  |  |  |  |
| Basil |  |  | X |  |  |  | X |  |  | X |  |  |  |  | X |  |  |  |  |  |  |  |  |
| Bay Leaves |  |  |  | X |  |  | X | X |  |  |  |  |  |  |  |  |  |  |  |  |  |  |  |
| Black Pepper |  |  | X |  |  |  | X | X |  | X |  |  |  |  |  |  |  | X |  |  | X | X |  |
| Bergamot |  |  |  |  |  |  | X |  |  |  |  |  |  |  |  |  |  |  |  |  |  |  |  |
| Cayenne |  | X |  |  |  |  | X |  |  |  |  |  |  |  | X |  |  | X |  | X | X | X | X |
| Chamomile |  |  | X |  |  |  | X |  |  |  |  |  |  | X |  | X | X |  |  |  |  |  | X |
| Chaparral | X |  |  |  |  |  | X |  |  |  |  |  |  |  |  |  |  |  |  |  |  |  |  |
| Cinnamon |  |  | X |  |  |  | X |  |  | X |  |  | X |  |  |  |  |  |  |  | X | X |  |
| Cranberry |  |  |  |  |  |  |  |  |  |  |  |  |  |  |  |  |  |  |  |  |  |  |  |
| Echinacea |  |  |  |  |  |  | X |  |  |  |  |  |  |  |  |  |  |  |  | X |  | X | X |
| Elecampane |  |  |  |  |  |  |  |  |  | X |  |  |  |  |  |  |  |  |  | X |  |  |  |
| Fennel Seeds |  |  | X |  |  |  | X | X | X | X |  |  |  |  |  |  |  |  |  |  | X |  |  |
| Garden Sage |  |  | X |  |  |  | X | X |  | X |  |  | X |  |  | X | X | X |  | X |  |  | X |
| Garlic |  |  | X | X |  |  | X |  |  |  |  |  | X |  | X |  |  | X |  | X |  | X | X |
| Gentian | X |  | X |  |  |  |  |  |  | X |  |  |  |  |  |  |  |  |  |  |  |  |  |
| Ginger |  | X | X | X |  |  | X | X | X |  |  |  | X |  | X |  |  | X |  | X | X | X | X |
| Goldenseal | X |  | X |  |  |  |  |  |  |  |  |  |  |  |  |  |  |  |  |  |  |  | X |
| Gumweed |  |  |  |  |  |  | X |  |  |  |  |  |  |  |  |  |  |  |  |  |  |  | X |
| Juniper |  |  | X |  |  |  |  | X |  |  |  |  |  |  |  |  |  |  |  | X | X |  |  |
| Juniper Berries |  |  | X |  |  |  |  | X |  |  |  |  |  |  |  |  |  |  |  | X | X |  |  |
| Lovage | X |  | X |  |  |  | X | X | X |  |  |  | X |  |  |  |  |  |  |  |  | X |  |
| Marjoram |  |  |  |  |  |  |  |  |  |  |  |  |  |  |  | X | X |  |  | X | X | X | X |
| Myrrh |  |  |  |  |  |  |  |  |  |  |  |  |  |  |  |  |  |  |  |  |  |  | X |
| Nasturtium |  |  |  |  |  |  | X |  |  |  |  |  |  |  |  |  |  |  |  |  |  |  | X |
| Neem |  |  |  |  |  |  |  |  |  |  |  |  |  |  |  |  |  |  |  |  |  |  |  |
| Olive Leaf |  |  |  |  |  |  | X |  |  |  |  |  | X |  |  |  |  |  |  |  |  | X |  |
| Onion |  |  |  |  |  |  | X |  |  |  |  |  |  |  | X |  |  |  |  |  |  |  |  |
| Oregano |  |  |  |  |  | X | X |  |  |  |  |  |  |  |  |  |  |  |  |  |  |  |  |
| Oregon Grape |  |  |  |  | X |  |  |  |  |  |  |  | X |  |  |  |  |  |  |  |  |  |  |
| Oregon Grape Root |  |  |  |  | X |  |  |  |  |  |  |  | X |  |  |  |  |  |  |  |  |  |  |
| Pau D'Arco |  |  |  |  |  |  |  |  |  | X |  |  |  |  |  |  |  |  |  |  |  |  |  |
| Peppermint |  |  |  |  |  |  | X |  |  | X |  |  |  |  |  |  |  |  |  |  | X | X | X |
| Plantain |  | X |  |  |  |  | X | X |  |  |  |  |  |  |  |  |  |  |  |  |  |  | X |
| Purslane |  |  |  |  |  | X | X | X |  |  |  |  |  |  |  |  |  |  |  |  |  |  | X |
| Rosemary |  |  | X |  |  |  | X |  |  |  |  |  | X |  |  | X |  | X |  | X |  | X | X |
| Rue |  |  |  |  |  |  |  |  |  |  |  |  | X |  |  |  |  | X |  |  |  |  |  |
| Sage |  |  | X |  |  |  | X |  |  |  |  |  | X |  |  | X | X |  |  |  | X | X | X |
| Savory | X | X | X | X | X | X | X | X | X | X | X |  |  |  |  | X | X | X |  | X | X | X | X |
| St. John's Wort |  |  |  |  |  |  |  |  |  |  |  |  |  |  |  | X | X |  |  |  |  |  | X |
| Sweet Cicely |  |  |  |  |  | X |  |  |  |  |  |  |  |  |  |  |  |  |  |  |  |  | X |
| Thyme |  |  | X |  |  |  | X |  |  | X |  |  |  |  |  |  |  |  |  |  |  |  | X |
| Turmeric |  | X |  |  | X |  |  |  |  |  |  |  | X |  |  |  |  |  |  |  |  | X |  |
| Usnea |  |  |  |  |  |  |  |  |  |  |  |  |  |  |  |  |  |  |  |  |  |  |  |
| Uva Ursi |  |  |  |  |  |  |  | X |  |  |  |  | X |  |  |  |  |  |  |  |  |  |  |
| Wormwood | X |  |  |  |  |  |  |  |  |  |  |  | X |  |  |  |  |  |  |  |  |  |  |
| Yarrow | X |  | X |  |  |  | X |  |  |  |  |  | X |  |  |  |  |  |  |  |  | X | X |

| Herbs By Classifications | Adaptogens | Alterative | Amphoteric | Analgesic | Anodyne | Antacid & Anti-ulcer | Anthelmintics | Antibiotic | Anticatarrhal | Antiemetics | Antifungal | Antihemorrhagic | Anti-Inflammatory | Antilithics-Gallstone | Antilithics-Urinary | Antiprotozoal | Antipyretic | Antirheumatic | Antispasmodic | Antiviral | Aperient | Astringent | Bitters | Cardiotonic | Carminative | Cathartic | Cholagogue | Demulcent | Diaphoretic | Diuretic | Emmenagogue | Expectorant | Galactogogue | Hematinic | Hepatic | Hypnotic | Hypotensive | Nervine Tonics | Nervine Relaxants | Nervine Stimulants | Oxytocic | Rubefacient | Sialogogue | Vasodilator | Vulnerary |
|---|---|---|---|---|---|---|---|---|---|---|---|---|---|---|---|---|---|---|---|---|---|---|---|---|---|---|---|---|---|---|---|---|---|---|---|---|---|---|---|---|---|---|---|---|---|
| **Anticatarrhal** |  |  |  |  |  |  |  |  |  |  |  |  |  |  |  |  |  |  |  |  |  |  |  |  |  |  |  |  |  |  |  |  |  |  |  |  |  |  |  |  |  |  |  |  |  |
| Cayenne |  |  | X | X | X |  |  | X | X |  |  | X | X |  |  |  |  | X |  |  |  |  |  | X |  |  |  |  | X |  |  |  |  |  |  |  | X |  |  | X |  | X | X | X | X |
| Chickweed |  |  |  |  |  |  |  |  | X |  |  |  | X |  |  |  | X |  |  |  |  |  |  |  |  |  |  |  |  |  |  |  |  | X |  |  |  |  |  |  |  |  |  |  |  |
| Coltsfoot |  |  |  |  |  |  |  |  | X |  |  |  |  |  |  |  |  |  |  |  |  |  |  |  |  |  |  | X |  |  |  | X |  |  |  |  |  |  |  |  |  |  |  |  |  |
| Elder |  |  |  |  |  |  |  |  | X |  |  |  |  |  |  |  | X |  |  | X |  |  |  |  |  |  |  |  | X | X |  | X |  |  |  |  |  |  |  |  |  |  |  |  | X |
| Elecampane |  |  |  |  |  |  | X | X | X |  |  |  |  |  |  |  |  |  |  |  |  |  |  |  |  |  |  |  |  |  |  | X |  |  |  |  |  |  |  |  |  |  |  | X |  |
| Eucalyptus |  |  |  |  |  |  |  |  | X |  |  |  |  |  |  |  |  |  |  |  |  |  |  |  |  |  |  |  |  |  |  | X |  |  |  |  |  |  |  |  |  | X |  |  |  |
| Fenugreek seeds |  |  |  |  |  | X |  |  | X |  |  |  |  |  |  |  |  |  |  |  | X |  |  |  |  |  |  | X |  |  |  | X | X | X |  |  |  |  |  |  |  |  |  |  |  |
| Garden Sage |  |  |  |  |  |  |  | X | X |  | X |  | X |  | X |  | X | X | X | X |  | X | X |  | X |  |  |  | X | X | X |  |  |  | X |  | X | X | X |  |  | X |  |  | X |
| Garlic |  | X |  |  |  |  | X | X | X |  | X |  |  |  |  | X |  |  |  | X |  |  |  | X | X |  |  |  |  |  |  | X |  |  |  |  | X |  |  | X |  | X |  | X | X |
| Ginger |  |  |  | X |  |  | X | X | X | X |  |  | X | X |  | X | X | X | X | X |  |  | X | X | X |  |  |  | X | X | X | X |  |  | X |  | X |  |  | X | X | X |  | X |  |
| Goldenrod |  |  |  |  |  |  |  |  | X |  |  |  |  |  | X |  |  |  |  |  |  |  |  |  |  |  |  |  | X |  |  |  |  |  |  |  |  |  |  |  |  |  |  |  |  |
| Hyssop |  |  |  |  |  |  | X |  | X |  |  |  | X |  |  |  |  |  | X |  |  |  |  |  |  |  |  |  | X |  |  | X |  |  |  |  |  |  | X |  |  |  |  |  |  |
| Irish Moss |  |  |  |  |  |  |  |  | X |  |  |  |  |  |  |  | X |  |  |  |  |  |  |  |  |  |  | X |  |  |  |  |  |  |  |  |  |  |  |  |  |  |  |  |  |
| Licorice | X | X | X |  |  | X |  |  | X |  |  |  | X |  |  | X |  | X |  | X | X |  |  |  |  | X | X | X |  |  |  | X |  |  | X |  |  |  |  |  |  |  |  | X |  |
| Licorice Root | X | X | X |  |  | X |  |  | X |  |  |  | X |  |  | X |  | X |  | X | X |  |  |  |  | X | X | X |  |  |  | X |  |  | X |  |  |  |  |  |  |  |  | X |  |
| Lovage |  | X |  |  |  |  |  | X | X | X |  |  |  |  |  |  |  |  |  |  |  |  | X |  | X |  |  | X | X | X |  | X |  |  | X |  |  |  |  |  |  |  |  |  | X |
| Marjoram |  |  |  | X | X |  |  | X | X |  |  |  | X |  |  |  |  |  | X | X | X | X | X |  | X |  |  |  |  |  |  |  |  |  |  |  | X | X | X | X |  | X | X | X | X |
| Marshmallow |  | X |  |  |  |  |  |  | X | X |  |  | X |  | X |  |  |  |  |  | X |  |  |  |  |  |  | X |  |  |  |  |  |  |  |  |  |  |  |  |  |  |  |  | X |
| Marshmallow Root |  | X |  |  |  |  |  |  | X | X |  |  | X |  | X |  |  |  |  |  | X |  |  |  |  |  |  | X |  |  |  |  |  |  |  |  |  |  |  |  |  |  |  |  | X |
| Mullein |  |  |  |  |  |  |  |  | X |  |  | X |  |  |  |  |  |  |  | X |  |  |  |  |  |  |  | X |  |  |  | X |  |  |  |  |  |  |  |  |  |  |  |  |  |
| Nasturtium | X | X | X |  |  |  |  | X | X | X | X | X | X | X | X |  | X | X | X | X | X | X | X |  |  |  |  |  | X |  |  |  |  |  |  |  |  |  |  |  |  |  |  |  | X |
| Nettle |  | X |  |  |  |  |  |  | X |  |  | X | X |  |  |  |  | X |  |  |  |  |  |  |  |  |  |  | X |  |  |  | X | X |  |  |  |  |  |  |  |  |  |  |  |
| Oregano |  |  |  |  |  |  |  | X | X |  | X |  | X |  |  |  |  |  |  | X |  |  |  |  |  |  |  | X |  |  |  | X |  |  |  |  |  |  |  |  |  |  |  |  |  |
| Peppermint |  |  |  |  |  |  |  | X | X | X |  |  |  | X |  |  | X |  | X |  |  |  |  |  | X |  |  |  | X |  | X |  |  |  |  |  |  |  |  |  |  |  | X | X |  |
| Purselane |  | X | X |  |  |  |  | X | X | X | X | X | X |  |  |  |  |  |  |  | X | X |  |  |  |  |  | X | X | X |  |  |  |  |  |  |  |  |  |  |  |  |  |  | X |
| Sage |  |  |  |  |  |  |  |  | X |  | X |  | X |  |  |  |  |  | X | X |  | X | X |  | X |  |  |  | X |  | X |  |  |  |  |  |  | X | X |  |  |  |  | X | X |
| Savory |  |  | X | X | X |  | X | X | X | X | X |  | X |  |  |  |  |  | X | X | X | X | X | X | X | X | X | X | X | X | X | X | X | X | X | X | X | X | X | X | X | X | X | X |  |
| Stinging Nettle |  | X |  |  |  |  |  |  | X |  |  | X |  |  |  |  |  | X |  |  |  |  |  |  |  |  |  |  |  | X |  |  | X | X |  |  |  |  |  |  |  |  |  |  |  |
| Uva Ursi |  | X |  |  |  |  |  | X | X |  |  | X |  |  | X |  |  | X |  |  |  | X |  |  |  |  |  |  |  | X |  |  |  |  |  |  |  |  |  |  |  |  |  |  |  |
| Yarrow |  |  |  | X | X |  |  | X | X |  |  | X | X |  |  |  | X |  |  |  |  | X |  | X |  |  |  |  | X |  |  |  |  |  |  |  | X |  |  | X |  |  |  | X | X |

**Columns 1–15**

| Herbs By Classifications | Adaptogens | Alterative | Amphoteric | Analgesic | Anodyne | Antacid & Anti-ulcer | Anthelmintics | Antibiotic | Anticatarrhal | Antiemetics | Antifungal | Antihemorrhagic | Anti-Inflammatory | Antilithics-Gallstone | Antilithics-Urinary |
|---|---|---|---|---|---|---|---|---|---|---|---|---|---|---|---|
| Antiemetics | | | | | | | | | | | | | | | |
| Basil | | | | | | | | | | X | | | | | |
| Black Horehound | | | | | | | | | | X | | | | | |
| Cannabis | | | | | | | | | | X | | | | | |
| Cardamom | | | | | | | | | | X | | | | | |
| Catnip | | | | | | | | | | X | | | | | |
| Chamomile | | | | X | X | X | | X | | X | X | | X | | |
| Cilantro | | | | | | | | | | X | | | | | |
| Cinnamon | | | | | | | | X | | X | X | | | | |
| Cinquefoil | | | | | | | | | | X | | | | | |
| Cloves | | | | X | X | | | X | | X | X | | | | |
| Coriander | | | | | | | | | | X | | | | | |
| Dill | | | | | | | | | | X | | | | | X |
| Dill Seed | | | | | | | | | | X | | | | | X |
| Fennel | | | | | | | | | | X | | | | | |
| Fennel Seeds | | | | | | | | | | X | | | | | |
| Ginger | | | | X | | | X | X | X | X | | | X | X | |
| Horehound | | | | | | | | | | X | | | | | |
| Lavendar | | | | X | X | | | | | X | | | | | |
| Lemon Balm | X | | | | | | | | | X | | | | | |
| Lovage | | X | | | | | | X | X | X | | | | | |
| Mallow | | X | | | | | | | X | X | | | X | | X |
| Marshmallow | | X | | | | | | | X | X | | | X | | X |
| Marshmallow Root | | X | | | | | | | X | X | | | X | | X |
| Meadowsweet | | | | | | X | | | | X | | | | | |
| Mint | | | | | | | | | | X | | | | | |
| Nasturtium | X | X | X | | | | | X | X | X | X | X | X | X | X |
| Peppermint | | | | | | | | X | X | X | | | X | X | |
| Purselane | | X | X | | | | | X | X | X | X | X | X | | |
| Savory | | | X | X | X | | X | X | X | X | X | | X | | |
| Spearmint | | | | | | | | | | X | | | | | |

**Columns 16–30**

| Herbs By Classifications | Antiprotozoal | Antipyretic | Antirheumatic | Antispasmodic | Antiviral | Aperient | Astringent | Bitters | Cardiotonic | Carminative | Cathartic | Cholagogue | Demulcent | Diaphoretic | Diuretic |
|---|---|---|---|---|---|---|---|---|---|---|---|---|---|---|---|
| Antiemetics | | | | | | | | | | | | | | | |
| Basil | | X | | | | | | | | | | | | X | |
| Black Horehound | | | | | | | | | | | | | | | |
| Cannabis | | | | | | | | | | | | | | | |
| Cardamom | | | | | | | | | | X | | | | | |
| Catnip | | X | | X | | | | | | X | | | | | |
| Chamomile | | X | X | X | | | | X | | X | | | | X | |
| Cilantro | | | | X | | | | | | | | | | | |
| Cinnamon | | | | | | | | | | | | | | | |
| Cinquefoil | | | | | | | | | | | | | | | |
| Cloves | | | | X | | | | | | | | | | | |
| Coriander | | | | | | | | | | X | | | | | |
| Dill | | | | | | | | | | X | | | | | |
| Dill Seed | | | | | | | | | | X | | | | | |
| Fennel | | | | X | | X | | | | X | | | | | |
| Fennel Seeds | | | | X | | X | | | | X | | | | | |
| Ginger | X | X | X | X | X | | | X | X | X | | | | X | X |
| Horehound | | | | | | | | X | | | | | | | |
| Lavendar | | | | X | | | | | | X | | | | | |
| Lemon Balm | | X | | X | X | | | X | X | X | | | | | |
| Lovage | | | | | | | | | X | X | | | | X | X |
| Mallow | | | | | | | | | | | | | X | | |
| Marshmallow | | | | | | | | | | | | | X | | |
| Marshmallow Root | | | | | | | | | | | | | X | | |
| Meadowsweet | | X | X | | | | X | | | | | | | | |
| Mint | | | | | | | | | | | | | | | |
| Nasturtium | X | X | X | X | X | X | X | | | | | | | | X |
| Peppermint | | | | X | | | | | | X | | | | X | |
| Purselane | | | | | | | X | X | | | | | X | X | X |
| Savory | | | | | | | | X | X | X | X | X | X | X | X |
| Spearmint | | | | | | | | | | | | | | | |

**Columns 31–45**

| Herbs By Classifications | Emmenagogue | Expectorant | Galactogogue | Hematinic | Hepatic | Hypnotic | Hypotensive | Nervine Tonics | Nervine Relaxants | Nervine Stimulants | Oxytocic | Rubefacient | Sialogogue | Vasodilator | Vulnerary |
|---|---|---|---|---|---|---|---|---|---|---|---|---|---|---|---|
| Antiemetics | | | | | | | | | | | | | | | |
| Basil | | | | | | | | | | | | | | | |
| Black Horehound | | | | | | | | | | | | | | | |
| Cannabis | | | | | | | | | | | | | | | |
| Cardamom | | | | | | | | | | X | | | X | | |
| Catnip | | | | | | X | | X | X | | | | | | |
| Chamomile | X | | | | | X | | X | X | | | | | | X |
| Cilantro | | | | | | | | | | | | | | | |
| Cinnamon | | | | | | | | | | X | | | X | X | X |
| Cinquefoil | | | | | | | | | | | | | | | |
| Cloves | | | | | | | | | | | | | X | | |
| Coriander | | | | | | | | | | | | | | | |
| Dill | | | X | | | | | | | | | | | | |
| Dill Seed | | | X | | | | | | | | | | | | |
| Fennel | | | X | | | | | | | | | | | | |
| Fennel Seeds | | | X | | | | | | | | | | | | |
| Ginger | X | X | | | | | | | | X | X | X | X | X | |
| Horehound | | | | | | | | | | | | | | | |
| Lavendar | | | | | | X | X | X | X | | | | | | X |
| Lemon Balm | | | | | | X | X | X | X | | | | | | |
| Lovage | X | X | | | | | | | | | | | | X | |
| Mallow | | | | | | | | | | | | | | | X |
| Marshmallow | | | | | | | | | | | | | | | X |
| Marshmallow Root | | | | | | | | | | | | | | | X |
| Meadowsweet | | | | | | | | | | | | | | | |
| Mint | | | | | | | | | | | | | | | |
| Nasturtium | | | | | | | | | | | | | | | X |
| Peppermint | X | | | | | | | | | | | | X | X | |
| Purselane | | | | | | | | | | | | | | | X |
| Savory | X | X | X | X | X | | | | | | | | | | |
| Spearmint | | | | | | | | | | | | | | | |

## Herbs By Classifications — Antifungal

| Herb | Adaptogens | Alterative | Amphoteric | Analgesic | Anodyne | Antacid & Anti-ulcer | Anthelmintics | Antibiotic | Anticatarrhal | Antiemetics | Antifungal | Antihemorrhagic | Anti-inflammatory | Antilithics-Gallstone | Antilithics-Urinary |
|---|---|---|---|---|---|---|---|---|---|---|---|---|---|---|---|
| **Antifungal** | | | | | | | | | | | | | | | |
| Aloe Vera | | X | | | | | | | | | X | | X | | |
| Anise seeds | | | | | | | | | X | | X | | | | |
| Basil | X | | | | | | | X | | X | X | | | | |
| Bay Leaves | | | | | | | | X | | | X | | | | |
| Bee Balm | | | | | | | | | | | X | | | | |
| Bergamot | | | | | | | | X | | | X | X | | | |
| Black Walnut Hull | | | | | | | X | | | | X | | | | |
| Burdock Root | | | | | | | | | | | X | | X | X | |
| Calendula | | X | | | | X | | X | | | X | X | X | | |
| Chamomile | | | | X | X | X | | X | | X | X | | X | | |
| Chaparral | | X | | | | | | X | | | X | | | | |
| Cinnamon | | | | | | | | X | | X | X | | | | |
| Cloves | | | | X | X | | X | | | X | X | | | | |
| Chamomile | | X | | | | | | X | | | X | | X | | |
| Fennel Seeds | | | | | | | | X | | X | X | | X | | |
| Fireweed | | | | | | | | | | | X | | | | |
| Garden Sage | | | | | | | | X | X | | X | | X | | X |
| Garlic | | X | | | | | | X | X | X | X | | | | |
| Goldenseal | | | | | | | | X | | | X | | | | |
| Lemon Grass | | | | | | | | | | | X | | | | |
| Myrrh | | | | | | | | X | | | X | | | | |
| Nasturtium | | | | | | | | X | X | X | X | | X | X | X |
| Neem | | | | | | | X | X | | | X | | X | | |
| Onion | | | | | | | | X | | | X | | X | | |
| Oregano | | | X | | | | | X | X | | X | | X | | |
| Oregon Grape | | X | | | | | | X | | | X | | X | X | |
| Oregon Grape Root | | X | | | | | | X | | | X | | X | X | |
| Pau D'Arco | | | | | | | | X | | | X | | | | |
| Purslane | | X | X | | | | | X | X | X | X | X | X | | |
| Rosemary | | | X | X | | | | X | | | X | | | | |
| Sage | | | X | | | | | X | X | | X | | X | | |
| Savory | | | X | X | X | | | X | X | X | X | | X | | |
| Sweet Cicely | | | | | | | | X | | | X | | | | |
| Sweet Root | | | | | | | | | | | X | | | | |
| Tea Tree Oil | | | | | | | | | | | X | | | | |
| Thyme | | | | | | | X | X | | | X | | | | |

| Herb | Antiprotozoal | Antipyretic | Antirheumatic | Antispasmodic | Antiviral | Aperient | Astringent | Bitters | Cardiotonic | Carminative | Cathartic | Cholagogue | Demulcent | Diaphoretic | Diuretic |
|---|---|---|---|---|---|---|---|---|---|---|---|---|---|---|---|
| Aloe Vera | | | | | | X | | | | | | | X | | |
| Anise seeds | | | | X | X | | | | | X | | | | | |
| Basil | | X | | | | | | | | X | | | | X | |
| Bay Leaves | | | | X | | | | | | | X | | | X | |
| Bee Balm | | | | | | | | | | | | | | | |
| Bergamot | | X | | | | | | | | | | | | X | |
| Black Walnut Hull | X | | | | | | | | | | | | | | |
| Burdock Root | | X | | | | | | | | | | | | | X |
| Calendula | | | | | | | | | | | | | | | |
| Chamomile | | X | X | X | | | | X | | X | | | | X | |
| Chaparral | X | | | | X | | | | | | | | | | |
| Cinnamon | | | | | X | | X | | | X | | | X | | |
| Cloves | | | | | X | | | | | X | | | | | |
| Chamomile | | X | | | X | | | | | | | | | X | |
| Fennel Seeds | | | | | X | X | X | | | X | | | | X | X |
| Fireweed | | | | | | | | | | | | | | | |
| Garden Sage | | X | X | X | X | | | X | X | X | | | | X | X |
| Garlic | X | | | | X | | | | X | X | | | | X | |
| Goldenseal | X | | | | | | X | X | | | | | | | |
| Lemon Grass | | | | | | | | | | | | | | | |
| Myrrh | X | | | | | | | | | | | | | | |
| Nasturtium | X | X | X | X | X | X | X | | | | | | | | |
| Neem | | | | | | | | | | | | | | | |
| Onion | | | | | | | | | | | | | | | |
| Oregano | | | | X | X | | | | | X | | | | | |
| Oregon Grape | | | | | | | | | | | | X | | | |
| Oregon Grape Root | | | | | | | | | | | | X | | | |
| Pau D'Arco | | | | | | | | | X | | | | | | |
| Purslane | | | | | | | | | | | | | X | X | X |
| Rosemary | | | | X | | | | | | | | X | | | |
| Sage | | | | | | | X | | | X | | | | X | |
| Savory | | | | | | | X | X | X | X | X | X | X | X | X |
| Sweet Cicely | | | | | | | | | | | | | | | |
| Sweet Root | | | | | | | | | | | | | | | |
| Tea Tree Oil | | | | | X | | | | | | | | | | |
| Thyme | | X | | X | X | | X | | | X | | | | X | |

| Herb | Emmenagogue | Expectorant | Galactogogue | Hematinic | Hepatic | Hypnotic | Hypotensive | Nervine Tonics | Nervine Relaxants | Nervine Stimulants | Oxytocic | Rubefacient | Sialagogue | Vasodilator | Vulnerary |
|---|---|---|---|---|---|---|---|---|---|---|---|---|---|---|---|
| Aloe Vera | | | | | | | | | | | | | | | X |
| Anise seeds | | X | X | | | | | | | | | | X | | |
| Basil | | X | | | | | | X | | | | | | | |
| Bay Leaves | X | | | | | | | | | | | | | | |
| Bee Balm | | | | | | | | | | | | | | | |
| Bergamot | | | | | | | | | | | | | | | |
| Black Walnut Hull | | | | | | | | | | | | | | | |
| Burdock Root | | | | | | | | | | | | | | | X |
| Calendula | X | | | | | | | | | | | | | | X |
| Chamomile | X | | | | | X | | X | X | | | | | | X |
| Chaparral | | | | | | | | | | | | | | | |
| Cinnamon | X | | | | | | X | | | X | | | X | X | |
| Cloves | | | | | | | | | | X | | | | | |
| Chamomile | | | | X | | | | | | | | | X | | X |
| Fennel Seeds | X | X | X | | | | | | | | | | X | | |
| Fireweed | | | | | | | | | | | | | | | |
| Garden Sage | X | | | | X | | X | X | X | X | | X | | | X |
| Garlic | | X | | | | | X | X | | X | X | | | X | X |
| Goldenseal | | | | | | | | | | | | | | | X |
| Lemon Grass | | | | | | | | | | | | | | | |
| Myrrh | | | | | | | | | | | | | | | X |
| Nasturtium | | | | | | | | | | | | | | | X |
| Neem | | | | | | | | | | | | | | | |
| Onion | | X | | | | | X | | | | | | | | |
| Oregano | X | X | | | | | | | | | | | | | |
| Oregon Grape | | | | | X | | | | | | | | | | |
| Oregon Grape Root | | | | | X | | | | | | | | | | |
| Pau D'Arco | | | | | | | | | | | | | | | |
| Purslane | | | | | | | | | | | | | | | X |
| Rosemary | X | | | | | | | X | | | | X | | X | |
| Sage | X | | | | | | | | X | X | | | | X | X |
| Savory | X | X | X | X | X | | | | | | | | | | |
| Sweet Cicely | | | | | | | | | | | | | | | X |
| Sweet Root | | | | | | | | | | | | | | | |
| Tea Tree Oil | | | | | | | | | | | | | | | |
| Thyme | | X | | | | | | | | | | | | | X |

**Herbs By Classifications — Antihemorrhagic & Hemostatic**

Herb columns 1–15:

| Classification | Blackberry | Black haw | Bloodroot | Calendula | Cayenne | Comfrey | Cranesbill | Cypress | Germander | Horsemint | Horsetail | Lady's Mantle | Lamb's Ear | Mullein | Nasturtium |
|---|---|---|---|---|---|---|---|---|---|---|---|---|---|---|---|
| Vulnerary | | | | X | X | X | | | | | | | | X | |
| Vasodilator | | | | | X | | | | | | | | | | |
| Sialogogue | | | | | X | | | | | | | | | | |
| Rubefacient | | | | | X | | | | | | | | | | |
| Oxytocic | | | | | | | | | | | | | | | |
| Nervine Stimulants | | | | | X | | | | | | | | | | |
| Nervine Relaxants | | | | | | | | | | | | | | | |
| Nervine Tonics | | | | | | | | | | | | | | | |
| Hypotensive | | | | | X | | | | | | | | | | |
| Hypnotic | | | | | | | | | | | | | | | |
| Hepatic | | | | | | | | | | | | | | | |
| Hematinic | | | | | | | | | | | | | | | |
| Galactogogue | | | | | | | | | | | | | | | |
| Expectorant | | | | | | X | | | | | | | | X | |
| Emmenagogue | | | | X | | | | | | | | | | | |
| Diuretic | | | | | | | | | | | X | | | | X |
| Diaphoretic | | | | | X | | | | | | | | | | |
| Demulcent | | | | | | X | | | | | | | | X | |
| Cholagogue | | | | | | | | | | | | | | | |
| Cathartic | | | | | | | | | | | | | | | |
| Carminative | | | | | | | | | | | | | | | |
| Cardiotonic | | | | | X | | | | | | | | | | |
| Bitters | | | | | | | | | | | | | | X | |
| Astringent | X | | | | | | X | | X | | | | | | |
| Aperient | | | | | | | | | | | | | | | |
| Antiviral | | | | | | | | | | | | | | | X |
| Antispasmodic | | X | | | | | | | | | | | | X | |
| Antirheumatic | | | | | X | | | | | | | | | | |
| Antipyretic | | | | | | | | | | | | | | | |
| Antiprotozoal | | | | | | | | | | | | | | | |
| Antilithics-Urinary | | | | | | | | | | | | | | | |
| Antilithics-Gallstone | | | | | | | | | | | | | | | |
| Anti-inflammatory | | | | X | X | X | | | | | | | | | |
| Antihemorrhagic | X | X | X | X | X | X | X | X | X | X | X | X | X | X | X |
| Antifungal | | | | X | | | | | | | | | | X | |
| Antiemetics | | | | | | | | | | | | | | X | |
| Anticatarrhal | | | | | | X | | | | | | | | X | X |
| Antibiotic | | | | X | X | | | | | | | | | | |
| Anthelmintics | | | | | | | | | | | | | | | |
| Antacid & Anti-ulcer | | | | X | | X | | | | | | | | | |
| Anodyne | | | | | X | | | | | | | | | | |
| Analgesic | | | | | X | | | | | | | | | | |
| Amphoteric | | | | | X | | | | | | | | | | |
| Alterative | | | | X | | X | | | X | | | | | | |
| Adaptogens | | | | | | | | | | | | | | | |

Herb columns 16–30:

| Classification | Nettle | Oak Moss | Plantain | purselane | Raspberry Leaf | Shepherd's Purse | Stinging Nettle | Tormentil | Uva Ursi | Weld | White Oak | White Oak Bark | Witch Hazel | Yarrow | Yellow Dock |
|---|---|---|---|---|---|---|---|---|---|---|---|---|---|---|---|
| Vulnerary | | X | X | | | | | | | | | | X | X | |
| Vasodilator | | | | | | | | | | | | | | X | |
| Sialogogue | | | | | | | | | | | | | | | |
| Rubefacient | | | | | | | | | | | | | | | |
| Oxytocic | | | | | X | X | | | | | | | | | |
| Nervine Stimulants | | | | | | | | | | | | | | X | |
| Nervine Relaxants | | | | | | | | | | | | | | | |
| Nervine Tonics | | | | | | | | | | | | | | | |
| Hypotensive | | | | | | | | | | | | | | X | |
| Hypnotic | | | | | | | | | | | | | | | |
| Hepatic | | | | | | | | | | | | | | | X |
| Hematinic | X | | | | | | X | | | | | | | | X |
| Galactogogue | X | | | | | | X | | | | | | | | |
| Expectorant | | | | | | | | | | | | | | | |
| Emmenagogue | | | | | | | | | | | | | | | |
| Diuretic | X | | X | X | | | | | X | | | | | | |
| Diaphoretic | | | X | | | | | | | | | | | X | |
| Demulcent | | | X | X | | | | | | | | | | | |
| Cholagogue | | | | | | | | | | | | | | | X |
| Cathartic | | | | | | | | | | | | | | | X |
| Carminative | | | | | | | | | | | | | | | |
| Cardiotonic | | | | | | | | | | | | | | X | |
| Bitters | | | | | | | | | | | | | | | |
| Astringent | X | X | X | X | | | | | X | | X | X | X | X | |
| Aperient | X | | X | | | | | | | | | | | | |
| Antiviral | X | | | | | | | | | | | | | | |
| Antispasmodic | | | | | | | | | | | | | | | |
| Antirheumatic | X | X | | | | | X | | X | | | | | | |
| Antipyretic | X | | | | X | | | | | | | | | X | |
| Antiprotozoal | | | | | | | | | | | | | | | |
| Antilithics-Urinary | X | | | | | | | | X | | | | | | |
| Antilithics-Gallstone | X | | | | | | | | | | | | | | |
| Anti-inflammatory | X | X | X | | | | X | | | | | | | X | |
| Antihemorrhagic | X | X | X | X | X | X | X | X | X | X | X | X | X | X | X |
| Antifungal | | | X | | | | | | | | | | | | |
| Antiemetics | | | X | | | | | | | | | | | | |
| Anticatarrhal | X | | X | | | | X | | X | | | | | X | |
| Antibiotic | X | | X | X | | | | | X | | | | | X | |
| Anthelmintics | | | | | | | | | | | | | | | |
| Antacid & Anti-ulcer | | | | | | | | | | | | | | | |
| Anodyne | | | | | | | | | | | | | | X | |
| Analgesic | | | | | | | | | | | | | | X | |
| Amphoteric | X | | X | | | | | | | | | | | | |
| Alterative | X | | X | | | | X | | X | | | | | | X |
| Adaptogens | X | | | | | | | | | | | | | | |

| Herbs By Classifications | Adaptogens | Alterative | Amphoteric | Analgesic | Anodyne | Antacid & Anti-ulcer | Anthelmintics | Antibiotic | Anticatarrhal | Antiemetics | Antifungal | Antihemorrhagic | Anti-Inflammatory | Antilithics-Gallstone | Antilithics-Urinary | Antiprotozoal | Antipyretic | Antirheumatic | Antispasmodic | Antiviral | Aperient | Astringent | Bitters | Cardiotonic | Carminative | Cathartic | Cholagogue | Demulcent | Diaphoretic | Diuretic | Emmenagogue | Expectorant | Galactogogue | Hematinic | Hepatic | Hypnotic | Hypotensive | Nervine Tonics | Nervine Relaxants | Nervine Stimulants | Oxytocic | Rubefacient | Sialogogue | Vasodilator | Vulnerary |
|---|---|---|---|---|---|---|---|---|---|---|---|---|---|---|---|---|---|---|---|---|---|---|---|---|---|---|---|---|---|---|---|---|---|---|---|---|---|---|---|---|---|---|---|---|---|
| **Anti-Inflammatory** | | | | | | | | | | | | | | | | | | | | | | | | | | | | | | | | | | | | | | | | | | | | | |
| Agrimony | | | | | | | | | | | | | X | | | | | | | | | X | X | | | | | | | X | | | | | | | | | | | | | | | |
| Arnica | | | | X | X | | | | | | | | X | | | | | X | | | | | | | | | | | | | | | | | | | | | | | | X | | | X |
| Aspen | | | | X | | | | | | | | | X | | | | X | | | | | | | | | | | | X | | | | | | | | | | | | | | | | |
| Bergamot | | | | | | | | X | | | X | | X | | | | X | | | | | | | | | | | | X | | | | | | | | | | | | | | | | |
| Birch | | | | X | | | | | | | | | X | | | | X | X | | | | | | | | | | | X | X | | | | | | | | | | | | | | | |
| Black Pepper | | | | | | | | X | | | | | X | | | | | | | | | | | | X | | | | X | X | | X | | | | | | | | | | X | X | X | |
| Boswellia | | | | X | X | | | | | | | | X | | | | | X | | | | | | | | | | | | | | | | | | | | | | | | | | | |
| Burdock Root | | | | | | | | | | | X | | X | X | | | | X | | | | | | | | | | | X | | | | | | | | | | | | | | | | |
| Calendula | | X | | | | X | | X | | | X | X | X | | | | | | | | | | | | | | | | X | | | | | | | | | | | | | | | | X |
| Cat's Claw | | | | | | | | | | | | | X | | | | | X | X | | | | | | | | | | X | | | | | | | | | | | | | | | | |
| Cayenne | | | X | X | X | | | X | X | | X | | X | | | | | X | | | | | | X | | | | | X | | | | | | | | X | | | | | X | X | X | X |
| Chamomile | | | | X | X | X | | X | | X | X | | X | | | | | | X | | | X | | | X | | | | X | | X | | | | X | | | X | X | | | | | | X |
| Chickweed | | | | | | | | | X | | | | X | | | X | | | | | | | | | | | | X | | | | | | | | | | | | | | | | | |
| Comfrey | | X | | | | X | | | | | | X | X | | | | | | | | | | | | | | | X | | X | | | | | | | | | | | | | | | X |
| Devil's Claw | | | | X | X | | | | | | | | X | | | | | X | | | | | | | | | | | | | | | | | | | | | | | | | | | |
| Echinacea | | X | | | | | | X | | | X | | X | | | | X | | | X | | | | | | | | | X | | | | | | X | | | | | | | | | X | |
| Fennel Seeds | | | | | | | | X | | X | X | | X | | | | | | X | X | X | | | | X | | | | X | X | X | X | X | | | | | | | | | | | X | |
| Frankincense | | | | X | X | | | | | | | | X | | | | | | | X | | | | | | | | | | | | | | | | | | | | | | | | | |
| Fringe Tree | | | | | | | | | | | | | X | | | | | | | | | | | | | | X | | | | | | | | | | | | | | | | | | |
| Chamomile | | | | | | | | X | X | | X | | X | | | X | X | X | X | X | X | X | X | X | | | | | X | X | X | | | | | X | X | X | X | X | | | X | | X |
| Ginger | | | | X | | | X | X | X | X | | | X | X | | X | X | X | X | X | | | | | X | X | X | | X | X | X | X | | | | | X | | | X | X | X | X | X | |
| Green Tea | | | | | | | | | | | | | X | | | | | | | | | | | | | | | | X | | | | | | | | | | | | | | | | |
| Gumweed | | | | | | | | | X | | | | X | | | | | | | | | | | | | | | | | | | X | | | | | | | | | | | | | X |
| Hyssop | | | | | | | X | X | | | | | X | | | | | X | | | | | | | | | | | X | | | X | | | | | | | X | | | | | | |
| Licorice | X | X | X | | | X | | X | | | | | X | | | X | | | X | | X | X | | | | X | X | X | | X | | X | | | | | | | | | | | | X | |
| Licorice Root | X | | X | | | X | | X | | | | | X | | | | X | | X | | X | X | | | | X | X | X | | X | | X | | | | | | | | | | | | X | |
| Mallow | | X | | | | | | X | X | | X | | X | | | X | | | | | X | | | | | | | X | | | | | | | | | | | | | | | | | X |
| Marjoram | | | | X | X | | | X | X | | | | X | | | | | | | | | X | X | X | X | | X | | | | | | | | | | | | X | X | | X | X | X | X |
| Marshmallow | | X | | | | | | X | X | | X | | X | | | | | X | | | | | | | | | | X | | | | | | | | | | | | | | | | | X |
| Marshmallow Root | | X | | | | | | X | X | | X | | X | | | | | X | | | | | | | | | | X | | | | | | | | | | | | | | | | | X |
| Nasturtium | X | X | X | | | | | X | X | X | X | X | X | X | X | X | X | X | X | X | X | X | | | | | | | X | | | | | | | | | | | | | | | | X |
| Nettle | | X | | | | | | | X | | | X | X | | | | | X | | | | | | | | | | | X | | | | X | X | | | | | | | | | | | |
| Onion | | | | | | | | X | | X | | | X | | | | | X | | | | | | | | | | | X | | | | | | | | X | | | | | | | | |
| Oregano | | | | X | | | | X | X | X | | | X | | | | X | X | X | | | | | | | | | | X | | X | | | | | | | | | | | | | X | X |
| Plantain | | X | | | | | | X | | | | X | X | | | | | | | | | X | | | | | | | X | X | | | | | | | | | | | | | | | X |
| Poplar | | | | X | | | | | | | | | X | | | X | | | | | | | | | | | | | X | | | | | | | | X | | | | | | | | |
| Purslane | | X | X | | | | | X | X | X | X | X | X | | | | | | | | | X | X | X | | | | | X | X | X | | | | | | | | | | | | | | X |
| Rosemary | | | | X | | | | | X | | | | X | | | | | X | X | | | | | | X | | | | X | | | | | | | | | | | X | | X | | X | |
| Sage | | | | X | | | | X | X | | | | X | | | | | X | X | | | X | X | | X | | | | X | | X | | | | | | | | X | X | | | X | | X |
| Savory | | | X | X | X | | X | X | X | X | X | | X | | | | | | | | | X | X | X | X | X | X | X | X | X | X | X | X | X | X | X | X | X | | | | | | | |
| Skullcap | | | | X | X | | | | | | | | X | | | | | | X | | | | | | | | | | X | | | | | | | | | X | X | X | | | | | X |
| St. John's Wort | | | | | | | | | X | | | | X | | | | | | X | | | | | | | | | | X | | | | | | | | | X | X | | | | | | X |
| Stinging Nettle | | X | | | | | | | X | | | X | X | | | | | X | | | | | | | | | | | X | | | | X | X | | | | | | | | | | | |
| Teasel Root | | | | | | | | | | | | | X | | | | X | X | X | | | | | | | | | | X | | | | | | X | | | | | | | | | | |
| Turmeric | X | | X | X | X | X | X | X | | | | | X | X | | | | X | | | | | | X | | | X | | X | X | | | | | | | X | | | | | X | | X | |
| White Willow | | | | X | X | | | | | | | | X | | | | X | X | | | | X | X | | | | | | X | | | | | | | | | | | | | | | | |
| White Willow Bark | | | | X | X | | | | | | | | X | | | | X | X | | | | X | X | | | | | | X | | | | | | | | | | | | | | | | |
| Willow | | | | X | X | | | | | | | | X | | | | X | X | | | | X | X | | | | | | X | | | | | | | | | | | | | | | | |
| Willow Bark | | | | X | X | | | | | | | | X | | | | X | X | | | | X | X | | | | | | X | | | | | | | | | | | | | | | | |
| Yarrow | | | | X | X | | | X | X | | | X | X | | | | | | X | | | X | | X | | | | | X | | | | | | | | X | | | | | X | | X | X |

| Herbs By Classifications | Adaptogens | Alterative | Amphoteric | Analgesic | Anodyne | Antacid & Anti-ulcer | Anthelmintics | Antibiotic | Anticatarrhal | Antiemetics | Antifungal | Antihemorrhagic | Anti-Inflammatory | Antilithics-Gallstone | Antilithics-Urinary | Antiprotozoal | Antipyretic | Antirheumatic | Antispasmodic | Antiviral | Aperient | Astringent | Bitters | Cardiotonic | Carminative | Cathartic | Cholagogue | Demulcent | Diaphoretic | Diuretic | Emmenagogue | Expectorant | Galactogogue | Hematinic | Hepatic | Hypnotic | Hypotensive | Nervine Tonics | Nervine Relaxants | Nervine Stimulants | Oxytocic | Rubefacient | Sialogogue | Vasodilator | Vulnerary |
|---|---|---|---|---|---|---|---|---|---|---|---|---|---|---|---|---|---|---|---|---|---|---|---|---|---|---|---|---|---|---|---|---|---|---|---|---|---|---|---|---|---|---|---|---|---|
| **Antilithic** | | | | | | | | | | | | | | | | | | | | | | | | | | | | | | | | | | | | | | | | | | | | | |
| **Gallstone Antilithics** | | | | | | | | | | | | | | | | | | | | | | | | | | | | | | | | | | | | | | | | | | | | | |
| Artichoke | | | | | | | | | | | | | | X | | | | | | | | | X | | | | X | | | | | | | | X | | | | | | | | | | |
| Barberry | | | | | | | | X | | | | | | X | | X | | | | | | | X | | | X | X | | | | | | | | X | | | | | | | | | | |
| Boldo | | | | | | | X | | | | | | | X | | | | | | | | | | | | | X | | | | | | | | X | | | | | | | | | | |
| Burdock Root | | | | | | | | | | | X | | X | X | | | | X | | | | | | | | | | | | | | | | | | | | | | | | | | | |
| Cascara sagrada | | | | | | | | | | | | | | X | | | | | | | X | | | | | X | | | | | | | | | | | | | | | | | | | |
| Chicory | | | | | | | | | | | | | | X | | | | | | | | | X | | | | | | | | | | | X | | | | | | | | | | | |
| Chicory Root | | | | | | | | | | | | | | X | | | | | | | | | X | | | | | | | | | | | X | | | | | | | | | | | |
| Dandelion | | X | | | | | | | | | | | | X | X | | | | | | X | | X | | | | X | | | X | | | | X | X | | | | | | | | | | |
| Dandelion Root | | X | | | | | | | | | | | | X | X | | | | | | X | | X | | | | X | | | X | | | | X | X | | | | | | | | | | |
| Ginger | | | | X | | | X | X | X | X | | | X | X | X | X | X | X | X | X | | | X | X | X | | | | | X | X | X | | | X | | X | | | X | X | X | | X | |
| Globe Artichoke | | | | | | | | | | | | | | X | | | | | | | | | | | | | | | | | | | | | | | | | | | | | | | |
| Greater Celandine | | | | | | | | | | | | | | X | | | | | X | | | X | | | | | X | | | | | | | | X | | | | | | | | | | |
| Lemon | | | | | | | | | | | | | | X | | | | | | | | | | | | | | | | | | | | | | | | | | | | | | | |
| Milk Thistle | X | | | | | X | | | | | | | | X | X | X | | | | | | | | | | | X | | | | | | | | X | | | | | | | | | | |
| Nasturtium | X | X | X | | | | | X | X | X | X | X | X | X | | | X | X | X | | X | X | X | | | | | | | X | | | | | | | | | | | | | | | X |
| Oregon Grape | | X | | | | | | X | | | X | | | X | | | | | | | | | | | | | X | | | | | | | | X | | | | | | | | | | |
| Oregon Grape Root | | X | | | | | | X | | | X | | | X | | | | | | | | | | | | | X | | | | | | | | X | | | | | | | | | | |
| Peppermint | | | | | | | | X | X | X | | | | X | | | X | | X | | | | | | X | | | | X | | X | | | | | | | | | | | X | X | | |
| Turkey Rhubarb | | | | | | | | | | | | | | X | | | | | | | | | | | | X | | | | | | | | | | | | | | | | | | | |
| Turmeric | X | | X | X | X | X | X | X | | | | | X | X | | | | X | | | | | | X | | | X | | | | | | | | X | | | | | | | X | | X | |
| Wild Cherry Bark | | | | | | | | | | | | | | X | | | | | X | | | | | | | | | | | | | X | | | | | | | | | | | | | |

| Herbs By Classifications | Adaptogens | Alterative | Amphoteric | Analgesic | Anodyne | Antacid & Anti-ulcer | Anthelmintics | Antibiotic | Anticatarrhal | Antiemetics | Antifungal | Antihemorrhagic | Anti-Inflammatory | Antilithics-Gallstone | Antilithics-Urinary | Antiprotozoal | Antipyretic | Antirheumatic | Antispasmodic | Antiviral | Aperient | Astringent | Bitters | Cardiotonic | Carminative | Cathartic | Cholagogue | Demulcent | Diaphoretic | Diuretic | Emmenagogue | Expectorant | Galactogogue | Hematinic | Hepatic | Hypnotic | Hypotensive | Nervine Tonics | Nervine Relaxants | Nervine Stimulants | Oxytocic | Rubefacient | Sialogogue | Vasodilator | Vulnerary |
|---|---|---|---|---|---|---|---|---|---|---|---|---|---|---|---|---|---|---|---|---|---|---|---|---|---|---|---|---|---|---|---|---|---|---|---|---|---|---|---|---|---|---|---|---|---|
| **Antilithic** | | | | | | | | | | | | | | | | | | | | | | | | | | | | | | | | | | | | | | | | | | | | | |
| **Urinary Antilithics** | | | | | | | | | | | | | | | | | | | | | | | | | | | | | | | | | | | | | | | | | | | | | |
| Bearberry | | | | | | | | | | | | | | | X | | | | | | | | | | | | | | | X | | | | | | | | | | | | | | | |
| Celery Seed | | | | | | | | | | | | | | | X | | | | | | | | | | X | | | | | | | | | | | | | | | | | | | | |
| Chanca Piedra | | | | | | | | | | | | | | | X | | | | | | | | | | | | | | | | | | | | | | | | | | | | | | |
| Cleavers | | X | | | | | | | | | | | | | X | | | | | | | | | | | | | | | X | | | | | X | | | | | | | | | | |
| Corn Silk | | | | | | | | | | | | | | | X | | | | | | | | | | | | | X | | X | | | | | | | | | | | | | | | |
| Couchgrass | | | | | | | | | | | | | | | X | | | | | | | | | | | | | | | X | | | | | | | | | | | | | | | |
| Dandelion | | X | | | | | | | | | | | | X | X | | | | | | X | | X | | | | X | | | X | | | | X | X | | | | | | | | | | |
| Dandelion Root | | X | | | | | | | | | | | | X | X | | | | | | X | | X | | | | X | | | X | | | | X | X | | | | | | | | | | |
| Dill | | | | | | | | | | X | | | | | X | | | | | | | | | | X | | | | | | | | X | | | | | | | | | | | | |
| Dill Seed | | | | | | | | | | X | | | | | X | | | | | | | | | | X | | | | | | | | X | | | | | | | | | | | | |
| Garden Sage | | | | | | | | X | X | | X | | X | | X | | X | X | X | X | | X | X | | X | | | | X | X | X | | | | X | | | X | X | X | | X | | | X |
| Goldenrod | | | | | | | | | X | | | | | | X | | | | | | | | | | | | | | | X | | | | | | | | | | | | | | | |
| Gravel Root | | | | | | | | | | | | | | | X | | | | | | | | | | | | | | | X | | | | | | | | | | X | | | | | |
| Horsetail | | X | | | | | | | | | | X | | | X | | | | | | | X | | | | | | | | X | | | | | | | | | | | | | | | X |
| Hydrangea Root | | | | | | | | | | | | | | | X | | | | | | | | | | | | | | | | | | | | | | | | | | | | | | |
| Juniper | | | | | | | | X | | | | | | | X | | | X | | | | | | | X | | | | | X | | | | | | | | | | | X | X | | | |
| Juniper Berries | | | | | | | | X | | | | | | | X | | | X | | | | | | | X | | | | | X | | | | | | | | | | | X | X | | | |
| Mallow | | X | | | | | | | X | X | | | X | | X | | | | | | X | | | | | | | X | | | | | | | | | | | | | | | | | X |
| Marshmallow | | X | | | | | | | X | X | | | X | | X | | | | | | X | | | | | | | X | | | | | | | | | | | | | | | | | X |
| Marshmallow Root | | X | | | | | | | X | X | | | X | | X | | | | | | X | | | | | | | X | | | | | | | | | | | | | | | | | X |
| Nasturtium | X | X | X | | | | | X | X | X | X | X | X | X | X | X | X | X | X | X | X | X | X | | | | | | | X | | | | | | | | | | | | | | | X |
| Parsley | | | | | | | | | | | | | | | X | | | | | | | | | | X | | | | | X | X | | | X | | | X | | | | | | | | |
| Parsley Root | | | | | | | | | | | | | | | X | | | | | | | | | | | | | | | X | | | | | | | | | | | | | | | |
| Uva Ursi | | X | | | | | | X | X | | | X | | | X | | | X | | | | X | | | | | | | | X | | | | | | | | | | | | | | | |

| Herbs By Classifications | Adaptogens | Alterative | Amphoteric | Analgesic | Anodyne | Antacid & Anti-ulcer | Anthelmintics | Antibiotic | Anticatarrhal | Antiemetics | Antifungal | Antihemorrhagic | Anti-Inflammatory | Antilithics-Gallstone | Antilithics-Urinary | Antiprotozoal | Antipyretic | Antirheumatic | Antispasmodic | Antiviral | Aperient | Astringent | Bitters | Cardiotonic | Carminative | Cathartic | Cholagogue | Demulcent | Diaphoretic | Diuretic | Emmenagogue | Expectorant | Galactogogue | Hematinic | Hepatic | Hypnotic | Hypotensive | Nervine Tonics | Nervine Relaxants | Nervine Stimulants | Oxytocic | Rubefacient | Sialogogue | Vasodilator | Vulnerary |
|---|---|---|---|---|---|---|---|---|---|---|---|---|---|---|---|---|---|---|---|---|---|---|---|---|---|---|---|---|---|---|---|---|---|---|---|---|---|---|---|---|---|---|---|---|---|
| **Antiprotozoals** | | | | | | | | | | | | | | | | | | | | | | | | | | | | | | | | | | | | | | | | | | | | | |
| Barberry | | | | | | | | X | | | | | | X | | X | | | | | | | X | | | X | X | | | | | | | | X | | | | | | | | | | |
| Black Walnut Hull | | | | | | | X | | | | X | | | | | X | | | | | | | | | | | | | | | | | | | | | | | | | | | | | |
| Chaparral | | X | | | | | | X | | | X | | | | | X | | | | X | | | | | | | | | | | | | | | | | | | | | | | | | |
| Garlic | | X | | | | | X | X | X | | X | | | | | X | | | | X | | | | X | X | | | | | | | X | | | | | X | | | X | | X | | X | X |
| Ginger | | | | X | | | X | X | X | X | | | X | X | | X | X | X | X | X | | | X | X | X | | | | | X | X | X | | | X | | X | | | X | X | X | | X | |
| Goldenseal | | | | | | | | X | | | X | | | | | X | | | | X | | | X | | | | | | | | | | | | | | | | | | | | | | X |
| Licorice | X | X | X | | | X | | | X | | | | X | | | X | | X | | X | X | | | | | X | X | X | | | | X | | | X | | | | | | | | X | | |
| Licorice Root | X | X | X | | | X | | | X | | | | X | | | X | | X | | X | X | | | | | X | X | X | | | | X | | | X | | | | | | | | X | | |
| Milk Thistle | X | | | | | X | | | | | | | | X | | X | | | | | | | | | | | X | | | | | | | | X | | | | | | | | | | |
| Myrrh | | | | | | | | X | | | X | | | | | X | | | | | | | | | | | | | | | | | | | | | | | | | | | | | X |
| Wormwood | | | | | | | X | X | | | | | | | | X | | | | | | | X | | | | | | | | | | | | X | | | | | | | | | | |

| Herbs By Classifications | Adaptogens | Alterative | Amphoteric | Analgesic | Anodyne | Antacid & Anti-ulcer | Anthelmintics | Antibiotic | Anticatarrhal | Antiemetics | Antifungal | Antihemorrhagic | Anti-Inflammatory | Antilithics-Gallstone | Antilithics-Urinary | Antiprotozoal | Antipyretic | Antirheumatic | Antispasmodic | Antiviral | Aperient | Astringent | Bitters | Cardiotonic | Carminative | Cathartic | Cholagogue | Demulcent | Diaphoretic | Diuretic | Emmenagogue | Expectorant | Galactogogue | Hematinic | Hepatic | Hypnotic | Hypotensive | Nervine Tonics | Nervine Relaxants | Nervine Stimulants | Oxytocic | Rubefacient | Sialogogue | Vasodilator | Vulnerary |
|---|---|---|---|---|---|---|---|---|---|---|---|---|---|---|---|---|---|---|---|---|---|---|---|---|---|---|---|---|---|---|---|---|---|---|---|---|---|---|---|---|---|---|---|---|---|
| **Antipyretic & Febrifuges** | | | | | | | | | | | | | | | | | | | | | | | | | | | | | | | | | | | | | | | | | | | | | |
| Alfalfa | | X | | | | | | | | | | | | | | | X | | | | X | | | | | | | | X | X | | | X | X | | | | | | | | | | | |
| Aspen | | | | X | | | | | | | | | X | | | | X | | | | | | | | | | | | | | | | | | | | | | | | | | | | |
| Basil | | | | | | | | | | X | | | | | | | X | | | | | | | | | | | | X | | | | | | | | | | | | | | | | |
| Bergamot | | | | | | | | X | | | X | | X | | | | X | | | | | | | | | | | | X | | | | | | | | | | | | | | | | |
| Bilberry | | | | | | X | | | | | | | | | | | X | | | | | | | | | | | | | | | | | X | | | | | | | | | | | |
| Birch | | | | X | | | | | | | | | X | | | | X | X | | | | | | | | | | | | | | | | | | | | | | | | | | | |
| Boneset | | | | | | | | | | | | | | | | | X | | | | | | | | | | | | X | | | | | | | | | | | | | | | | |
| Catnip | | | | | | | | | | X | | | | | | | X | | X | | | | | | | | | | X | | | | | | | X | | X | X | | | | | | |
| Chamomile | | | | X | X | X | | X | | X | X | | X | | | | X | X | X | | | | X | | X | | | | X | | X | | | | | X | | X | X | | | | | | X |
| Chickweed | | | | | | | | | X | | | | X | | | | X | | | | | | | | | | | | | | | | | X | | | | | | | | | | | |
| Echinacea | | X | | | | | | X | | | X | | X | | | | X | | | X | | | | | | | | | X | | | | | X | | | | | | | | | X | | X |
| Elder | | | | | | | | | X | | | | | | | | X | | | X | | | | | | | | | X | X | | X | | | | | | | | | | | | | X |
| Elderberry | | | | | | | | | | | | | | | | | X | | | X | | | | | | | | | X | X | | X | | | | | | | | | | | | | X |
| Elderflower | | | | | | | | | | | | | | | | | X | | | X | | | | | | | | | X | X | | X | | | | | | | | | | | | | X |
| Garden Sage | | | | | | | | X | X | | X | | X | | X | | X | X | X | X | | X | X | | X | | | | X | X | X | | | | X | | X | X | X | | | X | | | X |
| Ginger | | | | X | | | X | X | X | X | | | X | X | | X | X | X | X | X | | | X | X | X | | | | | X | X | X | | | X | | X | | | X | X | X | | X | |
| Gotu Kola | X | | X | | | X | | | | | | | | | | | X | | | | | | | | | | | | | | | | | | | | X | | X | | | | | | X |
| Irish Moss | | | | | | | | | X | | | | | | | | X | | | | | | | | | | | X | | | | | | | | | | | | | | | | | |
| Kelp | | | | | | | | | | | | | | | | | X | | | | | | | | | | | | | | | | | | | | | | | | | | | | |
| Lemon Balm | X | | | | | | | | | X | | | | | | | X | | X | X | | | | X | X | | X | | | | | | | | | X | X | X | X | | | | | | |
| Meadowsweet | | | | | X | | | | | X | | | | | | | X | X | | | | X | | | | | | | | | | | | | | | | | | | | | | | |
| Mistletoe | | | | | | | | | | | | | | | | | X | | | | | | | | | | | | | | | | | | | | X | | | | | | | X | |
| Nasturtium | X | X | X | | | | | X | X | X | X | X | X | X | X | | X | X | X | X | X | X | X | | | | | | | X | | | | | | | | | | | | | | | X |
| Oregano | | | | X | | | | X | X | | X | | X | | | | X | | X | X | | | | | | | | | X | | | X | | | | | | | | | | | | | |
| Peppermint | | | | X | | | | X | X | X | | | | X | | | X | | X | X | | | | | X | | | | X | | X | | | | | | | | | | | | X | X | |
| Poplar | | | | X | | | | | | | | | X | | | | X | | | | | | | | | | | | | X | | | | | | | | | | | | | | | |
| Raspberry Leaf | | | | | | | | | | | | X | | | | | X | | | | | X | | | | | | | | | | | | | | | | | | | X | | | | |
| Skullcap | | | | X | X | | | | | | | | X | | | | X | X | | | | | | | | | | | | | | | | | | X | X | X | X | | | | | | |
| Sweet Annie | | | | | | | | | | | | | | | | | X | | | | | | | | | | | | | | | | | | | | | | | | | | | | |
| Tansy | | | | | | | X | | | | | | | | | | X | | | | | | | | | | | | | | X | | | | | | | | | | | | | | |
| Teasel Root | | | | | | | | | | | | | X | | | | X | X | X | | | | | | | | | | X | | | | | | | | | | | | | | | | |
| Thyme | | | | | | | | X | X | | X | | | | | | X | | X | X | | X | | | X | | | | X | | | X | | | | | | | | | | | | | |
| White Willow | | | | X | X | | | | | | | | X | | | | X | X | | | | | | | | | | | | | | | | | | | | | | | | | | | |
| White Willow Bark | | | | X | X | | | | | | | | X | | | | X | X | | | | | | | | | | | | | | | | | | | | | | | | | | | |
| Willow | | | | X | X | | | | | | | | X | | | | X | X | | | | | | | | | | | | | | | | | | | | | | | | | | | |
| Willow Bark | | | | X | X | | | | | | | | X | | | | X | X | | | | | | | | | | | | | | | | | | | | | | | | | | | |
| Yarrow | | | | X | X | | | X | X | | | X | X | | | | X | | | | | X | | X | | | | | X | | | | | | | | X | | | X | | | | X | X |

Columns 1–15:

| Herbs By Classifications | Adaptogens | Alterative | Amphoteric | Analgesic | Anodyne | Antacid & Anti-ulcer | Anthelmintics | Antibiotic | Anticatarrhal | Antiemetics | Antifungal | Antihemorrhagic | Anti-Inflammatory | Antilithics-Gallstone | Antilithics-Urinary |
|---|---|---|---|---|---|---|---|---|---|---|---|---|---|---|---|
| **Antirheumatic** | | | | | | | | | | | | | | | |
| Angelica | | | | | | | | | | | | | | | |
| Arnica | | | | X | X | | | | | | | | X | | |
| Birch | | | | X | | | | | | | | | X | | |
| Black Current | | | | | | | | | | | | | | | |
| Borage | | | | | | | | | | | | | | | |
| Boswellia | | | | X | X | | | | | | | | X | | |
| Burdock | | X | | | | | | | | | | | | | |
| Burdock Root | | | | | | | | | | | X | | X | X | |
| Cat's Claw | | | | | | | | | | | | | X | | |
| Cayenne | | | X | X | X | | | X | X | | X | | X | | |
| Chamomile | | | | X | X | X | | X | | X | X | | X | | |
| Devil's Claw | | | | X | X | | | | | | | | X | | |
| Frankincense | | | | X | X | | | | | | | | X | | |
| Garden Sage | | | | | | | | X | X | | X | | X | X | X |
| Juniper | | | | | | | | X | | | | | | | X |
| Juniper Berries | | | | | | | | X | | | | | | | X |
| Licorice | X | X | X | | | X | | X | | | | | X | | |
| Licorice Root | X | X | X | | | X | | X | | | | | X | | |
| Meadowsweet | | | | X | | X | | | | | | | | | |
| Nasturtium | X | X | X | | | | | X | X | X | X | X | X | X | X |
| Nettle | | X | | | | | | | | | | X | X | | |
| Pineapple Bromelair | | | | | | | | | | | | | | | |
| Rosemary | | | | | | | | | | | | X | X | | |
| Stinging Nettle | | X | | | | | | | | | | X | X | | |
| Teasel Root | | | | | | | | | | | | | | | |
| Turmeric | X | | X | X | X | X | X | X | | | | X | X | | |
| Uva Ursi | | X | | | | | | X | X | | | | | | X |
| White Willow | | | | X | X | | | | | | | | X | | |
| White Willow Bark | | | | X | X | | | | | | | | X | | |
| Willow | | | | X | X | | | | | | | | X | | |
| Willow Bark | | | | X | X | | | | | | | | X | | |
| Wintergreen | | | | | | | | | | | | | | | |

Columns 16–30:

| Herbs By Classifications | Antiprotozoal | Antipyretic | Antirheumatic | Antispasmodic | Antiviral | Aperient | Astringent | Bitters | Cardiotonic | Carminative | Cathartic | Cholagogue | Demulcent | Diaphoretic | Diuretic |
|---|---|---|---|---|---|---|---|---|---|---|---|---|---|---|---|
| **Antirheumatic** | | | | | | | | | | | | | | | |
| Angelica | | | X | X | | | | X | | | | | | | |
| Arnica | | | X | | | | | | | | | | | | |
| Birch | X | | X | | | | | | | | | | | | |
| Black Current | | | X | | | | | | | | | | | | |
| Borage | | | X | | | | | | | | | | | | |
| Boswellia | | | X | | | | | | | | | | | | |
| Burdock | | | X | | | | | X | | | | | | X | |
| Burdock Root | | | X | | | | | | | | | | | | |
| Cat's Claw | | | X | | X | | | | | | | | | | |
| Cayenne | | | X | | | | | | X | | | | | X | |
| Chamomile | | X | X | X | | | | | | X | | | | X | |
| Devil's Claw | | | X | | | | | | | | | | | | |
| Frankincense | | | X | | | | | | | | | | | | |
| Garden Sage | X | X | X | X | X | | X | X | | X | | | | X | X |
| Juniper | | | X | | | | | | | | | | | | X |
| Juniper Berries | | | X | | | | | | | | | | | | X |
| Licorice | X | | X | | X | X | | | | | X | X | X | | |
| Licorice Root | X | | X | | X | X | | | | | X | X | X | | |
| Meadowsweet | | X | X | | | | X | | | | | | | X | |
| Nasturtium | | X | X | X | X | X | X | X | | | | | | | X |
| Nettle | | | X | | | | | | | | | | | | X |
| Pineapple Bromelair | | | X | | | | | | | | | | | | |
| Rosemary | | | X | X | | | | | X | | | X | | X | |
| Stinging Nettle | | | X | | | | | | | | | | | | X |
| Teasel Root | | | X | | X | | X | | | | | | | | X |
| Turmeric | | | X | | | | | | | | | X | | X | |
| Uva Ursi | | | X | | | | X | | | | | | | | X |
| White Willow | | X | X | | | | | | | | | | | | |
| White Willow Bark | | X | X | | | | | | | | | | | | |
| Willow | | X | X | | | | | | | | | | | | |
| Willow Bark | | X | X | | | | | | | | | | | | |
| Wintergreen | | | X | | | | | | | | | | | | |

Columns 31–45:

| Herbs By Classifications | Emmenagogue | Expectorant | Galactogogue | Hematinic | Hepatic | Hypnotic | Hypotensive | Nervine Tonics | Nervine Relaxants | Nervine Stimulants | Oxytocic | Rubefacient | Sialogogue | Vasodilator | Vulnerary |
|---|---|---|---|---|---|---|---|---|---|---|---|---|---|---|---|
| **Antirheumatic** | | | | | | | | | | | | | | | |
| Angelica | X | | | | | | | | | X | X | | | | |
| Arnica | | | | | | | | | | | | X | | | X |
| Birch | | | | | | | | | | | | | | | |
| Black Current | | | | | | | | | | | | | | | |
| Borage | | | X | | | | | | | | | | | | |
| Boswellia | | | | | | | | | | | | | | | |
| Burdock | | | | X | X | | | | | | | | | | |
| Burdock Root | | | | | | | | | | | | | | | |
| Cat's Claw | | | | | | | X | | | | | | | | |
| Cayenne | | | | | | | X | | | X | | X | X | X | X |
| Chamomile | X | | | | | X | | X | X | | | | | | X |
| Devil's Claw | | | | | | | | | | | | | | | |
| Frankincense | | | | | | | | | | | | | | | |
| Garden Sage | X | | | | X | | X | X | X | | | X | | | X |
| Juniper | | | | | | | | | | X | X | | | | |
| Juniper Berries | | | | | | | | | | X | X | | | | |
| Licorice | | X | | | X | | | | | | | | X | | |
| Licorice Root | | X | | | X | | | | | | | | X | | |
| Meadowsweet | | | | | | | | | | | | | | | |
| Nasturtium | | | | | | | | | | | | | | | X |
| Nettle | | | X | X | | | | | | | | | | | |
| Pineapple Bromelair | | | | | | | | | | | | | | | |
| Rosemary | | | | | | | | | | X | | X | | X | |
| Stinging Nettle | | | X | X | | | | | | | | | | | |
| Teasel Root | | | | | | | | | | | | | | | |
| Turmeric | | | | | | | | | | | | | | X | |
| Uva Ursi | | | | | | | | | | | | | | | |
| White Willow | | | | | | | | | | | | | | | |
| White Willow Bark | | | | | | | | | | | | | | | |
| Willow | | | | | | | | | | | | | | | |
| Willow Bark | | | | | | | | | | | | | | | |
| Wintergreen | | | | | | | | | | | | | | | |

| Herbs By Classifications | Adaptogens | Alterative | Amphoteric | Analgesic | Anodyne | Antacid & Anti-ulcer | Anthelmintics | Antibiotic | Anticatarrhal | Antiemetics | Antifungal | Antihemorrhagic | Anti-Inflammatory | Antilithics-Gallstone | Antilithics-Urinary | Antiprotozoal | Antipyretic | Antirheumatic | Antispasmodic | Antiviral | Aperient | Astringent | Bitters | Cardiotonic | Carminative | Cathartic | Cholagogue | Demulcent | Diaphoretic | Diuretic | Emmenagogue | Expectorant | Galactogogue | Hematinic | Hepatic | Hypnotic | Hypotensive | Nervine Tonics | Nervine Relaxants | Nervine Stimulants | Oxytocic | Rubefacient | Sialogogue | Vasodilator | Vulnerary |
|---|---|---|---|---|---|---|---|---|---|---|---|---|---|---|---|---|---|---|---|---|---|---|---|---|---|---|---|---|---|---|---|---|---|---|---|---|---|---|---|---|---|---|---|---|---|
| **Antispasmodic** | | | | | | | | | | | | | | | | | | | | | | | | | | | | | | | | | | | | | | | | | | | | | |
| Allspice | | | | | | | | X | | | | | | | | | | | X | X | | | | | X | | | | | | | | | | | | | | | | | X | | X | |
| Angelica | | | | | | | | | | | | | | | | | | X | X | | | | X | | | | | | | | X | | | | | | | | | X | X | | | | |
| Anise seeds | | | | | | | | | X | | X | | | | | | | | X | X | | | | | X | | | | | | | X | X | | | | | | | | | | X | | |
| Baneberry | | | | X | | | | | | | | | | | | | | | X | | | | | | | | | | | | | | | | | | | | | | | | | | |
| Black Cohosh | X | | | X | X | | | | | | | | | | | | | | X | | | | | | | | | | | | X | | | | | | | | X | | X | | | | |
| Black haw | | | | | | | | | | | | X | | | | | | | X | | | | | | | | | | | | | | | | | | | | | | | | | | |
| Caraway | | | | | | | X | | | | | | | | | | | | X | | | | | | X | | | | | | | | X | | | | | X | | | | | | | |
| Catnip | | | | | | | | | | X | | | | | | | X | | X | | | | | | | | | | X | | | | | | | X | | X | X | | | | | | |
| Chamomile | | | | X | X | X | | X | | X | X | | X | | | | X | X | X | | | | X | | X | | | | X | | X | | | | | X | | X | X | | | | | | X |
| Cinnamon | | | | | | | | X | | X | X | | | | | | | | X | | | X | | | X | | | X | | | X | | | | | | X | | | X | | | X | X | |
| Cramp Bark | | | | | | | | | | | | | | | | | | | X | | | | | | | | | | | | X | | | | | | X | | X | | X | | | | |
| Fennel Seeds | | | | | | | | X | | X | X | | X | | | | | | X | X | X | | | | X | | | | X | X | X | X | X | | | | | | | | | | X | | |
| Garden Sage | | | | | | | | X | X | | X | | X | | X | | X | X | X | X | | X | X | | X | | | | X | X | X | | | | X | | X | X | X | | | X | | | X |
| Ginger | | | | X | | | X | X | X | X | | | X | X | | X | X | X | X | X | | | X | X | X | | | | | X | X | X | | | X | | X | | | X | X | X | | X | |
| Hyssop | | | | | | | X | | X | | | | X | | | | | | X | | | | | | | | | | X | | | X | | | | | | | X | | | | | | |
| Lavender | | | | X | X | | | | | X | | | | | | | | | X | | | | | | X | | | | | | | | | | | X | X | X | X | | | | | | X |
| Lemon Balm | X | | | | | | | | | X | | | | | | | X | | X | X | | | | X | X | | X | | | | | | | | | X | X | X | X | | | | | | |
| Lemon Verbana | | | | | | | | | | | | | | | | | | | X | | | | X | | | | | | | | | | | | | | | | X | | | | | | |
| Lobelia | | | | | | | | | | | | | | | | | | | X | | | | | | | | | | | | | X | | | | | | | X | | | | | | |
| Marjoram | | | | X | X | | | X | X | | | | X | | | | | | X | X | X | X | X | | X | | | | | | | | | | | | | X | X | | X | X | X | X | X |
| Motherwort | | | | | | | | | | | | | | | | | | | X | | | | | X | X | | | | | | X | | | | | X | X | X | X | | | | | | |
| Nasturtium | X | X | X | | | | | X | X | X | X | X | X | X | X | | X | X | X | X | X | X | X | | | | | | | X | | | | | | | | | | | | | | | X |
| Oregano | | | | X | | | | X | X | | X | | X | | | | X | | X | X | | | | | | | | | X | | | X | | | | | | | | | | | | | |
| Passionflower | X | | | | | | | | | | | | | | | | | | X | | | | | | | | | | | | | | | | | X | X | X | X | | | | | | |
| Peppermint | | | | X | | | | X | X | X | | | | X | | | X | | X | X | | | | | X | | | | X | | X | | | | | | | | | | | X | X | | |
| Rosemary | | | | X | | | | | | | X | | X | | | | | X | X | | | | | | | | X | | X | | | | | | | | | | | X | | X | | X | |
| Sage | | | | X | | | | X | X | | X | | X | | | | | | X | X | | X | X | | X | | | | X | | X | | | | | | | X | X | | | | X | | X |
| Savory | | | X | X | X | | X | X | X | X | X | | X | | | | | | X | X | X | X | X | X | X | X | X | X | X | X | X | X | X | X | X | | | | | | | | | | |
| Skullcap | | | | X | X | | | | | | | | X | | | | X | | X | | | | | | | | | | | | | | | | | X | X | X | X | | | | | | |
| St. John's Wort | | | | | | | | X | | | | | X | | | | | | X | X | | | | | | | | | | | | | | | | | | X | X | | | | | | X |
| Teasel Root | | | | | | | | | | | | | X | | | | X | X | X | | | | | | | | | | X | | | | | | | | | | | | | | | | |
| Thyme | | | | | | | X | X | | | X | | | | | | X | | X | X | | X | | | X | | | | X | | | X | | | | | | | | | | | | | X |
| Valerian | X | | | | | | | | | | | | | | | | | | X | | | | | | | | | | | | | | | | | X | X | X | X | | | | | | |
| Wild Cherry Bark | | | | | | | | | | | | | | X | | | | | X | | | | | | | | | | | | | X | | | | | | | | | | | | | |
| Wild Yam | | | | | | | | | | | | | | | | | | | X | | | | | | | | X | | | | | | | | X | | | | | | | | | | |

| Herbs By Classifications | Adaptogens | Alterative | Amphoteric | Analgesic | Anodyne | Antacid & Anti-ulcer | Anthelmintics | Antibiotic | Anticatarrhal | Antiemetics | Antifungal | Antihemorrhagic | Anti-Inflammatory | Antilithics-Gallstone | Antilithics-Urinary | Antiprotozoal | Antipyretic | Antirheumatic | Antispasmodic | Antiviral | Aperient | Astringent | Bitters | Cardiotonic | Carminative | Cathartic | Cholagogue | Demulcent | Diaphoretic | Diuretic | Emmenagogue | Expectorant | Galactogogue | Hematinic | Hepatic | Hypnotic | Hypotensive | Nervine Tonics | Nervine Relaxants | Nervine Stimulants | Oxytocic | Rubefacient | Sialogogue | Vasodilator | Vulnerary |
|---|---|---|---|---|---|---|---|---|---|---|---|---|---|---|---|---|---|---|---|---|---|---|---|---|---|---|---|---|---|---|---|---|---|---|---|---|---|---|---|---|---|---|---|---|---|
| **Antiviral** |  |  |  |  |  |  |  |  |  |  |  |  |  |  |  |  |  |  |  |  |  |  |  |  |  |  |  |  |  |  |  |  |  |  |  |  |  |  |  |  |  |  |  |  |  |
| Allspice |  |  |  |  |  |  |  | X |  |  |  |  |  |  |  |  |  |  | X | X |  |  |  |  | X |  |  |  |  |  |  |  |  |  |  | X |  |  |  |  |  | X |  | X |  |
| Andrographis |  |  |  |  |  |  |  | X |  |  |  |  |  |  |  |  |  |  |  | X |  |  |  |  |  |  |  |  |  |  |  |  |  |  |  |  |  |  |  |  |  |  |  |  |  |
| Anise seeds |  |  |  |  |  |  |  |  | X |  | X |  |  |  |  |  |  |  | X | X |  |  |  |  | X |  |  |  |  |  |  | X | X |  |  |  |  |  |  |  |  |  |  | X |  |  |
| Astragalus | X |  | X |  |  |  |  |  |  |  |  |  |  |  |  |  |  |  |  | X |  |  |  | X |  |  |  |  |  |  |  |  |  | X | X |  |  |  |  |  |  |  |  | X |  |
| Bay Leaves |  |  |  |  |  |  |  | X |  |  | X |  |  |  |  |  |  |  |  | X |  |  |  |  |  | X |  |  | X |  | X |  |  |  |  |  |  |  |  |  |  |  |  |  |  |
| Cat's Claw |  |  |  |  |  |  |  |  |  |  |  |  | X |  |  |  |  | X |  | X |  |  |  |  |  |  |  |  |  |  |  |  |  |  |  |  | X |  |  |  |  |  |  |  |  |
| Chaparral |  | X |  |  |  |  |  | X |  |  | X |  |  |  |  | X |  |  |  | X |  |  |  | X |  |  |  |  |  |  |  |  |  |  |  |  |  |  |  |  |  |  |  |  |  |
| Cloves |  |  |  | X | X |  | X |  |  | X | X |  |  |  |  |  |  |  |  | X |  |  |  |  | X |  |  |  |  |  |  |  |  |  |  |  |  |  |  |  |  | X |  |  |  |
| Echinacea |  | X |  |  |  |  |  | X |  |  | X |  | X |  |  |  |  |  |  | X |  |  |  |  |  |  |  |  | X |  |  |  |  |  |  |  | X |  |  |  |  |  |  | X | X |
| Elder |  |  |  |  |  |  |  |  | X |  |  |  |  |  |  |  | X |  |  | X |  |  |  |  |  |  |  |  | X | X | X |  |  |  |  |  |  |  |  |  |  |  |  |  | X |
| Elderberry |  |  |  |  |  |  |  |  |  |  |  |  |  |  |  |  | X |  |  | X |  |  |  |  |  |  |  |  | X | X | X |  |  |  |  |  |  |  |  |  |  |  |  |  | X |
| Fennel Seeds |  |  |  |  |  |  |  |  | X | X | X |  | X |  |  |  |  |  | X | X |  |  |  |  | X |  |  |  | X | X | X | X | X |  |  |  |  |  |  |  |  |  |  |  |  |
| Elderflower |  |  |  |  |  |  |  |  |  |  |  |  |  |  |  |  | X |  |  | X |  |  |  |  |  |  |  |  | X | X |  |  |  |  |  |  |  |  |  |  |  |  |  |  | X |
| Garden Sage |  |  |  | X |  |  |  | X | X |  | X |  | X |  |  | X |  | X | X | X |  | X | X |  | X |  |  |  | X | X | X |  |  |  | X |  |  | X | X | X |  |  |  |  | X |
| Garlic |  | X |  |  |  |  | X | X | X |  | X |  |  |  |  | X |  |  |  | X |  |  |  | X | X |  |  |  | X |  |  |  |  |  |  |  | X |  |  |  |  | X |  | X | X |
| Ginger |  |  |  | X |  |  |  | X | X | X | X |  | X |  |  | X | X | X | X | X |  |  |  |  | X | X | X |  | X | X | X |  |  |  |  |  |  |  |  | X |  | X | X | X |  |
| Goldenseal |  |  |  |  |  |  |  | X |  |  | X |  |  |  |  | X |  |  |  | X |  |  |  | X |  |  |  |  |  |  |  |  |  |  |  |  |  |  |  |  |  |  |  |  | X |
| Japanese Knotweed |  |  |  |  |  |  |  |  |  |  |  |  |  |  |  |  |  |  |  | X |  |  |  |  |  |  |  |  |  |  |  |  |  |  |  |  |  |  |  |  |  |  |  |  |  |
| Lemon Balm | X |  |  |  |  |  |  |  | X |  |  |  |  |  |  |  | X |  | X | X |  | X | X |  | X |  |  |  |  |  |  |  |  |  |  | X | X | X | X |  |  |  |  |  |  |
| Licorice | X | X | X |  |  | X |  |  |  |  | X |  | X |  |  |  |  |  |  | X | X |  |  |  |  |  |  | X | X | X |  |  | X |  | X |  |  |  |  |  |  |  |  | X |  |
| Licorice Root | X | X | X |  |  | X |  |  |  |  | X |  | X |  |  |  |  |  |  | X | X |  |  |  |  |  |  | X | X | X |  |  | X |  | X |  |  |  |  |  |  |  |  |  |  |
| Lomatium |  |  |  |  |  |  |  |  |  |  |  |  |  |  |  |  |  |  |  | X |  |  |  |  |  |  |  |  |  |  |  |  |  |  |  |  |  |  |  |  |  |  |  |  |  |
| Marjoram |  |  |  | X | X |  |  | X | X |  |  |  | X |  |  |  | X | X | X | X |  |  |  |  | X |  |  |  |  |  |  |  |  |  |  |  |  | X | X |  | X | X | X | X | X |
| Mullein |  |  |  |  |  |  |  | X |  |  |  | X |  |  |  |  |  |  |  | X |  |  |  |  |  |  |  | X |  |  |  |  |  |  |  |  |  |  |  |  |  |  |  |  |  |
| Nasturtium | X | X | X |  |  |  |  | X | X | X | X | X | X | X | X | X | X | X | X | X |  |  |  |  |  |  |  |  | X |  |  |  |  |  |  |  |  |  |  |  |  |  |  |  | X |
| Olive Leaf |  |  |  |  |  |  |  | X |  |  |  |  |  |  |  |  |  |  |  | X |  |  |  | X |  |  |  |  |  |  |  |  |  |  |  |  | X |  |  |  |  |  |  |  |  |
| Onion |  |  |  |  |  |  |  | X |  |  | X |  | X |  |  |  |  |  |  | X |  |  |  |  |  |  |  |  |  | X |  |  |  |  |  |  | X |  |  |  |  |  |  |  |  |
| Oregano |  |  |  | X |  |  |  | X | X |  | X |  | X |  |  |  |  |  |  | X |  |  |  |  |  |  |  |  | X |  | X |  |  |  |  |  |  |  |  |  |  |  |  |  |  |
| Pau D'Arco |  |  |  |  |  |  |  | X |  |  | X |  |  |  |  |  |  |  |  | X |  |  |  |  |  |  |  |  |  |  |  |  |  |  |  |  |  |  |  |  |  |  |  |  |  |
| Peppermint |  |  |  | X |  |  |  | X | X | X |  |  | X |  |  |  |  |  | X | X |  |  |  |  | X |  |  |  | X |  | X |  |  |  |  |  |  |  |  |  |  | X | X |  |  |
| Rosemary |  |  |  | X |  |  |  | X |  |  | X |  | X |  |  |  |  | X | X | X |  |  |  |  | X |  | X |  | X |  | X |  |  |  |  |  |  |  |  | X |  | X |  | X |  |
| Sage |  |  |  | X |  |  |  | X | X |  | X |  | X |  |  |  |  |  | X | X |  |  |  | X | X |  |  |  | X |  | X |  |  |  |  |  |  | X | X |  |  |  |  | X | X |
| Savory |  | X |  | X | X |  | X | X | X | X | X |  | X |  |  |  |  |  |  | X | X | X | X | X | X | X | X | X | X | X | X | X | X | X | X | X | X | X | X | X | X |  |  |  |  |
| Shiitake Mushroom |  |  |  |  |  |  |  |  |  |  |  |  |  |  |  |  |  |  |  | X |  |  |  |  |  |  |  |  |  |  |  |  |  |  |  |  |  |  |  |  |  |  |  |  |  |
| St. John's Wort |  |  |  |  |  |  |  | X |  |  |  |  | X |  |  |  |  |  |  | X |  |  |  |  |  |  |  |  |  |  |  |  |  |  |  |  |  | X | X |  |  |  |  |  | X |
| Tea Tree Oil |  |  |  |  |  |  |  |  | X |  |  |  |  |  |  |  |  |  |  | X |  |  |  |  |  |  |  |  |  |  |  |  |  |  |  |  |  |  |  |  |  |  |  |  |  |
| Thuja |  |  |  |  |  |  |  |  |  |  |  |  |  |  |  |  |  |  |  | X |  |  |  |  |  |  |  |  |  |  |  |  |  |  |  |  |  |  |  |  |  |  |  |  |  |
| Thyme |  |  |  |  |  |  |  | X | X |  | X |  |  |  |  |  |  |  | X | X |  | X |  |  | X |  |  |  | X |  | X |  |  |  |  |  |  |  |  |  |  |  |  |  | X |

| Herbs By Classifications | Adaptogens | Alterative | Amphoteric | Analgesic | Anodyne | Antacid & Anti-ulcer | Anthelmintics | Antibiotic | Anticatarrhal | Antiemetics | Antifungal | Antihemorrhagic | Anti-Inflammatory | Antilithics-Gallstone | Antilithics-Urinary | Antiprotozoal | Antipyretic | Antirheumatic | Antispasmodic | Antiviral | Aperient | Astringent | Bitters | Cardiotonic | Carminative | Cathartic | Cholagogue | Demulcent | Diaphoretic | Diuretic | Emmenagogue | Expectorant | Galactogogue | Hematinic | Hepatic | Hypnotic | Hypotensive | Nervine Tonics | Nervine Relaxants | Nervine Stimulants | Oxytocic | Rubefacient | Sialogogue | Vasodilator | Vulnerary |
|---|---|---|---|---|---|---|---|---|---|---|---|---|---|---|---|---|---|---|---|---|---|---|---|---|---|---|---|---|---|---|---|---|---|---|---|---|---|---|---|---|---|---|---|---|---|
| **Aperient** |  |  |  |  |  |  |  |  |  |  |  |  |  |  |  |  |  |  |  |  |  |  |  |  |  |  |  |  |  |  |  |  |  |  |  |  |  |  |  |  |  |  |  |  |  |
| Alfalfa |  | X |  |  |  |  |  |  |  |  |  |  |  |  |  |  | X |  |  |  | X |  |  |  |  |  |  |  |  | X |  |  | X | X |  |  |  |  |  |  |  |  |  |  |  |
| Aloe Vera |  | X |  |  |  |  |  |  |  |  | X |  | X |  |  |  |  |  |  |  | X |  |  |  |  |  |  | X |  |  |  |  |  |  |  |  |  |  |  |  |  |  |  |  | X |
| Buckthorn |  |  |  |  |  |  |  |  |  |  |  |  |  |  |  |  |  |  |  |  | X |  |  |  |  | X |  |  |  |  |  |  |  |  |  |  |  |  |  |  |  |  |  |  |  |
| Cascara sagrada |  |  |  |  |  |  |  |  |  |  |  |  |  | X |  |  |  |  |  |  | X |  |  |  |  | X |  |  |  |  |  |  |  |  |  |  |  |  |  |  |  |  |  |  |  |
| Cilantro |  |  |  |  |  |  |  |  |  | X |  |  |  |  |  |  |  |  |  |  | X |  |  |  | X |  |  |  |  |  |  |  |  |  |  |  |  |  |  |  |  |  |  |  |  |
| Coriander |  |  |  |  |  |  |  |  |  | X |  |  |  |  |  |  |  |  |  |  | X |  |  |  | X |  |  |  |  |  |  |  |  |  |  |  |  |  |  |  |  |  |  |  |  |
| Dandelion |  | X |  |  |  |  |  |  |  |  |  |  |  | X | X |  |  |  |  |  | X |  | X |  |  |  | X |  |  | X |  |  |  | X | X |  |  |  |  |  |  |  |  |  |  |
| Dandelion Root |  | X |  |  |  |  |  |  |  |  |  |  |  | X | X |  |  |  |  |  | X |  | X |  |  |  | X |  |  | X |  |  |  | X | X |  |  |  |  |  |  |  |  |  |  |
| Fennel |  |  |  |  |  |  |  |  |  | X |  |  |  |  |  |  |  |  | X |  | X |  |  |  | X |  |  |  |  |  |  |  | X |  |  |  |  |  |  |  |  |  | X |  |  |
| Fennel Seeds |  |  |  |  |  |  |  |  |  | X |  |  |  |  |  |  |  |  | X |  | X |  |  |  | X |  |  |  |  |  |  |  | X |  |  |  |  |  |  |  |  |  | X |  |  |
| Fenugreek seeds |  |  |  |  |  | X |  |  | X |  |  |  |  |  |  |  |  |  |  |  | X |  |  |  |  |  |  | X |  |  |  | X | X | X |  |  |  |  |  |  |  |  |  |  |  |
| Flax |  |  |  |  |  |  |  |  |  |  |  |  |  |  |  |  |  |  |  |  | X |  |  |  |  |  |  | X |  |  |  |  |  |  |  |  |  |  |  |  |  |  |  |  |  |
| Licorice | X | X | X |  |  | X |  |  | X |  |  |  | X |  |  | X |  | X | X | X | X |  |  |  |  | X | X | X |  |  |  | X |  |  | X |  |  |  |  |  |  |  | X |  |  |
| Licorice Root | X | X | X |  |  | X |  |  | X |  |  |  | X |  |  | X |  | X | X | X | X |  |  |  |  | X | X | X |  |  |  | X |  |  | X |  |  |  |  |  |  |  | X |  |  |
| Mallow |  | X |  |  |  |  |  |  | X | X |  |  | X |  | X |  |  |  |  |  | X |  |  |  |  |  |  | X |  |  |  |  |  |  |  |  |  |  |  |  |  |  |  |  | X |
| Marjoram |  |  |  | X | X |  |  | X | X |  |  |  | X |  |  |  |  |  |  | X | X | X | X | X | X |  |  |  |  |  |  |  |  |  |  |  |  | X | X |  | X | X | X | X | X |
| Marshmallow |  | X |  |  |  |  |  |  | X | X |  |  | X |  | X |  |  |  |  |  | X |  |  |  |  |  |  | X |  |  |  |  |  |  |  |  |  |  |  |  |  |  |  |  | X |
| Marshmallow Root |  | X |  |  |  |  |  |  | X | X |  |  | X |  | X |  |  |  |  |  | X |  |  |  |  |  |  | X |  |  |  |  |  |  |  |  |  |  |  |  |  |  |  |  | X |
| Nasturtium | X | X | X |  |  |  |  | X | X | X | X | X | X | X | X |  | X |  | X | X | X | X | X |  |  |  |  | X |  |  |  |  |  |  |  |  |  |  |  |  |  |  |  |  | X |
| Psyllium |  |  |  |  |  |  |  |  |  |  |  |  |  |  |  |  |  |  |  |  | X |  |  |  |  |  |  |  |  |  |  |  |  |  |  |  |  |  |  |  |  |  |  |  |  |
| Pumpkin |  |  |  |  |  |  |  |  |  |  |  |  |  |  |  |  |  |  |  |  | X |  |  |  |  |  |  |  |  |  |  |  |  |  |  |  |  |  |  |  |  |  |  |  |  |
| purselane |  | X | X |  |  |  |  |  | X | X | X | X | X |  |  |  |  |  |  |  | X | X |  |  |  |  |  | X | X | X |  |  |  |  |  |  |  |  |  |  |  |  |  |  | X |
| Rhubarb |  |  |  |  |  |  |  |  |  |  |  |  |  |  |  |  |  |  |  |  | X |  |  |  |  | X |  |  |  |  |  |  |  |  |  |  |  |  |  |  |  |  |  |  |  |
| Savory |  |  | X | X | X |  | X | X | X | X | X |  | X |  |  |  |  |  |  | X | X | X | X | X | X | X | X | X | X | X | X | X | X | X | X |  |  |  |  |  |  |  |  |  |  |
| Senna |  |  |  |  |  |  |  |  |  |  |  |  |  |  |  |  |  |  |  |  | X |  |  |  |  | X |  |  |  |  |  |  |  |  |  |  |  |  |  |  |  |  |  |  |  |
| Slippery Elm |  |  |  |  |  |  |  |  |  |  |  |  |  |  |  |  |  |  |  |  | X |  |  |  |  |  |  | X |  |  |  |  |  |  |  |  |  |  |  |  |  |  |  |  |  |

**Herbs By Classifications — Astringent (part 1 of 3)**

| Herbs By Classifications | Adaptogens | Alterative | Amphoteric | Analgesic | Anodyne | Antacid & Anti-ulcer | Anthelmintics | Antibiotic | Anticatarrhal | Antiemetics | Antifungal | Antihemorrhagic | Anti-Inflammatory | Antilithics-Gallstone | Antilithics-Urinary |
|---|---|---|---|---|---|---|---|---|---|---|---|---|---|---|---|
| Astringent |  |  |  |  |  |  |  |  |  |  |  |  |  |  |  |
| Agrimony |  |  |  |  |  |  |  |  |  |  |  |  | X |  |  |
| Alum |  |  |  |  |  |  |  |  |  |  |  |  |  |  |  |
| Blackberry |  |  |  |  |  |  |  |  |  |  |  | X |  |  |  |
| Blackberry Leaf |  |  |  |  |  |  |  |  |  |  |  |  |  |  |  |
| Cinnamon |  |  |  |  |  |  |  | X | X | X |  |  |  |  |  |
| Cranesbill |  |  |  |  |  |  |  |  |  |  |  | X |  |  |  |
| Garden Sage |  |  |  |  |  |  |  | X | X |  | X |  | X |  |  |
| Geranium |  |  |  |  |  |  |  |  |  |  |  |  |  |  |  |
| Horsetail |  | X |  |  |  |  |  |  |  |  |  |  | X |  | X |
| Marjoram |  |  |  | X | X |  |  | X | X |  |  |  | X |  |  |
| Meadowsweet |  |  |  |  |  | X |  |  |  |  |  |  |  |  |  |
| Nasturtium | X | X | X |  |  |  |  | X | X | X | X |  | X | X | X |
| Oak Bark |  |  |  |  |  |  |  |  |  |  |  |  |  |  |  |
| Plantain |  | X |  |  |  |  |  | X |  |  |  |  | X |  |  |
| Purslane |  | X | X |  |  |  |  | X | X | X | X |  | X |  |  |
| Raspberry Leaf |  |  |  |  |  |  |  |  |  |  |  |  | X |  |  |
| Rose |  |  |  |  |  |  |  |  |  |  |  |  |  |  |  |
| Sage |  |  |  | X |  |  |  | X | X |  |  |  |  |  |  |
| Savory |  |  | X | X | X |  | X | X | X | X | X | X | X | X | X |
| Shepherd's Purse |  |  |  |  |  |  |  |  |  |  |  | X |  |  |  |
| Thyme |  |  |  |  |  |  |  | X | X |  |  |  |  |  |  |
| Turkey Rhubarb |  |  |  |  |  |  |  |  |  |  |  |  |  | X |  |
| Uva Ursi |  | X |  |  |  |  |  | X | X |  |  |  |  |  | X |
| White Oak |  |  |  |  |  |  |  |  |  |  |  | X |  |  |  |
| White Oak Bark |  |  |  |  |  |  |  |  |  |  |  | X |  |  |  |
| Witch Hazel |  |  |  |  |  |  |  |  |  |  |  | X |  |  |  |
| Yarrow |  |  |  | X | X |  |  | X | X |  | X | X | X |  |  |

**Herbs By Classifications — Astringent (part 2 of 3)**

| Herbs By Classifications | Antiprotozoal | Antipyretic | Antirheumatic | Antispasmodic | Antiviral | Aperient | Astringent | Bitters | Cardiotonic | Carminative | Cathartic | Cholagogue | Demulcent | Diaphoretic | Diuretic |
|---|---|---|---|---|---|---|---|---|---|---|---|---|---|---|---|
| Astringent |  |  |  |  |  |  |  |  |  |  |  |  |  |  |  |
| Agrimony |  |  |  |  |  |  | X | X |  |  |  |  |  |  | X |
| Alum |  |  |  |  |  |  | X |  |  |  |  |  |  |  |  |
| Blackberry |  |  |  |  |  |  | X |  |  |  |  |  |  |  |  |
| Blackberry Leaf |  |  |  |  |  |  | X |  |  |  |  |  |  |  |  |
| Cinnamon |  |  | X |  |  |  | X |  |  | X |  |  | X |  |  |
| Cranesbill |  |  |  |  |  |  | X |  |  |  |  |  |  |  |  |
| Garden Sage |  | X | X | X | X | X | X | X |  | X |  |  |  | X | X |
| Geranium |  |  |  |  |  |  | X |  |  |  |  |  |  |  |  |
| Horsetail |  |  |  |  |  |  | X |  |  |  |  |  |  |  | X |
| Marjoram |  | X | X | X |  |  | X | X |  | X |  |  |  |  |  |
| Meadowsweet |  | X | X |  |  |  | X |  |  |  |  |  |  |  |  |
| Nasturtium | X | X | X | X | X | X | X |  |  |  |  |  |  |  | X |
| Oak Bark |  |  |  |  |  |  | X |  |  |  |  |  |  |  |  |
| Plantain |  |  |  |  |  |  | X |  |  |  |  |  | X |  | X |
| Purslane |  |  |  |  |  | X | X |  |  |  |  |  | X | X | X |
| Raspberry Leaf |  | X |  |  |  |  | X |  |  |  |  |  |  |  |  |
| Rose |  |  |  |  |  |  | X |  |  |  |  |  |  |  |  |
| Sage |  |  |  |  | X |  | X | X |  | X |  |  |  | X |  |
| Savory | X | X | X | X | X | X | X | X | X | X | X | X | X | X | X |
| Shepherd's Purse |  |  |  |  |  |  | X |  |  |  |  |  |  |  |  |
| Thyme |  |  |  |  | X |  | X |  |  | X |  |  |  | X |  |
| Turkey Rhubarb |  |  |  |  |  |  | X |  |  |  |  |  |  |  |  |
| Uva Ursi |  |  |  |  |  |  | X |  |  |  |  |  |  |  | X |
| White Oak |  |  |  |  |  |  | X |  |  |  |  |  |  |  |  |
| White Oak Bark |  |  |  |  |  |  | X |  |  |  |  |  |  |  |  |
| Witch Hazel |  |  |  |  |  |  | X |  |  |  |  |  |  |  |  |
| Yarrow |  | X |  |  |  |  | X |  | X |  |  |  |  | X |  |

**Herbs By Classifications — Astringent (part 3 of 3)**

| Herbs By Classifications | Emmenagogue | Expectorant | Galactogogue | Hematinic | Hepatic | Hypnotic | Hypotensive | Nervine Tonics | Nervine Relaxants | Nervine Stimulants | Oxytocic | Rubefacient | Sialogogue | Vasodilator | Vulnerary |
|---|---|---|---|---|---|---|---|---|---|---|---|---|---|---|---|
| Astringent |  |  |  |  |  |  |  |  |  |  |  |  |  |  |  |
| Agrimony |  |  |  |  |  |  |  |  |  |  |  |  |  |  |  |
| Alum |  |  |  |  |  |  |  |  |  |  |  |  |  |  |  |
| Blackberry |  |  |  |  |  |  |  |  |  |  |  |  |  |  |  |
| Blackberry Leaf |  |  |  |  |  |  |  |  |  |  |  |  |  |  |  |
| Cinnamon | X |  |  |  |  |  | X |  |  | X |  | X | X | X |  |
| Cranesbill |  |  |  |  |  |  |  |  |  |  |  |  |  |  |  |
| Garden Sage | X |  |  |  | X |  | X | X | X |  |  |  | X |  | X |
| Geranium |  |  |  |  |  |  |  |  |  |  |  |  |  |  |  |
| Horsetail |  |  |  |  |  |  |  |  |  |  |  |  |  |  |  |
| Marjoram |  |  |  |  |  |  |  | X | X |  |  | X | X | X | X |
| Meadowsweet | X |  |  |  |  |  |  |  |  |  |  |  |  |  |  |
| Nasturtium |  |  |  |  |  |  |  |  |  |  |  |  |  |  | X |
| Oak Bark |  |  |  |  |  |  |  |  |  |  |  |  |  |  |  |
| Plantain |  |  |  |  |  |  |  |  |  |  |  |  |  |  | X |
| Purslane |  |  |  |  |  |  |  |  |  |  |  |  |  |  | X |
| Raspberry Leaf |  |  |  |  |  |  |  |  |  |  | X |  |  |  |  |
| Rose |  |  |  |  |  |  |  |  |  |  |  |  |  |  |  |
| Sage | X |  |  |  |  |  |  | X | X |  |  |  | X |  | X |
| Savory | X | X | X | X |  |  |  |  |  |  |  |  |  |  |  |
| Shepherd's Purse |  |  |  |  |  |  |  |  |  |  |  |  |  |  |  |
| Thyme |  | X |  |  |  |  |  |  |  |  | X |  |  |  | X |
| Turkey Rhubarb |  |  |  |  |  |  |  |  |  |  |  |  |  |  |  |
| Uva Ursi |  |  |  |  |  |  |  |  |  |  |  |  |  |  |  |
| White Oak |  |  |  |  |  |  |  |  |  |  |  |  |  |  |  |
| White Oak Bark |  |  |  |  |  |  |  |  |  |  |  |  |  |  |  |
| Witch Hazel |  |  |  |  |  |  |  |  |  |  |  |  |  |  | X |
| Yarrow |  |  |  |  |  |  | X |  |  | X |  | X |  | X | X |

| Herbs By Classifications | Adaptogens | Alterative | Amphoteric | Analgesic | Anodyne | Antacid & Anti-ulcer | Anthelmintics | Antibiotic | Anticatarrhal | Antiemetics | Antifungal | Antihemorrhagic | Anti-Inflammatory | Antilithics-Gallstone | Antilithics-Urinary | Antiprotozoal | Antipyretic | Antirheumatic | Antispasmodic | Antiviral | Aperient | Astringent | Bitters | Cardiotonic | Carminative | Cathartic | Cholagogue | Demulcent | Diaphoretic | Diuretic | Emmenagogue | Expectorant | Galactogogue | Hematinic | Hepatic | Hypnotic | Hypotensive | Nervine Tonics | Nervine Relaxants | Nervine Stimulants | Oxytocic | Rubefacient | Sialogogue | Vasodilator | Vulnerary |
|---|---|---|---|---|---|---|---|---|---|---|---|---|---|---|---|---|---|---|---|---|---|---|---|---|---|---|---|---|---|---|---|---|---|---|---|---|---|---|---|---|---|---|---|---|---|
| **Bitters** | | | | | | | | | | | | | | | | | | | | | | | | | | | | | | | | | | | | | | | | | | | | | |
| Agrimony | | | | | | | | | | | | | X | | | | | | | | | X | X | | | | | | | X | | | | | | | | | | | | | | | |
| Angelica | | | | | | | | | | | | | | | | | | X | X | | | | X | | | | | | | | X | | | | | | | | | X | X | | | | |
| Artichoke | | | | | | | | | | | | | | X | | | | | | | | | X | | | | X | | | | | | | | X | | | | | | | | | | |
| Barberry | | | | | | | | X | | | | | | X | | X | | | | | | | X | | | X | X | | | | | | | | X | | | | | | | | | | |
| Bitter Melon | | | | | | | | | | | | | | | | | | | | | | | X | | | | | | | | | | | | | | | | | | | | | | |
| Burdock | | X | | | | | | | | | | | | | | | | X | | | | | X | | | | | | X | | | | | X | X | | | | | | | | | | |
| Centaury | | | | | | | | | | | | | | | | | | | | | | | X | | | | | | | | | | | | | | | | | | | | | | |
| Chamomile | | | | X | X | X | | X | | X | X | | X | | | | X | X | X | | | | X | | X | | | | X | | X | | | | | X | | X | X | | | | | | X |
| Chicory | | | | | | | | | | | | | X | | | | | | | | | | X | | | | | | | | | | | X | | | | | | | | | | | |
| Chicory Root | | | | | | | | | | | | | X | | | | | | | | | | X | | | | | | | | | | | X | | | | | | | | | | | |
| Dandelion | | X | | | | | | | | | | | | X | X | | | | | | X | | X | | | | X | | | X | | | | X | X | | | | | | | | | | |
| Dandelion Root | | X | | | | | | | | | | | | X | X | | | | | | X | | X | | | | X | | | X | | | | X | X | | | | | | | | | | |
| Garden Sage | | | | | | | | X | X | | X | | X | | X | | X | X | X | X | | X | X | | X | | | | X | | | | | | X | | X | X | X | X | | X | | | X |
| Gentian | | | | | | | | X | | | | | | | | | | | | | | | X | | | | X | | | | | | | | X | | | | | | | | | | |
| Ginger | | | | X | | | X | X | X | X | | | X | X | | X | X | X | X | X | | | X | X | X | | | | | X | X | X | | | X | | X | | | | X | X | | X | |
| Goldenseal | | | | | | | | X | | X | | | | | | X | | | | X | | | X | | | | | | | | | | | | | | | | | | | | | | X |
| Horehound | | | | | | | | | | X | | | | | | | | | | | | | X | | | | | | | | | | | | | | | | | | | | | | |
| Lemon Verbana | | | | | | | | | | | | | | | | | | X | | | | | X | | | | | | | | | | | | | | | | X | | | | | | |
| Lovage | | X | | | | | | X | X | X | | | | | | | | | | | | | X | | X | | | X | X | X | | X | | | X | | | | | | | | X | | |
| Marjoram | | | | X | X | | | X | X | | | | X | | | | | | X | X | X | X | X | | X | | | | | | | | | | | | | X | X | | X | X | X | X | X |
| Nasturtium | X | X | X | | | | | X | X | X | X | X | X | X | X | X | | X | X | X | X | X | X | | | | | | X | | | | | | | | | | | | | | | | X |
| Sage | | | | | | | | | X | | X | | X | | | | | | X | X | | X | X | | X | | | | X | | | | | | | | | X | X | | | X | | X |
| Savory | | | | X | X | X | X | X | X | X | X | | X | | | | | | X | X | X | X | X | X | X | X | X | X | X | X | X | X | X | X | X | | | | | | | | | | |
| Wormwood | | | | | | | X | X | | | | | | | | X | | | | | | | X | | | | | | | | | | | | X | | | | | | | | | | |

**Herbs By Classifications**

**Cardiotonic & Cardioactive**

Columns 1–15:

| Herbs By Classifications | Adaptogens | Alterative | Amphoteric | Analgesic | Anodyne | Antacid & Anti-ulcer | Anthelmintics | Antibiotic | Anticatarrhal | Antiemetics | Antifungal | Antihemorrhagic | Anti-Inflammatory | Antilithics-Gallstone | Antilithics-Urinary |
|---|---|---|---|---|---|---|---|---|---|---|---|---|---|---|---|
| Astragalus | X | | X | | | | | | | | | | | | |
| Cayenne | | | X | X | X | | | X | X | | | X | X | | |
| Coleus Forskohlii | | | | | | | | | | | | | | | |
| Danshen | | | | | | | | | | | | | | | |
| Garlic | | X | | | | | X | X | X | | X | | | X | |
| Ginger | | | | X | | | X | X | X | X | | | X | | |
| Ginkgo | X | | | | | | | | | | | | | | |
| Ginkgo Biloba | X | | | | | | | | | | | | | | |
| Hawthorn | X | | | | | | | | | | | | | | |
| Lemon Balm | X | | | | | | | | | X | | | | | |
| Lily of the Valley | | | | | | | | | | | | | | | |
| Linden | | | | | | | | | | | | | | | |
| Motherwort | | | | | | | | | | | | | | | |
| Olive Leaf | | | | | | | | X | | | | | | | |
| Savory | | | X | X | X | X | X | X | X | X | X | | X | | |
| Turmeric | X | | X | X | X | X | X | X | | | | | X | X | |
| Yarrow | | | | X | X | | | X | X | | | X | X | | |

Columns 16–30:

| Herbs By Classifications | Antiprotozoal | Antipyretic | Antirheumatic | Antispasmodic | Antiviral | Aperient | Astringent | Bitters | Cardiotonic | Carminative | Cathartic | Cholagogue | Demulcent | Diaphoretic | Diuretic |
|---|---|---|---|---|---|---|---|---|---|---|---|---|---|---|---|
| Astragalus | | | | | X | | | | X | | | | | | |
| Cayenne | | | X | | | | | | X | | | | | X | |
| Coleus Forskohlii | | | | | | | | | X | | | | | | |
| Danshen | | | | | | | | | X | | | | | | |
| Garlic | X | X | | | X | | | | X | X | | | | X | |
| Ginger | X | X | X | X | X | | | X | X | X | | | | X | X |
| Ginkgo | | | | | | | | | X | | | | | | |
| Ginkgo Biloba | | | | | | | | | X | | | | | | |
| Hawthorn | | | | | | | | | X | | | | | | X |
| Lemon Balm | | X | | | X | | | | X | X | | X | | | |
| Lily of the Valley | | | | | | | | | X | | | | | | |
| Linden | | | | | | | | | X | | | | | | |
| Motherwort | | | | X | | | | | X | X | | | | | |
| Olive Leaf | | | | | X | | | | X | | | | | | |
| Savory | | | X | X | X | X | X | X | X | X | X | X | X | X | X |
| Turmeric | | | X | | | | | | X | | | X | | | |
| Yarrow | | X | | X | X | | X | | X | | | | | X | |

Columns 31–45:

| Herbs By Classifications | Emmenagogue | Expectorant | Galactogogue | Hematinic | Hepatic | Hypnotic | Hypotensive | Nervine Tonics | Nervine Relaxants | Nervine Stimulants | Oxytocic | Rubefacient | Sialogogue | Vasodilator | Vulnerary |
|---|---|---|---|---|---|---|---|---|---|---|---|---|---|---|---|
| Astragalus | | | | X | X | | X | | | | | | | X | |
| Cayenne | | | | | | | X | | | X | | X | X | X | X |
| Coleus Forskohlii | | | | | | | | | | | | | | | |
| Danshen | | | | | | | | | | | | | | | |
| Garlic | | | | | | | X | | | X | | X | | X | X |
| Ginger | X | X | | | | | X | | | X | X | X | | X | |
| Ginkgo | | | | | | | | | | X | | | | X | |
| Ginkgo Biloba | | | | | | | | | | X | | | | X | |
| Hawthorn | | | | | | | | | | | | | | X | |
| Lemon Balm | | | | | | X | X | X | X | | | | | | |
| Lily of the Valley | | | | | | | | | | | | | | | |
| Linden | | | | | | X | X | X | X | | | | | X | |
| Motherwort | X | | | | | X | X | X | X | | | | | | |
| Olive Leaf | | | | | | | X | | | | | | | | |
| Savory | X | X | X | X | X | | | | | | | | | | |
| Turmeric | | | | | X | | | | | | | | | X | |
| Yarrow | | | | | | | X | | | X | | | | X | X |

## Herbs By Classifications

**Carminative**

Columns 1–15:

| Herbs By Classifications | Adaptogens | Alterative | Amphoteric | Analgesic | Anodyne | Antacid & Anti-ulcer | Anthelmintics | Antibiotic | Anticatarrhal | Antiemetics | Antifungal | Antihemorrhagic | Anti-Inflammatory | Antilithics-Gallstone | Antilithics-Urinary |
|---|---|---|---|---|---|---|---|---|---|---|---|---|---|---|---|
| Allspice | | | | | | | | X | | | | | | | |
| Anise seeds | | | | | | | | | X | | X | | | | |
| Basil | X | | | | | | | X | | X | X | | | | |
| Black Pepper | | | | | | | | X | | | | | X | | |
| Caraway | | | | X | | | | | | | | | | | |
| Cardamom | | | X | | | | | | | X | | | | | |
| Celery Seed | | | | | | | | | | | | | | | X |
| Chamomile | | | | X | X | X | | X | | X | X | | X | | |
| Cilantro | | | | | | | | X | | | | | | | |
| Cinnamon | | | | | | | | X | | X | X | | | | |
| Cloves | | | | X | X | | X | | | X | X | | | | |
| Coriander | | | | | | | | X | | | | | | | |
| Cumin | | | | | | | | | | | | | | | |
| Dill | | | | | | | | X | | | | | | | X |
| Dill Seed | | | | | | | | X | | | | | | | X |
| Fennel Seeds | | | | | | | | X | | X | X | | X | | |
| Garden Sage | | | | | | | | X | X | | X | | X | | X |
| Garlic | | X | | | | | X | X | X | | X | | | | |
| Ginger | | | | X | | | X | X | X | X | | | X | | |
| Juniper | | | | | | | | X | | | | | | | X |
| Juniper Berries | | | | | | | | X | | | | | | | X |
| Lavender | | | | X | X | | | | | | | | | | |
| Lemon Balm | X | | | | | | | | | | X | | | | |
| Lovage | | X | | | | | | | | | X | X | X | | |
| Marjoram | | | | X | X | | | | | | X | | X | | |
| Motherwort | | | | | | | | | | | | | | | |
| Parsley | | | | | | | | | | | | | | | X |
| Peppermint | | | | X | | | X | X | X | | | | X | | |
| Rosemary | | | | X | | | | X | | | X | | X | | |
| Sage | | | | X | | | | X | | | X | | X | | |
| Savory | | | X | X | X | | X | X | X | X | X | | X | | |
| Thyme | | | | | | | X | X | | | X | | | | |

Columns 16–30:

| Herbs By Classifications | Antiprotozoal | Antipyretic | Antirheumatic | Antispasmodic | Antiviral | Aperient | Astringent | Bitters | Cardiotonic | Carminative | Cathartic | Cholagogue | Demulcent | Diaphoretic | Diuretic |
|---|---|---|---|---|---|---|---|---|---|---|---|---|---|---|---|
| Allspice | | | | X | X | | | | | X | | | | | |
| Anise seeds | | | | X | X | | | | | X | | | | | |
| Basil | | X | | | | | | | | X | | | | X | |
| Black Pepper | | | | | | | | | | X | | | | X | X |
| Caraway | | | | | | | | | | X | | | | | |
| Cardamom | | | | | | | | | | X | | | | | |
| Celery Seed | | | | | | | | | | X | | | | | |
| Chamomile | | X | X | X | | | | X | | X | | | | X | |
| Cilantro | | | | | | X | | | | X | | | | | |
| Cinnamon | | X | | X | | | X | | | X | | | X | | |
| Cloves | | | | X | | | | | | X | | | | | |
| Coriander | | | | | | | X | | | X | | | | | |
| Cumin | | | | | | | | | | X | | | | | |
| Dill | | | | | | | | | | X | | | | | |
| Dill Seed | | | | | | | | | | X | | | | | |
| Fennel Seeds | | X | X | X | | | | | | X | | | | X | X |
| Garden Sage | | X | X | X | | | X | | | X | | | | X | X |
| Garlic | X | | | X | | | | X | X | X | | | | | |
| Ginger | X | X | X | X | X | | X | X | | X | | | | X | X |
| Juniper | | | | X | | | | | | X | | | | | X |
| Juniper Berries | | | | X | | | | | | X | | | | | X |
| Lavender | | | | | | | | | | X | | | | | |
| Lemon Balm | | | X | | X | | | X | X | X | | | | X | |
| Lovage | | | | | | | | | X | X | | | X | X | X |
| Marjoram | | X | X | X | | | | | | X | | | | | |
| Motherwort | | | | | | | | X | X | X | | | | | |
| Parsley | | | | | | | | | | X | | | | | X |
| Peppermint | | | | X | | | | X | | X | | | | X | |
| Rosemary | | | X | X | | | X | X | | X | | X | | X | X |
| Sage | | | X | X | | | X | X | | X | | | | X | |
| Savory | | | | | | | X | X | X | X | X | X | X | X | X |
| Thyme | | | | X | | | X | X | | X | | | | X | |

Columns 31–45:

| Herbs By Classifications | Emmenagogue | Expectorant | Galactogogue | Hematinic | Hepatic | Hypnotic | Hypotensive | Nervine Tonics | Nervine Relaxants | Nervine Stimulants | Oxytocic | Rubefacient | Sialogogue | Vasodilator | Vulnerary |
|---|---|---|---|---|---|---|---|---|---|---|---|---|---|---|---|
| Allspice | | | | | | | | | | | | X | | X | |
| Anise seeds | | X | X | | | | | | | | | | X | | |
| Basil | | X | | | | | | X | | | | | | | |
| Black Pepper | | X | | | | | | | | | | X | | X | |
| Caraway | | | X | | | | | | | | | | X | | |
| Cardamom | | | | | | | | | | | | | X | X | |
| Celery Seed | | | | | | | | | | | | | | | |
| Chamomile | X | | | | | X | | X | X | | | | | | X |
| Cilantro | | | | | | | | | | | | | | | |
| Cinnamon | X | | | | | | | X | | | | X | | X | X |
| Cloves | | | | | | | | | | X | | | | | |
| Coriander | | | | | | | | | | | | | | | |
| Cumin | | | X | | | | | | | | | | | | |
| Dill | | | X | | | | | | | | | | | | |
| Dill Seed | | | X | | | | | | | | | | | | |
| Fennel Seeds | X | X | X | | | | | | | | | | | X | |
| Garden Sage | X | | | | X | | | X | X | | | X | | | X |
| Garlic | | X | | | | | X | | | | | X | | X | X |
| Ginger | X | | | | X | | X | | | X | X | X | | X | |
| Juniper | | | | | | | | | | | X | X | | | |
| Juniper Berries | | | | | | | | | | | X | X | | | |
| Lavender | | | | | | X | X | X | X | | | | | | X |
| Lemon Balm | | | | | | X | X | X | X | | | | | | |
| Lovage | | X | | | | | X | | | | | | X | | |
| Marjoram | X | | | | | | | X | X | | | X | X | X | X |
| Motherwort | X | | | | | | X | X | X | X | | | | | |
| Parsley | X | | | | | | X | | | | | | | | |
| Peppermint | X | | | | | | | | | | | | | X | X |
| Rosemary | | | | | | | | | | X | | X | | X | |
| Sage | X | | | | | | | | | X | | | | X | X |
| Savory | X | X | X | X | X | X | X | X | X | X | | | | | |
| Thyme | | X | | | | | | | | | | | | | X |

| Herbs By Classifications | Adaptogens | Alterative | Amphoteric | Analgesic | Anodyne | Antacid & Anti-ulcer | Anthelmintics | Antibiotic | Anticatarrhal | Antiemetics | Antifungal | Antihemorrhagic | Anti-Inflammatory | Antilithics-Gallstone | Antilithics-Urinary | Antiprotozoal | Antipyretic | Antirheumatic | Antispasmodic | Antiviral | Aperient | Astringent | Bitters | Cardiotonic | Carminative | Cathartic | Cholagogue | Demulcent | Diaphoretic | Diuretic | Emmenagogue | Expectorant | Galactogogue | Hematinic | Hepatic | Hypnotic | Hypotensive | Nervine Tonics | Nervine Relaxants | Nervine Stimulants | Oxytocic | Rubefacient | Sialogogue | Vasodilator | Vulnerary |
|---|---|---|---|---|---|---|---|---|---|---|---|---|---|---|---|---|---|---|---|---|---|---|---|---|---|---|---|---|---|---|---|---|---|---|---|---|---|---|---|---|---|---|---|---|---|
| **Cathartic** | | | | | | | | | | | | | | | | | | | | | | | | | | | | | | | | | | | | | | | | | | | | | |
| Alder Buckthorn | | | | | | | | | | | | | | | | | | | | | | | | | | X | | | | | | | | | | | | | | | | | | | |
| Aloe Vera Leaf | | | | | | | | | | | | | | | | | | | | | | | | | | X | | | | | | | | | | | | | | | | | | | |
| Barberry | | | | | | | | X | | | | | | X | | X | | | | | | | X | | | X | X | | | | | | | | X | | | | | | | | | | |
| Bay Leaves | | | | | | | | X | | | X | | | | | | | | | X | | | | | | X | | | X | | X | | | | | | | | | | | | | | |
| Black hellebore | | | | | | | | | | | | | | | | | | | | | | | | | | X | | | | | | | | | | | | | | | | | | | |
| Buckthorn | | | | | | | | | | | | | | | | | | | | | X | | | | | X | | | | | | | | | | | | | | | | | | | |
| Cascara amarga | | | | | | | | | | | | | | | | | | | | | | | | | | X | | | | | | | | | | | | | | | | | | | |
| Cascara sagrada | | | | | | | | | | | | | | X | | | | | | | X | | | | | X | | | | | | | | | | | | | | | | | | | |
| Cassia | | | | | | | | | | | | | | | | | | | | | | | | | | X | | | | | | | | | | | | | | | | | | | |
| Licorice | X | X | X | | | X | | | X | | | | X | | | X | | X | | X | X | | | | | X | X | X | | | | X | | | X | | | | | | | | X | | |
| Licorice Root | X | X | X | | | X | | | X | | | | X | | | X | | X | | X | X | | | | | X | X | X | | | | X | | | X | | | | | | | | X | | |
| Prune | | | | | | | | | | | | | | | | | | | | | | | | | | X | | | | | | | | | | | | | | | | | | | |
| Rhubarb | | | | | | | | | | | | | | | | | | | | | X | | | | | X | | | | | | | | | | | | | | | | | | | |
| Savory | | | X | X | X | | X | X | X | X | X | | X | | | | | | X | X | X | X | X | X | X | X | X | X | X | X | X | X | X | X | X | | | | | | | | | | |
| Senna | | | | | | | | | | | | | | | | | | | | | X | | | | | X | | | | | | | | | | | | | | | | | | | |
| Yellow Dock | | X | | | | | | | | | | X | | | | | | | | | | | | | | X | X | | | | | | | X | X | | | | | | | | | | |

**Herbs By Classifications — Cholagogue**

| Classification | Artichoke | Barberry | Boldo | Bupleurum | Dandelion | Dandelion Root | Fringe Tree | Gentian | Greater Celandine | Lemon Balm | Licorice | Licorice Root | Milk Thistle | Oregon Grape | Oregon Grape Root | Rosemary | Savory | Tinospora Cordifolia | Turmeric | Wild Yam | Yellow Dock |
|---|---|---|---|---|---|---|---|---|---|---|---|---|---|---|---|---|---|---|---|---|---|
| Adaptogens | | | | | | | | | | X | X | X | X | | | | | | X | | |
| Alterative | | | | | X | X | | | | | | | | X | X | | | | | | X |
| Amphoteric | | | | | | | | | | | X | X | | | | X | | | X | | |
| Analgesic | | | | | | | | | | X | | | | | | X | X | | | | |
| Anodyne | | | | | | | | | | X | | | | | | X | X | | | | |
| Antacid & Anti-ulcer | | | | | X | X | X | | | | | | | | | X | X | | | | |
| Anthelmintics | | | X | | | | | | | | | | | | | X | X | | | | |
| Antibiotic | | X | | | | | | | X | | | | | X | X | X | | | | | |
| Anticatarrhal | | | | | | | | | | | X | X | | | | X | | | | | |
| Antiemetics | | | | | | | | | | X | | | | | | X | | | | | |
| Antifungal | | | | | | | | | | | | | | X | X | X | X | | | | |
| Antihemorrhagic | | | | | | | | | | | | | | | | | | | | | X |
| Anti-Inflammatory | | | | | | | X | | | | X | X | | | | X | X | | X | | |
| Antilithics-Gallstone | X | X | X | | X | X | | | X | | | X | X | | | X | | | X | | |
| Antilithics-Urinary | | | | | X | X | | | | | | | | | | | | | | | |
| Antiprotozoal | | X | | | | | | | | | X | X | X | | | | | | | | |
| Antipyretic | | | | | | | | | | X | | | | | | | | | | | |
| Antirheumatic | | | | | | | | | | | X | X | | | | X | | | X | | |
| Antispasmodic | | | | | | | | | | X | | | | | | X | X | | X | | |
| Antiviral | | | | | | | | | | | X | X | X | | | X | | | | | |
| Aperient | | | | | X | X | | | | | | | | | | X | | | | | |
| Astringent | | | | | | | | | | | | | | | | X | | | | | |
| Bitters | X | X | | | X | X | | X | | | | | | | | X | | | | | |
| Cardiotonic | | | | | | | | | | X | | | | | | X | | | X | | |
| Carminative | | | | | | | | | | X | | | | | | X | | | | | |
| Cathartic | | X | | | | | | | | | X | X | | | | X | | | | | X |
| Cholagogue | X | X | X | X | X | X | X | X | X | X | X | X | X | X | X | X | X | X | X | X | X |
| Demulcent | | | | | | | | | | | X | X | | | | X | | | | | |
| Diaphoretic | | | | | | | | | | | | | | | | X | X | | | | |
| Diuretic | | | | | X | X | | | | | | | | | | X | | | | | |
| Emmenagogue | | | | | | | | | | | | | | | | X | | | | | |
| Expectorant | | | | | | | | | | | X | X | | | | X | | | | | |
| Galactogogue | | | | | | | | | | | | | | | | X | | | | | |
| Hematinic | | | | | X | X | | | | | | | | | | X | | | | | X |
| Hepatic | X | X | X | X | X | X | | X | X | | X | X | X | X | X | | X | | X | X | X |
| Hypnotic | | | | | | | | | | X | | | | | | | | | | | |
| Hypotensive | | | | | | | | | | X | | | | | | | | | | | |
| Nervine Tonics | | | | | | | | | | X | | | | | | | | | | | |
| Nervine Relaxants | | | | | | | | | | X | | | | | | | | | | | |
| Nervine Stimulants | | | | | | | | | | | | | | | | X | | | | | |
| Oxytocic | | | | | | | | | | | | | | | | | | | | | |
| Rubefacient | | | | | | | | | | | | | | | | X | | | | | |
| Sialogogue | | | | | | | | | | | X | X | | | | | | | | | |
| Vasodilator | | | | | | | | | | | | | | | | X | | | X | | |
| Vulnerary | | | | | | | | | | | | | | | | | | | | | |

Columns 1–15:

| Herbs By Classifications | Adaptogens | Alterative | Amphoteric | Analgesic | Anodyne | Antacid & Anti-ulcer | Anthelmintics | Antibiotic | Anticatarrhal | Antiemetics | Antifungal | Antihemorrhagic | Anti-Inflammatory | Antilithics-Gallstone | Antilithics-Urinary |
|---|---|---|---|---|---|---|---|---|---|---|---|---|---|---|---|
| **Demulcent** | | | | | | | | | | | | | | | |
| Aloe Vera | | X | | | | | | | | | X | | X | | |
| Chia Seeds | | | | | | | | | | | | | | | |
| Cinnamon | | | | | | | | X | | X | X | | | | |
| Coltsfoot | | | | | | | | | X | | | | | | |
| Comfrey | | X | | | | X | | | | | | X | X | | |
| Corn Silk | | | | | | | | | | | | | | | X |
| Fenugreek seeds | | | | | | X | | | X | | | | | | |
| Flax | | | | | | | | | | | | | | | |
| Hollyhock | | | | | | | | | | | | | | | |
| Irish Moss | | | | | | | | | X | | | | | | |
| Licorice | X | X | X | | | X | | | X | | | | X | | |
| Licorice Root | X | X | X | | | X | | X | X | | | | X | | |
| Lovage | | X | | | | | | | X | X | | | | | |
| Mallow | | X | | | | | | | X | X | | | X | | X |
| Marshmallow | | X | | | | | | | X | X | | | X | | X |
| Marshmallow Root | | X | | | | | | | X | X | | | X | | X |
| Mullein | | | | | | | | | X | | | X | | | |
| Oats | | | | | | | | | | | | | | | |
| Okra | | | | | | | | | | | | | | | |
| Plantain | | X | | | | | | X | X | X | X | X | X | | |
| Purslane | | X | X | | | | | X | X | X | X | X | X | | |
| Savory | | | X | X | X | | X | X | X | | | | X | | |
| Slippery Elm | | | | | | | | | | | | | | | |

Columns 16–30:

| Herbs By Classifications | Antiprotozoal | Antipyretic | Antirheumatic | Antispasmodic | Antiviral | Aperient | Astringent | Bitters | Cardiotonic | Carminative | Cathartic | Cholagogue | Demulcent | Diaphoretic | Diuretic |
|---|---|---|---|---|---|---|---|---|---|---|---|---|---|---|---|
| **Demulcent** | | | | | | | | | | | | | | | |
| Aloe Vera | | | | | | X | | | | | | | X | | |
| Chia Seeds | | | | | | | | | | | | | X | | |
| Cinnamon | | | | X | | | X | | | X | | | X | | |
| Coltsfoot | | | | | | | | | | | | | X | | |
| Comfrey | | | | | | | | | | | | | X | | |
| Corn Silk | | | | | | | | | | | | | X | | X |
| Fenugreek seeds | | | | | | X | | | | | | | X | | |
| Flax | | | | | | X | | | | | | | X | | |
| Hollyhock | | | | | | | | | | | | | X | | |
| Irish Moss | | X | | | | | | | | | | | X | | |
| Licorice | X | | X | | X | X | | | | | X | X | X | | |
| Licorice Root | X | | X | | X | X | | | | | X | X | X | | |
| Lovage | | | | | | | | X | | X | | | X | X | X |
| Mallow | | | | | | X | | | | | | | X | | |
| Marshmallow | | | | | | X | | | | | | | X | | |
| Marshmallow Root | | | | | | X | | | | | | | X | | |
| Mullein | | | | | X | | | | | | | | X | | |
| Oats | | | | | | | | | | | | | X | | |
| Okra | | | | | | | | | | | | | X | | |
| Plantain | | | | | | | X | | | | | | X | | X |
| Purslane | | | | | | X | X | | | | | | X | X | X |
| Savory | | | | X | | X | X | X | X | X | X | X | X | X | X |
| Slippery Elm | | | | | | X | | | | | | | X | | |

Columns 31–45:

| Herbs By Classifications | Emmenagogue | Expectorant | Galactogogue | Hematinic | Hepatic | Hypnotic | Hypotensive | Nervine Tonics | Nervine Relaxants | Nervine Stimulants | Oxytocic | Rubefacient | Sialogogue | Vasodilator | Vulnerary |
|---|---|---|---|---|---|---|---|---|---|---|---|---|---|---|---|
| **Demulcent** | | | | | | | | | | | | | | | |
| Aloe Vera | | | | | | | | | | | | | | | X |
| Chia Seeds | | | | | | | | | | | | | | | |
| Cinnamon | X | | | | | | X | | | X | | | X | X | |
| Coltsfoot | | X | | | | | | | | | | | | | |
| Comfrey | | X | | | | | | | | | | | | | X |
| Corn Silk | | | | | | | | | | | | | | | |
| Fenugreek seeds | | X | X | X | | | | | | | | | | | |
| Flax | | | | | | | | | | | | | | | |
| Hollyhock | | | | | | | | | | | | | | | |
| Irish Moss | | | | | | | | | | | | | | | |
| Licorice | | X | | | X | | | | | | | | X | | |
| Licorice Root | | X | | | X | | | | | | | | X | | |
| Lovage | | X | | | X | | | | | | | | | | X |
| Mallow | | | | | | | | | | | | | | | X |
| Marshmallow | | | | | | | | | | | | | | | X |
| Marshmallow Root | | | | | | | | | | | | | | | X |
| Mullein | | X | | | | | | | | | | | | | |
| Oats | | | | | | | | | | | | | | | |
| Okra | | | | | | | | | | | | | | | |
| Plantain | | | | | | | | | | | | | | | X |
| Purslane | | | | | | | | | | | | | | | X |
| Savory | X | X | X | X | X | | | | | | | | | | |
| Slippery Elm | | | | | | | | | | | | | | | |

| Herbs By Classifications | Adaptogens | Alterative | Amphoteric | Analgesic | Anodyne | Antacid & Anti-ulcer | Anthelmintics | Antibiotic | Anticatarrhal | Antiemetics | Antifungal | Antihemorrhagic | Anti-Inflammatory | Antilithics-Gallstone | Antilithics-Urinary | Antiprotozoal | Antipyretic | Antirheumatic | Antispasmodic | Antiviral | Aperient | Astringent | Bitters | Cardiotonic | Carminative | Cathartic | Cholagogue | Demulcent | Diaphoretic | Diuretic | Emmenagogue | Expectorant | Galactogogue | Hematinic | Hepatic | Hypnotic | Hypotensive | Nervine Tonics | Nervine Relaxants | Nervine Stimulants | Oxytocic | Rubefacient | Sialogogue | Vasodilator | Vulnerary |
|---|---|---|---|---|---|---|---|---|---|---|---|---|---|---|---|---|---|---|---|---|---|---|---|---|---|---|---|---|---|---|---|---|---|---|---|---|---|---|---|---|---|---|---|---|---|
| Diaphoretic | | | | | | | | | | | | | | | | | | | | | | | | | | | | | | | | | | | | | | | | | | | | | |
| Basil | | | | | | | | | | X | | | | | | | X | | | | | | | | | | | | X | | | | | | | | | | | | | | | | |
| Bay Leaves | | | | | | | | X | | | X | | | | | | | | | X | | | | | | X | | | X | | X | | | | | | | | | | | | | | |
| Bergamot | | | | | | | | X | | | X | | X | | | | X | | | | | | | | | | | | X | | | | | | | | | | | | | | | | |
| Black Pepper | | | | | | | | X | | | | | X | | | | | | | | | | | | X | | | | X | X | | X | | | | | | | | X | | X | X | | |
| Blessed Thistle | | | | | | | | | | | | | | | | | | | | | | | | | | | | | X | | | | X | | | | | | | | | | | | |
| Boneset | | | | | | | | | | | | | | | | | X | | | | | | | | | | | | X | | | | | | | | | | | | | | | | |
| Catnip | | | | | | | | | | X | | | | | | | X | | X | | | | | | | | | | X | | | | | | | X | | X | X | | | | | | |
| Cayenne | | | X | X | X | | | X | X | | | X | X | | | | | X | | | | | | X | | | | | X | | | | | | | | X | | | | | X | X | X | X |
| Chamomile | | | X | X | X | | | X | | X | | | X | | | | X | X | X | | | | X | | X | | | | X | | X | | | | | X | | X | X | | | | | | X |
| Echinacea | | X | | | | | | X | | | | | X | | | | X | | | X | | | | | | | | | X | | | | | X | | | | | | | | | | X | X |
| Elder | | | | | | | | | X | | | | | | | | X | | | X | | | | | | | | | X | X | | X | | | | | | | | | | | | | X |
| Elderberry | | | | | | | | | | | | | | | | | X | | | X | | | | | | | | | X | X | | X | | | | | | | | | | | | | X |
| Elderflower | | | | | | | | | | | | | | | | | X | | | X | | | | | | | | | X | X | | X | | | | | | | | | | | | | X |
| Fennel Seeds | | | | | | | | X | | X | X | | X | | | | | | X | X | X | | | | X | | | | X | X | X | X | X | | | | | | | | | | X | | |
| Garden Sage | | | | | | | | X | X | | X | | X | | X | | X | X | X | X | | X | X | | X | | | | X | X | X | | | | X | | X | X | X | | | | X | | X |
| Hyssop | | | | X | | | | X | | | | | X | | | | | | X | | | | | | | | | | X | | | X | | | | | | | X | | | | | | |
| Lovage | | X | | | | | | X | X | X | | | | | | | | | | | | X | | | X | | | X | X | X | | X | | | X | | | | | | | | X | | |
| Oregano | | | X | | | | | X | X | | | | X | | | | X | | X | X | | | | | X | | | | X | | X | | | | | | | | | X | | | | X | |
| Peppermint | | | X | | | | | X | X | X | | | | X | | | X | | X | X | | | | | X | | | | X | | | | | | | | | | | X | | X | | X | |
| Purslane | X | X | | | | | | X | X | X | X | X | X | | | | | | | | | | | | | | | X | X | X | | | | | | | | | | | | | | | X |
| Rosemary | | | X | | | | | | X | | | | X | | | | | | | | | X | X | | | | X | | X | | | | | | | | | | | X | | X | | X | |
| Sage | | | X | | | | | X | X | | | | X | | | | | | X | X | | X | X | | X | | | X | X | | X | | | | | | | X | X | | | X | X | | X |
| Savory | | | X | X | X | | X | X | X | X | | | X | | | | | | X | X | X | X | X | X | X | X | X | X | X | X | X | X | X | X | X | | | | | | | | | | |
| Teasel Root | | | | | | | | | | | | | | | | | X | X | X | | | | | | | | | | X | | | | | | | | | | | | | X | X | X | |
| Thyme | | | | | | | | X | | | | | | | | | X | | X | X | | | | | X | | | | X | | | X | | | | | | | | | | | | | X |
| Yarrow | | | | X | X | | | X | X | | | X | X | | | | X | | | | | X | | X | | | | | X | | | | | | | | X | | | X | | | | X | X |

## Herbs By Classifications

**Diuretic**

| Herbs By Classifications | Adaptogens | Alterative | Amphoteric | Analgesic | Anodyne | Antacid & Anti-ulcer | Anthelmintics | Antibiotic | Anticatarrhal | Antiemetics | Antifungal | Antihemorrhagic | Anti-Inflammatory | Antilithics-Gallstone | Antilithics-Urinary |
|---|---|---|---|---|---|---|---|---|---|---|---|---|---|---|---|
| Agrimony | | | | | | | | | | | | | X | | |
| Alfalfa | | X | | | | | | | | | | | | | |
| Black Pepper | | | | | | | | X | | | | | X | | |
| Buchu | | | | | | | | | | | | | | | |
| Burdock | | X | | | | | | | | | | | | | |
| Celery | | | | | | | | | | | | | | | |
| Cleavers | | X | | | | | | | | | | | | | X |
| Corn Silk | | | | | | | | | | | | | | | X |
| Couchgrass | | | | | | | | | | | | | | | X |
| Dandelion | | X | | | | | | | | | | | | X | X |
| Dandelion Root | | X | | | | | | | | | | | | X | X |
| Elder | | | | | | | | | X | | | | | | |
| Elderberry | | | | | | | | | | | | | | | |
| Elderflower | | | | | | | | | | | | | | | |
| Fennel Seeds | | | | | | | | X | | X | X | | X | | |
| Garden Sage | | | | | | | | X | X | | X | | X | | |
| Ginger | | | | X | | | X | X | X | X | | | X | | |
| Goldenrod | | | | | | | | | X | | | | | | X |
| Gravel Root | | | | | | | | | | | | | | | X |
| Green Tea | | | | | | | | | | | | | X | | |
| Hawthorn | X | | | | | | | | | | | | | | |
| Hibiscus | | | | | | | | | | | | | | | |
| Horsetail | | X | | | | | | | | | | X | | | |
| Juniper | | | | | | | | X | | | | | | | X |
| Juniper Berries | | | | | | | | X | | | | | | | X |
| Lovage | | X | | | | | | X | X | X | | | | | |
| Nasturtium | X | X | X | | | | | X | X | X | X | | X | | X |
| Nettle | | X | | | | | | X | | | | | X | | |
| Parsley | | | | | | | | | | | | | | | X |
| Pumpkin | | | | | | | X | | | | | | | | |
| Purslane | | X | X | | | | | X | X | X | X | | X | | |
| Rosemary | | | X | | | | | X | | X | | | X | | |
| Savory | | | | X | X | | X | X | X | X | X | | X | | |
| Stinging Nettle | | X | | | | | | X | | | | X | | | |
| Uva Ursi | | X | | | | | | X | X | | | | | | X |

| Herbs By Classifications | Antiprotozoal | Antipyretic | Antirheumatic | Antispasmodic | Antiviral | Aperient | Astringent | Bitters | Cardiotonic | Carminative | Cathartic | Cholagogue | Demulcent | Diaphoretic | Diuretic |
|---|---|---|---|---|---|---|---|---|---|---|---|---|---|---|---|
| Agrimony | | | | | | | X | X | | | | | | | X |
| Alfalfa | | X | | | | X | | | | | | | | | X |
| Black Pepper | | | | | | | | | | X | | | | X | X |
| Buchu | | | | | | | | | | | | | | | X |
| Burdock | | | X | | | | | | | | | | | | X |
| Celery | | | | | | | | | | | | | | | X |
| Cleavers | | | | | | | | | | | | | | | X |
| Corn Silk | | | | | | | | | | | | | X | | X |
| Couchgrass | | | | | | | | | | | | | | | X |
| Dandelion | | | | | | X | | X | | | | X | | | X |
| Dandelion Root | | | | | | X | | X | | | | X | | | X |
| Elder | | X | | X | X | | | | | | | | | X | X |
| Elderberry | | X | | X | X | | | | | | | | | X | X |
| Elderflower | | X | | X | X | | | | | | | | | X | X |
| Fennel Seeds | | | X | X | X | X | | | | X | | | | X | X |
| Garden Sage | | X | X | X | X | | X | X | | X | | | | X | X |
| Ginger | X | X | X | X | X | | | X | X | X | | | | X | X |
| Goldenrod | | | | | | | | | | | | | | | X |
| Gravel Root | | | | | | | | | | | | | | | X |
| Green Tea | | | | | | | | | | | | | | | X |
| Hawthorn | | | | | | | | | X | | | | | | X |
| Hibiscus | | | | | | | | | | | | | | | X |
| Horsetail | | | | | | X | X | | | | | | | | X |
| Juniper | | | | X | | | | | | X | | | | | X |
| Juniper Berries | | | | X | | | | | | X | | | | | X |
| Lovage | | | | | | X | | X | | X | | X | X | X | X |
| Nasturtium | X | X | X | X | X | X | X | X | | | | | | | X |
| Nettle | | | X | | | | | | | | | | | | X |
| Parsley | | | | | | | | | | X | | | | | X |
| Pumpkin | | | | | X | | | | | | | | | | X |
| Purslane | | | | | | X | X | | | | | X | X | | X |
| Rosemary | | | | X | X | | | | | X | X | | | X | X |
| Savory | | | | X | X | X | X | X | X | X | X | X | X | X | X |
| Stinging Nettle | | | X | | | | | | | | | | | | X |
| Uva Ursi | | | | X | | | X | | | | | | | | X |

| Herbs By Classifications | Emmenagogue | Expectorant | Galactogogue | Hematinic | Hepatic | Hypnotic | Hypotensive | Nervine Tonics | Nervine Relaxants | Nervine Stimulants | Oxytocic | Rubefacient | Sialogogue | Vasodilator | Vulnerary |
|---|---|---|---|---|---|---|---|---|---|---|---|---|---|---|---|
| Agrimony | | | | | | | | | | | | | | | |
| Alfalfa | | | X | X | | | | | | | | | | | |
| Black Pepper | | X | | | | | | | | X | | X | X | | |
| Buchu | | | | | | | | | | | | | | | |
| Burdock | | | | X | X | | | | | | | | | | |
| Celery | | | | | | | X | | | | | | | | |
| Cleavers | | | | | X | | | | | | | | | | |
| Corn Silk | | | | | | | | | | | | | | | |
| Couchgrass | | | | | | | | | | | | | | | |
| Dandelion | | | | X | X | | | | | | | | | | |
| Dandelion Root | | | | X | X | | | | | | | | | | |
| Elder | | X | | | | | | | | | | | | | X |
| Elderberry | | X | | | | | | | | | | | | | X |
| Elderflower | | X | | | | | | | | | | | | | X |
| Fennel Seeds | X | X | X | | | | | | | | | | X | | |
| Garden Sage | X | | | | X | | X | X | X | | | X | | | X |
| Ginger | X | X | | | X | | X | | | X | X | X | | X | |
| Goldenrod | | | | | | | | | | | | | | | |
| Gravel Root | | | | | | | | | | X | | | | | |
| Green Tea | | | | | | | | | | | | | | | |
| Hawthorn | | | | | | | X | | | | | | | X | |
| Hibiscus | | | | | | | | | | | | | | | |
| Horsetail | | | | | | | | | | | | | | | |
| Juniper | | | | | | | | | | X | X | | | | |
| Juniper Berries | | | | | | | | | | X | X | | | | |
| Lovage | | X | | | X | | | | | | | | X | | |
| Nasturtium | | | | | | | | | | | | | | | X |
| Nettle | | | X | X | | | | | | | | | | | |
| Parsley | X | | | | X | | X | | | | | | | | |
| Pumpkin | | | | | | | | | | | | | | | |
| Purslane | | | | | | | | | | | | | | | X |
| Rosemary | | | | | | | | | | X | | X | | X | |
| Savory | X | X | X | X | X | | | | | | | | | | |
| Stinging Nettle | | | X | X | | | | | | | | | | | |
| Uva Ursi | | | | | | | | | | | | | | | |

| Herbs By Classifications | Adaptogens | Alterative | Amphoteric | Analgesic | Anodyne | Antacid & Anti-ulcer | Anthelmintics | Antibiotic | Anticatarrhal | Antiemetics | Antifungal | Antihemorrhagic | Anti-Inflammatory | Antilithics-Gallstone | Antilithics-Urinary | Antiprotozoal | Antipyretic | Antirheumatic | Antispasmodic | Antiviral | Aperient | Astringent | Bitters | Cardiotonic | Carminative | Cathartic | Cholagogue | Demulcent | Diaphoretic | Diuretic | Emmenagogue | Expectorant | Galactogogue | Hematinic | Hepatic | Hypnotic | Hypotensive | Nervine Tonics | Nervine Relaxants | Nervine Stimulants | Oxytocic | Rubefacient | Sialogogue | Vasodilator | Vulnerary |
|---|---|---|---|---|---|---|---|---|---|---|---|---|---|---|---|---|---|---|---|---|---|---|---|---|---|---|---|---|---|---|---|---|---|---|---|---|---|---|---|---|---|---|---|---|---|
| **Emmenagogue** | | | | | | | | | | | | | | | | | | | | | | | | | | | | | | | | | | | | | | | | | | | | | |
| Angelica | | | | | | | | | | | | | | | | | | X | X | | | | X | | | | | | | | X | | | | | | | | | X | X | | | | |
| Bay Leaves | | | | | | | | X | | | X | | | | | | | | | X | | | | | | X | | | X | | X | | | | | | | | | | | | | | |
| Black Cohosh | X | | | X | X | | | | | | | | | | | | | X | | | | | | | | | | | | | X | | | | | | | | X | | X | | | | |
| Blue Cohosh | | | | | | | | | | | | | | | | | | | | | | | | | | | | | | | X | | | | | | | | | | X | | | | |
| Calendula | | X | | | | X | | X | | | X | X | X | | | | | | | | | | | | | | | | | | X | | | | | | | | | | | | | | X |
| Chamomile | | | | X | X | X | | X | | X | X | | X | | | | X | X | X | | | | | | X | | | | X | | X | | | | | X | | X | X | | | | | | X |
| Cinnamon | | | | | | | | X | | X | X | | | | | | | | X | | | X | | | X | | | X | | | X | | | | | | X | | | X | | | X | X | |
| Cramp Bark | | | | | | | | | | | | | | | | | | | X | | | | | | | | | | | | X | | | | | | X | | X | | X | | | | |
| Dong Quai | | | | | | | | | | | | | | | | | | | | | | | | | | | | | | | X | | X | X | | | | | | | | | | | |
| Fennel Seeds | | | | | | | | X | | X | X | | X | | | | | | X | X | | X | X | | X | | | | X | X | X | X | X | | | | | | | | | | X | | |
| Garden Sage | | | | | | | | X | X | | X | | X | | X | | X | X | X | X | | X | X | | X | | | | X | X | X | | | | X | | X | X | X | | | X | | | X |
| Ginger | | | | X | | | X | X | X | X | | | X | X | | X | X | X | X | X | | X | | X | X | | | | X | X | X | X | | | X | | X | | | X | X | X | | X | |
| Motherwort | | | | | | | | | | | | | | | | | | | X | | | | | X | X | | | | | | X | | | | | X | X | X | X | | | | | | |
| Parsley | | | | | | | | | | | | | | | | X | | | | | | | | X | X | | | | | X | X | | | X | | | X | | | | | | | | |
| Pennyroyal | | | | | | | | | | | | | | | | | | | | | | | | | | | | | | | X | | | | | | | | | | X | | | | |
| Peppermint | | | | X | | | | | X | X | X | | | X | | | | X | | X | X | | | | | X | | | | X | | X | | | | | | | | | | | X | X | | |
| Rue | | | | X | X | | | | | | | | | | | | | | | | | | | | | | | | | | X | | | | | | | | | | X | | | | |
| Sage | | | | X | | | | | X | X | | X | | X | | | | | X | X | X | | X | X | | X | | | | X | | X | | | | | | | X | X | | | | X | | X |
| Savory | | | X | X | X | | | | X | X | X | X | | X | | | | | X | X | X | X | X | X | X | X | X | X | X | X | X | X | X | X | X | X | | | | | | | | | |
| Tansy | | | | | | | | X | | | | | | | | | X | | | | | | | | | | | | | | | X | | | | | | | | | | | | | | |
| Yarrow | | | | X | X | | | | X | X | | | X | X | | | | | | X | | | X | | X | | | | | X | | X | | | | | | X | | | X | | | | X | X |

**Herbs By Classifications**

| Herbs By Classifications | Anise seeds | Basil | Black Pepper | Black Seed | Caraway | Coltsfoot | Comfrey | Elder | Elderberry | Elderflower | Elecampane | Eucalyptus | Fennel Seeds | Fenugreek seeds | Garlic |
|---|---|---|---|---|---|---|---|---|---|---|---|---|---|---|---|
| Vulnerary | | | | | | | X | X | X | X | | | X | | X |
| Vasodilator | | | | | | | | | | | | | | | X |
| Sialogogue | X | | X | | | | | | | | | | X | | |
| Rubefacient | | | X | | | | | | | | X | | | | X |
| Oxytocic | | | | | | | | | | | | | | | |
| Nervine Stimulants | | | X | | | | | | | | | X | | | X |
| Nervine Relaxants | | | | | | | | | | | | | | | |
| Nervine Tonics | | X | | | X | | | | | | | | | | |
| Hypotensive | | | | | | | | | | | | | | | X |
| Hypnotic | | | | | | | | | | | | | | | |
| Hepatic | | | | | | | | | | | | | | | X |
| Hematinic | | | | | | | | | | | | | | X | |
| Galactogogue | X | | | | X | | | | | | | | | | X |
| Expectorant | X | X | X | X | | X | X | X | X | X | X | X | X | X | X |
| Emmenagogue | | | | | | | | | | | | | | | X |
| Diuretic | | X | | | | | | X | X | X | | | | | X |
| Diaphoretic | | X | X | | | | | X | X | X | | | | | X |
| Demulcent | | | | | | X | X | | | | | | | X | |
| Cholagogue | | | | | | | | | | | | | | | |
| Cathartic | | | | | | | | | | | | | | | |
| Carminative | X | X | X | | X | | | | | | | | | | X |
| Cardiotonic | | | | | | | | | | | | | | | X |
| Bitters | | | | | | | | | | | | | | | X |
| Astringent | | | | | | | | | | | | | | | X |
| Aperient | | | | | | | | | | | | | | | X |
| Antiviral | X | | | | | | | X | X | X | | | | | X |
| Antispasmodic | X | | | | X | | | | | | | | | | X |
| Antirheumatic | | | | | | | | | | | | | | | X |
| Antipyretic | | X | | | | | | X | X | X | | | | | X |
| Antiprotozoal | | | | | | | | | | | | | | | X |
| Antilithics-Urinary | | | | | | | | | | | | | | | |
| Antilithics-Gallstone | | | | | | | | | | | | | | | X |
| Anti-Inflammatory | | X | | | X | | | | | | | | | | X |
| Antihemorrhagic | | | | | | | X | | | | | | | | |
| Antifungal | X | X | | | | | | | | | | | | | X |
| Antiemetics | | X | | | | | | | | | | | | | X |
| Anticatarrhal | X | | | | X | | X | | | X | | | | | X |
| Antibiotic | | X | X | | | | | | | | | | | | X |
| Anthelmintics | | | | | X | | | | | | X | | | | X |
| Antacid & Anti-ulcer | | | | | | | X | | | | | | | X | |
| Anodyne | | | | | | | | | | | | | | | |
| Analgesic | | | | | | | X | | | | | | | | |
| Amphoteric | | | | | | | | X | X | | | | | | |
| Alterative | | | | | | | X | | | | | | | | X |
| Adaptogens | | X | | | | | | | | | | | | | X |

| Herbs By Classifications | Ginger | Gumweed | Hyssop | Licorice | Licorice Root | Lobelia | Lovage | Mullein | Onion | Oregano | Pleurisy Root | Savory | Thyme | Wild Cherry Bark | Yerba Santa |
|---|---|---|---|---|---|---|---|---|---|---|---|---|---|---|---|
| Vulnerary | | X | | | | | | | | | | | X | | |
| Vasodilator | X | | | | | | | | | | | | | | |
| Sialogogue | X | | | | X | | X | | | | | | | | X |
| Rubefacient | X | | | | | | | | | | | | | | |
| Oxytocic | X | | | | | | | | | | | | | | |
| Nervine Stimulants | X | | | | | | | | | | | | | | |
| Nervine Relaxants | | | X | | | | X | | | | | | | | |
| Nervine Tonics | | | | | | | | | | | | | | | |
| Hypotensive | X | | | | | | | | X | | | | | | |
| Hypnotic | | | | | | | | | | | | | | X | |
| Hepatic | | | | X | X | | X | | | X | | | | | |
| Hematinic | | | | | | | | | | X | | | | | |
| Galactogogue | X | | | | | | | | | X | | | | | |
| Expectorant | X | X | X | X | X | X | X | X | X | X | X | X | X | X | X |
| Emmenagogue | X | | | | | | | | | X | | | | | |
| Diuretic | X | | | | | | X | | | X | | | | | |
| Diaphoretic | | X | | | | | X | | X | | | X | X | | |
| Demulcent | | | | X | X | | X | X | | | | X | | | |
| Cholagogue | | | | X | X | | | | | X | | | | | |
| Cathartic | | | | X | X | | | | | X | | | | | |
| Carminative | X | | | | | | X | | | | | X | X | | |
| Cardiotonic | X | | | | | | | | | X | | | | | |
| Bitters | | | | | | | X | | | X | | | | | |
| Astringent | X | | | | | | | | | | | | | | |
| Aperient | X | | | X | X | | | | | X | | | | | |
| Antiviral | X | | | X | X | | | | X | X | X | X | X | | |
| Antispasmodic | X | | X | | | | X | | | X | | X | X | X | |
| Antirheumatic | | | | X | X | X | | | | | | | | | |
| Antipyretic | | | | | | | | | X | | | X | | | |
| Antiprotozoal | X | | | X | X | | | | | | | | | | |
| Antilithics-Urinary | | | | | | | | | | | | | | | |
| Antilithics-Gallstone | | | | | | | | | | | | | | X | |
| Anti-Inflammatory | X | X | X | X | | | | X | X | X | | | | | |
| Antihemorrhagic | | | | | | | | X | | | | | | | |
| Antifungal | | | | | | | | | X | X | | X | X | | |
| Antiemetics | X | | | | | | X | | | X | | | | | |
| Anticatarrhal | X | X | X | X | | | | | X | X | | X | | | |
| Antibiotic | X | X | | X | | | | | X | X | | X | X | | |
| Anthelmintics | X | | X | | | | | | X | X | | | | | |
| Antacid & Anti-ulcer | | | | X | X | | | | | | | | | | |
| Anodyne | | | | | | X | | | | | | | | | |
| Analgesic | X | | | | | | | | | X | X | | | | |
| Amphoteric | | | | | | | | | X | X | | | | | |
| Alterative | | | | X | X | | X | | | | | | | | |
| Adaptogens | X | | | X | X | | | | | | | | | | |

| Herbs By Classifications | Adaptogens | Alterative | Amphoteric | Analgesic | Anodyne | Antacid & Anti-ulcer | Anthelmintics | Antibiotic | Anticatarrhal | Antiemetics | Antifungal | Antihemorrhagic | Anti-Inflammatory | Antilithics-Gallstone | Antilithics-Urinary | Antiprotozoal | Antipyretic | Antirheumatic | Antispasmodic | Antiviral | Aperient | Astringent | Bitters | Cardiotonic | Carminative | Cathartic | Cholagogue | Demulcent | Diaphoretic | Diuretic | Emmenagogue | Expectorant | Galactogogue | Hematinic | Hepatic | Hypnotic | Hypotensive | Nervine Tonics | Nervine Relaxants | Nervine Stimulants | Oxytocic | Rubefacient | Sialogogue | Vasodilator | Vulnerary |
|---|---|---|---|---|---|---|---|---|---|---|---|---|---|---|---|---|---|---|---|---|---|---|---|---|---|---|---|---|---|---|---|---|---|---|---|---|---|---|---|---|---|---|---|---|---|
| **Galactogogue** | | | | | | | | | | | | | | | | | | | | | | | | | | | | | | | | | | | | | | | | | | | | | |
| Alfalfa | | X | | | | | | | | | | | | | | | X | | | | | | | | | | | | | | | | X | X | | | | | | | | | | | |
| Anise Seed | | | | | | | | | | | | | | | | | | | | | | | | | | | | | | | | | X | | | | | | | | | | X | | |
| Blessed Thistle | | | | | | | | | | | | | | | | | | | | | | | | | | | | | X | | | | X | | | | | | | | | | | | |
| Borage | | | | | | | | | | | | | | | | | | X | | | | | | | | | | | | | | | X | | | | | | | | | | | | |
| Caraway | | | | | | | | | | | | | | | | | | | X | | | | | | X | | | | | | | | X | | | | | | | | | | | | |
| Chaste Tree | | | | | | | | | | | | | | | | | | | | | | | | | | | | | | | | | X | | | | | | | | | | | | |
| Cumin | | | | | | | | | | | | | | | | | | | | | | | | | X | | | | | | | | X | | | | | | | | | | | | |
| Dill | | | | | | | | | | X | | | | | X | | | | | | | | | | X | | | | | | | | X | | | | | | | | | | | | |
| Dill Seed | | | | | | | | | | X | | | | | X | | | | | | | | | | X | | | | | | | | X | | | | | | | | | | | | |
| Fennel | | | | | | | | | | X | | | | | | | | | X | | X | | | | X | | | | | | | | X | | | | | | | | | | | X | |
| Fennel Seeds | | | | | | | | | | X | | | | | | | | | X | | X | | | | X | | | | | | | | X | | | | | | | | | | | X | |
| Fenugreek seeds | | | | | | X | | | X | | | | | | | | | | | | X | | | | | | | X | | | | X | X | X | | | | | | | | | | | |
| Goat's Rue | | | | | | | | | | | | | | | | | | | | | | | | | | | | | | | | | X | | | | | | | | | | | | |
| Nettle | | X | | | | | | | X | | | X | X | | | | | X | | | | | | | | | | | | X | | | X | X | | | | | | | | | | | |
| Savory | | | X | X | X | | X | X | X | X | X | | X | | | | | | X | X | X | X | X | X | X | X | X | X | X | X | X | X | X | X | X | | | | | | | | | | |
| Shatavari | | | | | | | | | | | | | | | | | | | | | | | | | | | | | | | | | X | | | | | | | | | | | | |
| Stinging Nettle | | X | | | | | | | X | | | X | X | | | | | X | | | | | | | | | | | | X | | | X | X | | | | | | | | | | | |
| Vervain | | | | | | | | | | | | | | | | | | | | | | | | | | | | | | | | | X | | | X | | | X | | | | | | |

## Herbs By Classifications — Hematinic

**Part 1 of 3 (columns Adaptogens – Antilithics-Urinary)**

| Herbs By Classifications | Adaptogens | Alterative | Amphoteric | Analgesic | Anodyne | Antacid & Anti-ulcer | Anthelmintics | Antibiotic | Anticatarrhal | Antiemetics | Antifungal | Antihemorrhagic | Anti-Inflammatory | Antilithics-Gallstone | Antilithics-Urinary |
|---|---|---|---|---|---|---|---|---|---|---|---|---|---|---|---|
| **Hematinic** | | | | | | | | | | | | | | | |
| Albizia | | | | | | | | | | | | | | | |
| Alfalfa | | X | | | | | | | | | | | | | |
| Ashwagandha | X | | X | | | | | | | | | | | | |
| Astragalus | X | | X | | | | | | | | | | | | |
| Bilberry | | | | | | X | | | | | | | | | |
| Burdock | | X | | | | | | | | | | | | | |
| Chickpeas | | | | | | | | | | | | | | | |
| Chickweed | | | | | | | | | X | | | | X | | |
| Chicory | | | | | | | | | | | | | | X | |
| Chicory Root | | | | | | | | | | | | | | X | |
| Dandelion | | X | | | | | | | | | | | | X | X |
| Dandelion Root | | X | | | | | | | | | | | | X | X |
| Dong Quai | | | | | | | | | | | | | | | |
| Echinacea | | X | | | | | | X | | | X | | X | | |
| Fenugreek seeds | | | | | | X | | | X | | | | | | |
| Nettle | | X | | | | | | | X | | | X | X | | |
| Parsley | | | | | | | | | | | | | | | X |
| Rehmannia | | | | | | | | | | | | | | | |
| Savory | | | X | X | X | | | X | X | X | X | | X | | |
| Stinging Nettle | | X | | | | | | | X | | | X | X | | |
| Yellow Dock | | X | | | | | | | | | | X | | | |

**Part 2 of 3 (columns Antiprotozoal – Diuretic)**

| Herbs By Classifications | Antiprotozoal | Antipyretic | Antirheumatic | Antispasmodic | Antiviral | Aperient | Astringent | Bitters | Cardiotonic | Carminative | Cathartic | Cholagogue | Demulcent | Diaphoretic | Diuretic |
|---|---|---|---|---|---|---|---|---|---|---|---|---|---|---|---|
| **Hematinic** | | | | | | | | | | | | | | | |
| Albizia | | | | | | | | | | | | | | | |
| Alfalfa | | X | | | | | | | | | | | | | |
| Ashwagandha | | | | | | | | | | | | | | | |
| Astragalus | | | | | X | | | | X | | | | | | |
| Bilberry | | X | | | | | | | | | | | | | |
| Burdock | | | X | | | | | X | | | | | | | X |
| Chickpeas | | | | | | | | | | | | | | | |
| Chickweed | | X | | | | | | | | | | | | | |
| Chicory | | | | | | | | X | | | | | | | |
| Chicory Root | | | | | | | | X | | | | | | | |
| Dandelion | | | | | | X | | X | | | | X | | | X |
| Dandelion Root | | | | | | X | | X | | | | X | | | X |
| Dong Quai | | | | | | | | | | | | | | | |
| Echinacea | | X | | | X | | | | | | | | | X | |
| Fenugreek seeds | | | X | | | | | | | | | | X | | |
| Nettle | | | X | | | | | | | | | | | | X |
| Parsley | | | | | | | | | | X | | | | | X |
| Rehmannia | | | | | | | | | | | | | | | |
| Savory | | | X | X | X | X | X | X | X | X | X | X | X | X | X |
| Stinging Nettle | | | X | | | | | | | | | | | | X |
| Yellow Dock | | | | | | | | | | | X | X | | | |

**Part 3 of 3 (columns Emmenagogue – Vulnerary)**

| Herbs By Classifications | Emmenagogue | Expectorant | Galactogogue | Hematinic | Hepatic | Hypnotic | Hypotensive | Nervine Tonics | Nervine Relaxants | Nervine Stimulants | Oxytocic | Rubefacient | Sialogogue | Vasodilator | Vulnerary |
|---|---|---|---|---|---|---|---|---|---|---|---|---|---|---|---|
| **Hematinic** | | | | | | | | | | | | | | | |
| Albizia | | | | X | | | | | | | | | | | |
| Alfalfa | | | X | X | | | | | | | | | | | |
| Ashwagandha | | | | X | | X | | X | X | X | | | | | |
| Astragalus | | | | X | X | | X | | | | | | | X | |
| Bilberry | | | | X | | | | | | | | | | | |
| Burdock | | | | X | X | | | | | | | | | | |
| Chickpeas | | | | X | | | | | | | | | | | |
| Chickweed | | | | X | | | | | | | | | | | |
| Chicory | | | | X | | | | | | | | | | | |
| Chicory Root | | | | X | | | | | | | | | | | |
| Dandelion | | | | X | X | | | | | | | | | | |
| Dandelion Root | | | | X | X | | | | | | | | | | |
| Dong Quai | X | | | X | | | | | | | | | | | |
| Echinacea | | | | X | | | | | | | | | X | | X |
| Fenugreek seeds | | X | X | X | | | | | | | | | | | |
| Nettle | | | X | X | | | | | | | | | | | |
| Parsley | X | | | X | | | X | | | | | | | | |
| Rehmannia | | | | X | | | | | | | | | | | |
| Savory | X | X | X | X | X | | | | | | | | | | |
| Stinging Nettle | | | X | X | | | | | | | | | | | |
| Yellow Dock | | | | X | X | | | | | | | | | | |

| Herbs By Classifications | Adaptogens | Alterative | Amphoteric | Analgesic | Anodyne | Antacid & Anti-ulcer | Anthelmintics | Antibiotic | Anticatarrhal | Antiemetics | Antifungal | Antihemorrhagic | Anti-Inflammatory | Antilithics-Gallstone | Antilithics-Urinary | Antiprotozoal | Antipyretic | Antirheumatic | Antispasmodic | Antiviral | Aperient | Astringent | Bitters | Cardiotonic | Carminative | Cathartic | Cholagogue | Demulcent | Diaphoretic | Diuretic | Emmenagogue | Expectorant | Galactogogue | Hematinic | Hepatic | Hypnotic | Hypotensive | Nervine Tonics | Nervine Relaxants | Nervine Stimulants | Oxytocic | Rubefacient | Sialogogue | Vasodilator | Vulnerary |
|---|---|---|---|---|---|---|---|---|---|---|---|---|---|---|---|---|---|---|---|---|---|---|---|---|---|---|---|---|---|---|---|---|---|---|---|---|---|---|---|---|---|---|---|---|---|
| **Hepatic** | | | | | | | | | | | | | | | | | | | | | | | | | | | | | | | | | | | | | | | | | | | | | |
| Artichoke | | | | | | | | | | | | | | X | | | | | | | | | X | | | | X | | | | | | | | X | | | | | | | | | | |
| Astragalus | X | | X | | | | | | | | | | | | | | | | | X | | | | X | | | | | | | | | | X | X | | X | | | | | | | X | |
| Barberry | | | | | | | | X | | | | | | X | | X | | | | | | | X | | | X | X | | | | | | | | X | | | | | | | | | | |
| Boldo | | | | | | | X | | | | | | | X | | | | | | | | | | | | | X | | | | | | | | X | | | | | | | | | | |
| Bupleurum | | | | | | | | | | | | | | | | | | | | | | | | | | | X | | | | | | | | X | | | | | | | | | | |
| Burdock | | X | | | | | | | | | | | | | | | | X | | | | | X | | | | | | | X | | | | X | X | | | | | | | | | | |
| Cleavers | | X | | | | | | | | | | | | | X | | | | | | | | | | | | | | | X | | | | | X | | | | | | | | | | |
| Dandelion | | X | | | | | | | | | | | | X | X | | | | | | X | | X | | | | X | | | X | | | | X | X | | | | | | | | | | |
| Dandelion Root | | X | | | | | | | | | | | | X | X | | | | | | X | | X | | | | X | | | X | | | | X | X | | | | | | | | | | |
| Garden Sage | | | | | | | | X | X | | X | | X | X | | | X | X | X | X | | X | X | | X | | | | X | X | X | | | | X | | | X | X | X | | X | | | X |
| Gentian | | | | | | | | X | | | | | | | | | | | | | | | X | | | | X | | | | | | | | X | | | | | | | | | | |
| Ginger | | | X | X | | X | X | X | X | | | | X | X | | X | X | X | X | X | | | X | X | X | | | | | X | X | X | | | X | | X | | | X | X | X | | X | |
| Greater Celandine | | | | | | | | | | | | | | X | | | | | | | | | | | | | X | | | | | | | | X | | | | | | | | | | |
| Horseradish | | | | | | | | | | | | | | | | | | | | | | | | | | | | | | | | X | | | X | | | | | X | | X | | | |
| Licorice | X | X | X | | | X | | X | | | | | X | | | X | | X | X | | | | | | | X | X | X | | | | X | | | X | | | | | | | | X | | |
| Licorice Root | X | X | X | | | X | | X | | | | | X | | | X | | X | X | | | | | | | X | X | X | | | | X | | | X | | | | | | | | X | | |
| Lovage | | X | | | | | | X | X | X | | | | | | | | | | | | | | | X | | X | X | X | | | X | | | X | | | | | | | | X | | |
| Milk Thistle | X | | | | | X | | | | | | | | X | X | | | | | | | | | | | | X | | | | | | | | X | | | | | | | | | | |
| Oregon Grape | | X | | | | | | X | | | X | | | X | | | | | | | | | | | | | X | | | | | | | | X | | | | | | | | | | |
| Oregon Grape Root | | X | | | | | | X | | | X | | | X | | | | | | | | | | | | | X | | | | | | | | X | | | | | | | | | | |
| Savory | | | X | X | X | | | X | X | X | X | | X | | | | | | X | | | X | X | | X | X | X | X | X | X | X | X | X | X | X | | | | | | | | | | |
| Schisandra | X | | X | | | | | | | | | | | | | | | | | | | | | | | | | | | | | | | | X | | | | | | | | | | |
| Turmeric | X | | X | X | X | X | X | X | | | | | X | | | X | | X | | | | | X | | | | X | | | | | | | | X | | | | | | | | | X | |
| Wild Yam | | | | | | | | | | | | | | | | | | | X | | | | | | | | | | | | | | | | X | | | | | | | | | | |
| Wormwood | | | | | | | X | X | | | | | | | | | | | | | | | X | | | | | | | | | | | | X | | | | | | | | | | |
| Yellow Dock | | X | | | | | | | | | | X | | | | X | | | | | | | | | | X | X | | | | | | | X | X | | | | | | | | | | |

| Herbs By Classifications | Adaptogens | Alterative | Amphoteric | Analgesic | Anodyne | Antacid & Anti-ulcer | Anthelmintics | Antibiotic | Anticatarrhal | Antiemetics | Antifungal | Antihemorrhagic | Anti-Inflammatory | Antilithics-Gallstone | Antilithics-Urinary | Antiprotozoal | Antipyretic | Antirheumatic | Antispasmodic | Antiviral | Aperient | Astringent | Bitters | Cardiotonic | Carminative | Cathartic | Cholagogue | Demulcent | Diaphoretic | Diuretic | Emmenagogue | Expectorant | Galactogogue | Hematinic | Hepatic | Hypnotic | Hypotensive | Nervine Tonics | Nervine Relaxants | Nervine Stimulants | Oxytocic | Rubefacient | Sialogogue | Vasodilator | Vulnerary |
|---|---|---|---|---|---|---|---|---|---|---|---|---|---|---|---|---|---|---|---|---|---|---|---|---|---|---|---|---|---|---|---|---|---|---|---|---|---|---|---|---|---|---|---|---|---|
| **Hypnotic** | | | | | | | | | | | | | | | | | | | | | | | | | | | | | | | | | | | | | | | | | | | | | |
| Ashwagandha | X | | X | | | | | | | | | | | | | | | | | | | | | | | | | | | | | | | X | | X | | X | X | X | | | | | |
| Blue Vervain | | | | | | | | | | | | | | | | | | | | | | | | | | | | | | | | | | | | X | | X | X | | | | | | |
| California Poppy | | | | | | | | | | | | | | | | | | | | | | | | | | | | | | | | | | | | X | | X | X | | | | | | |
| Catnip | | | | | | | | | | X | | | | | | | X | | X | | | | | | | | | | X | | | | | | | X | | X | X | | | | | | |
| Chamomile | | | | X | X | X | | X | | X | X | | X | | | | X | X | X | | | | X | | X | | | | X | | X | | | | | X | | X | X | | | | | | X |
| Hops | | | | | | | | | | | | | | | | | | | | | | | | | | | | | | | | | | | | X | | | X | | | | | | |
| Jamaican Dogwood | | | | | | | | | | | | | | | | | | | | | | | | | | | | | | | | | | | | X | | | | | | | | | |
| Kava Kava | X | | | X | X | | | | | | | | | | | | | | | | | | | | | | | | | | | | | | | X | | X | X | | | | | | |
| Kratom | | | | | | | | | | | | | | | | | | | | | | | | | | | | | | | | | | | | X | | | | | | | | | |
| Lavendar | | | | X | X | | | | | X | | | | | | | | | X | | | | | | X | | | | | | | | | | | X | X | X | X | | | | | | X |
| Lemon Balm | X | | | | | | | | | X | | | | | | | | | X | X | | | | X | X | X | | | | | | | | | | X | X | X | X | | | | | | |
| Linden | | | | | | | | | | | | | | | | | | | | | | | | X | | | | | | | | | | | | X | X | X | X | | | | | X | |
| Motherwort | | | | | | | | | | | | | | | | | | | X | | | | | X | X | | | | | | X | | | | | X | X | X | X | | | | | | |
| Passionflower | X | | | | | | | | | | | | | | | | | | X | | | | | | | | | | | | | | | | | X | X | X | X | | | | | | |
| Skullcap | | | | X | X | | | | | | | | X | | | | X | | X | | | | | | | | | | | | | | | | | X | X | X | X | | | | | | |
| Valerian | X | | | | | | | | | | | | | | | | | | X | | | | | | | | | | | | | | | | | X | X | X | X | | | | | | |
| Vervain | | | | | | | | | | | | | | | | | | | | | | | | | | | | | | | | | X | | | X | | | X | | | | | | |

| Herbs By Classifications | Adaptogens | Alterative | Amphoteric | Analgesic | Anodyne | Antacid & Anti-ulcer | Anthelmintics | Antibiotic | Anticatarrhal | Antiemetics | Antifungal | Antihemorrhagic | Anti-Inflammatory | Antilithics-Gallstone | Antilithics-Urinary | Antiprotozoal | Antipyretic | Antirheumatic | Antispasmodic | Antiviral | Aperient | Astringent | Bitters | Cardiotonic | Carminative | Cathartic | Cholagogue | Demulcent | Diaphoretic | Diuretic | Emmenagogue | Expectorant | Galactogogue | Hematinic | Hepatic | Hypnotic | Hypotensive | Nervine Tonics | Nervine Relaxants | Nervine Stimulants | Oxytocic | Rubefacient | Sialogogue | Vasodilator | Vulnerary |
|---|---|---|---|---|---|---|---|---|---|---|---|---|---|---|---|---|---|---|---|---|---|---|---|---|---|---|---|---|---|---|---|---|---|---|---|---|---|---|---|---|---|---|---|---|---|
| **Hypotensive** |  |  |  |  |  |  |  |  |  |  |  |  |  |  |  |  |  |  |  |  |  |  |  |  |  |  |  |  |  |  |  |  |  |  |  |  |  |  |  |  |  |  |  |  |  |
| Arjuna |  |  |  |  |  |  |  |  |  |  |  |  |  |  |  |  |  |  |  |  |  |  |  |  |  |  |  |  |  |  |  |  |  |  |  |  | X |  |  |  |  |  |  |  |  |
| Astragalus | X |  | X |  |  |  |  |  |  |  |  |  |  |  |  |  |  |  |  | X |  |  |  | X |  |  |  |  |  |  |  |  |  | X | X |  | X |  |  |  |  |  |  | X |  |
| Cat's Claw |  |  |  |  |  |  |  |  |  |  |  |  | X |  |  |  |  | X |  | X |  |  |  |  |  |  |  |  |  |  |  |  |  |  |  |  | X |  |  |  |  |  |  |  |  |
| Cayenne |  |  | X | X | X |  |  | X | X |  |  | X | X |  |  |  |  | X |  |  |  |  |  | X |  |  |  |  | X |  |  |  |  |  |  |  | X |  |  | X |  | X | X | X | X |
| Celery |  |  |  |  |  |  |  |  |  |  |  |  |  |  |  |  |  |  |  |  |  |  |  |  |  |  |  |  |  | X |  |  |  |  |  |  | X |  |  |  |  |  |  |  |  |
| Cinnamon |  |  |  |  |  |  |  | X |  | X | X |  |  |  |  |  |  |  | X |  |  | X |  | X | X |  |  | X |  |  | X |  |  |  |  |  | X |  |  | X |  |  | X | X |  |
| Cramp Bark |  |  |  |  |  |  |  |  |  |  |  |  |  |  |  |  |  |  | X |  |  |  |  |  |  |  |  |  |  |  |  |  |  |  |  |  | X |  | X |  | X |  |  |  |  |
| French Lavender |  |  |  |  |  |  |  |  |  |  |  |  |  |  |  |  |  |  |  |  |  |  |  |  |  |  |  |  |  |  |  |  |  |  |  |  | X |  |  |  |  |  |  |  |  |
| Garden Sage |  |  |  |  |  |  |  | X | X |  | X |  | X |  | X |  | X | X | X | X |  | X | X | X | X |  |  |  | X |  | X | X |  |  | X |  | X | X | X |  |  | X |  |  | X |
| Garlic |  | X |  |  |  |  | X | X | X |  | X |  |  |  |  | X |  |  | X |  |  |  |  | X | X |  |  |  |  |  |  |  |  |  |  |  | X |  |  | X |  | X |  | X | X |
| Ginger |  |  | X |  |  |  | X | X | X | X |  | X | X | X |  | X | X | X | X | X |  |  | X | X | X |  | X |  | X | X |  | X |  |  | X |  | X |  |  | X | X | X |  | X |  |
| Hawthorn | X |  |  |  |  |  |  |  |  |  |  |  |  |  |  |  |  |  |  |  |  |  |  | X |  |  |  |  |  |  |  |  |  |  |  |  | X |  |  |  |  |  |  | X |  |
| Lavender |  |  |  | X | X |  |  |  |  | X |  |  |  |  |  |  |  |  | X |  |  |  |  |  | X |  |  |  |  |  |  |  |  |  |  | X | X | X | X |  |  |  |  |  | X |
| Lemon Balm | X |  |  |  |  |  |  |  |  | X |  |  |  |  |  |  | X |  | X | X |  |  |  | X | X |  |  |  |  |  |  |  |  |  |  | X | X | X | X |  |  |  |  |  |  |
| Linden |  |  |  |  |  |  |  |  |  |  |  |  |  |  |  |  |  |  |  |  |  |  |  | X |  |  |  |  |  |  |  |  |  |  |  | X | X | X | X |  |  |  |  | X |  |
| Mistletoe |  |  |  |  |  |  |  |  |  |  |  |  |  |  |  | X |  |  |  |  |  |  |  |  |  |  |  |  |  |  |  |  |  |  |  |  | X |  |  |  |  |  |  | X |  |
| Motherwort |  |  |  |  |  |  |  |  |  |  |  |  |  |  |  |  |  | X |  |  |  |  |  | X | X |  |  |  |  |  | X |  |  |  |  |  | X | X | X | X |  |  |  |  |  |
| Olive |  |  |  |  |  |  |  |  |  |  |  |  |  |  |  |  |  |  |  |  |  |  |  |  |  |  |  |  |  |  |  |  |  |  |  |  | X |  |  |  |  |  |  |  |  |
| Olive Leaf |  |  |  |  |  |  |  | X |  |  |  |  |  |  |  |  | X |  |  |  |  |  |  | X |  |  |  |  |  |  |  |  |  |  |  |  | X |  |  |  |  |  |  |  |  |
| Onion |  |  |  |  |  |  |  |  |  |  |  |  |  |  |  |  |  |  |  |  |  |  |  |  |  |  |  |  |  |  |  |  |  |  |  |  | X |  |  |  |  |  |  |  |  |
| Parsley |  |  |  |  |  |  |  |  |  |  |  |  |  |  | X |  |  |  |  |  |  |  |  |  | X |  |  |  |  | X | X |  |  | X |  |  | X |  |  |  |  |  |  |  |  |
| Passionflower | X |  |  |  |  |  |  |  |  |  |  |  |  |  |  |  |  |  | X |  |  |  |  |  |  |  |  |  |  |  |  |  |  |  |  | X | X | X | X |  |  |  |  |  |  |
| Siberian Ginseng | X |  |  |  |  |  |  |  |  |  |  |  |  |  |  |  |  |  |  |  |  |  |  |  |  |  |  |  |  |  |  |  |  |  |  |  | X | X | X | X |  |  |  |  |  |
| Skullcap |  |  |  | X | X |  |  |  |  |  |  |  | X |  |  |  |  |  | X |  |  |  |  |  |  |  |  |  |  |  |  |  |  |  |  | X | X | X | X |  |  |  |  |  |  |
| Valerian | X |  |  |  |  |  |  |  |  |  |  |  |  |  |  |  |  |  | X |  |  |  |  |  |  |  |  |  |  |  |  |  |  |  |  | X | X | X | X |  |  |  |  |  |  |
| Yarrow |  |  |  | X | X |  |  | X | X |  |  | X | X |  |  |  | X |  |  | X |  | X |  | X |  |  |  |  | X |  |  |  |  |  |  |  | X |  |  | X |  |  |  | X | X |

| Herbs By Classifications | Adaptogens | Alterative | Amphoteric | Analgesic | Anodyne | Antacid & Anti-ulcer | Anthelmintics | Antibiotic | Anticatarrhal | Antiemetics | Antifungal | Antihemorrhagic | Anti-Inflammatory | Antilithics-Gallstone | Antilithics-Urinary | Antiprotozoal | Antipyretic | Antirheumatic | Antispasmodic | Antiviral | Aperient | Astringent |
|---|---|---|---|---|---|---|---|---|---|---|---|---|---|---|---|---|---|---|---|---|---|---|
| **Nervine** | | | | | | | | | | | | | | | | | | | | | | |
| **Nervine Tonics** | | | | | | | | | | | | | | | | | | | | | | |
| Ashwagandha | X | | X | | | | | | | | | | | | | | | | | | | |
| Basil | X | | | | | | | X | | X | X | | | | | | X | | | | | |
| Blue Vervain | | | | | | | | | | | | | | | | | | | | | | |
| California Poppy | | | | | | | | | | | | | | | | | | | | | | |
| Caraway | | | | | | | X | | | | | | | | | | | | X | | | |
| Catnip | | | | | | | | | | X | | | | | | | X | | X | | | |
| Chamomile | | | | X | X | X | | X | | X | X | | X | | | | X | X | X | | | |
| Garden Sage | | | | | | | | X | X | | X | | X | | X | | X | X | X | X | | X |
| Gotu Kola | X | | X | | | X | | | | | | | | | | | X | | | | | |
| Holy Basil | X | | X | | | | | | | | | | | | | | | | | | | |
| Kava Kava | X | | | X | X | | | | | | | | | | | | | | | | | |
| Lavender | | | | X | X | | | | | X | | | | | | | | | X | | | |
| Lemon Balm | X | | | | | | | | | X | | | | | | | X | | X | X | | |
| Linden | | | | | | | | | | | | | | | | | | | | | | |
| Marjoram | | | | X | X | | | X | X | | | | X | | | | | | X | X | X | X |
| Motherwort | | | | | | | | | | | | | | | | | | | X | | | |
| Oat Straw | | | | | | | | | | | | | | | | | | | | | | |
| Panax ginseng | X | | | | | | | | | | | | | | | | | | | | | |
| Passionflower | X | | | | | | | | | | | | | | | | | | X | | | |
| Sage | | | | X | | | | X | X | | X | | X | | | | | | X | X | | X |
| Siberian Ginseng | X | | | | | | | | | | | | | | | | | | | | | |
| Skullcap | | | | X | X | | | | | | | | X | | | | X | | X | | | |
| St. John's Wort | | | | | | | | X | | | | | X | | | | | | X | X | | |
| Tulsi | X | | X | | | | | | | | | | | | | | | | | | | |
| Valerian | X | | | | | | | | | | | | | | | | | | X | | | |
| Wood Betony | | | | | | | | | | | | | | | | | | | | | | |

| Herbs By Classifications | Bitters | Cardiotonic | Carminative | Cathartic | Cholagogue | Demulcent | Diaphoretic | Diuretic | Emmenagogue | Expectorant | Galactogogue | Hematinic | Hepatic | Hypnotic | Hypotensive | Nervine Tonics | Nervine Relaxants | Nervine Stimulants | Oxytocic | Rubefacient | Sialogogue | Vasodilator | Vulnerary |
|---|---|---|---|---|---|---|---|---|---|---|---|---|---|---|---|---|---|---|---|---|---|---|---|
| **Nervine** | | | | | | | | | | | | | | | | | | | | | | | |
| **Nervine Tonics** | | | | | | | | | | | | | | | | | | | | | | | |
| Ashwagandha | | | | | | | | | | | | X | | X | | X | X | X | | | | | |
| Basil | | | X | | | | X | | | X | | | | | | X | | | | | | | |
| Blue Vervain | | | | | | | | | | | | | | X | | X | X | | | | | | |
| California Poppy | | | | | | | | | | | | | | X | | X | X | | | | | | |
| Caraway | | | X | | | | | | | | X | | | | | X | | | | | | | |
| Catnip | | | | | | | X | | | | | | | X | | X | X | | | | | | |
| Chamomile | X | | X | | | | X | | X | | | | | X | | X | X | | | | | | X |
| Garden Sage | X | | X | | | | X | X | X | | | | X | | X | X | X | | | X | | | X |
| Gotu Kola | | | | | | | | | | | | | | | | X | | X | | | | | X |
| Holy Basil | | | | | | | | | | | | | | | | X | X | | | | | | |
| Kava Kava | | | | | | | | | | | | | | X | | X | X | | | | | | |
| Lavender | | | X | | | | | | | | | | | X | X | X | X | | | | | | X |
| Lemon Balm | | X | X | | X | | | | | | | | | X | X | X | X | | | | | | |
| Linden | | X | | | | | | | | | | | | X | X | X | X | | | | | X | |
| Marjoram | X | | X | | | | | | | | | | | | | X | X | | X | X | X | X | X |
| Motherwort | | X | X | | | | | | X | | | | | X | X | X | X | | | | | | |
| Oat Straw | | | | | | | | | | | | | | | | X | | | | | | | |
| Panax ginseng | | | | | | | | | | | | | | | | X | | | | | | | |
| Passionflower | | | | | | | | | | | | | | X | X | X | X | | | | | | |
| Sage | X | | X | | | | X | | X | | | | | | | X | X | | | | X | | X |
| Siberian Ginseng | | | | | | | | | | | | | | | X | X | | X | | | | | |
| Skullcap | | | | | | | | | | | | | | X | X | X | X | | | | | | |
| St. John's Wort | | | | | | | | | | | | | | | | X | X | | | | | | X |
| Tulsi | | | | | | | | | | | | | | | | X | X | | | | | | |
| Valerian | | | | | | | | | | | | | | X | X | X | X | | | | | | |
| Wood Betony | | | | | | | | | | | | | | | | X | X | | | | | | |

| Herbs By Classifications | Adaptogens | Alterative | Amphoteric | Analgesic | Anodyne | Antacid & Anti-ulcer | Anthelmintics | Antibiotic | Anticatarrhal | Antiemetics | Antifungal | Antihemorrhagic | Anti-Inflammatory | Antilithics-Gallstone | Antilithics-Urinary | Antiprotozoal | Antipyretic | Antirheumatic | Antispasmodic | Antiviral | Aperient | Astringent | Bitters | Cardiotonic | Carminative | Cathartic | Cholagogue | Demulcent | Diaphoretic | Diuretic | Emmenagogue | Expectorant | Galactogogue | Hematinic | Hepatic | Hypnotic | Hypotensive | Nervine Tonics | Nervine Relaxants | Nervine Stimulants | Oxytocic | Rubefacient | Sialogogue | Vasodilator | Vulnerary |
|---|---|---|---|---|---|---|---|---|---|---|---|---|---|---|---|---|---|---|---|---|---|---|---|---|---|---|---|---|---|---|---|---|---|---|---|---|---|---|---|---|---|---|---|---|---|
| **Nervine** | | | | | | | | | | | | | | | | | | | | | | | | | | | | | | | | | | | | | | | | | | | | | |
| **Nervine Relaxants** | | | | | | | | | | | | | | | | | | | | | | | | | | | | | | | | | | | | | | | | | | | | | |
| Ashwagandha | X | | X | | | | | | | | | | | | | | | | | | | | | | | | | | | | | | | X | | X | | X | X | X | | | | | |
| Black Cohosh | X | | | X | X | | | | | | | | | | | | | | X | | | | | | | | | | | | X | | | | | | | | X | | X | | | | |
| Blue Vervain | | | | | | | | | | | | | | | | | | | | | | | | | | | | | | | | | | | | X | | X | X | | | | | | |
| California Poppy | | | | | | | | | | | | | | | | | | | | | | | | | | | | | | | | | | | | X | | X | X | | | | | | |
| Catnip | | | | | | | | | | X | | | | | | | X | | X | | | | | | | | | | X | | | | | | | X | | X | X | | | | | | |
| Chamomile | | | | X | X | X | | X | | X | X | | X | | | | X | X | X | | | | X | | X | | | | X | | X | | | | | X | | X | X | | | | | | X |
| Cramp Bark | | | | | | | | | | | | | | | | | | | X | | | | | | | | | | X | | | | | | | | X | | X | | | X | | | |
| Garden Sage | | | | | | | | X | X | | X | | X | | X | | X | X | X | X | X | X | X | | X | | | | X | X | X | | | | X | X | X | X | X | | | | X | | X |
| Holy Basil | X | | X | | | | | | | | | | | | | | | | | | | | | | | | | | | | | | | | | X | | | X | | | | | | |
| Hops | | | | | | | | | | | | | | | | | | | | | | | | | | | | | | | | | | | | X | | | X | | | | | | |
| Hyssop | | | | | | | X | | X | | | | X | | | | | | X | | | | | | | | | | X | | | X | | | | | | | X | | | | | | |
| Kava Kava | X | | | X | X | | | | | | | | | | | | | | | | | | | | | | | | | | | | | | | X | | X | X | | | | | | |
| Lavendar | | | | X | X | | | | | X | | | | | | | | | X | | | | | | X | | | | | | | | | | | X | X | X | X | | | | | | X |
| Lemon Balm | X | | | | | | | | | X | | | | | | | | | X | X | | | | X | X | | X | | | | | | | | | X | X | X | X | | | | | | |
| Lemon Verbana | | | | | | | | | | | | | | | | | | | X | | | X | | | | | | | | | | | | | | | | | X | | | | | | |
| Linden | | | | | | | | | | | | | | | | | | | | | | | | X | | | | | | | | | | | | X | X | X | X | | | | | X | |
| Lobelia | | | | | | | | | | | | | | | | | | | X | | | | | | | | | | | | | X | | | | | | | X | | | | | | |
| Marjoram | | | | X | X | | | X | X | | | | X | | | | | | X | X | X | X | X | | X | | | | | | | | | | | X | X | X | X | | X | X | X | X | X |
| Motherwort | | | | | | | | | | | | | | | | | | | X | | | | | X | X | | | | | | X | | | | | X | X | X | X | | | | | | |
| Passionflower | X | | | | | | | | | | | | | | | | | | X | | | | | | | | | | | | | | | | | X | X | X | X | | | | | | |
| Passionvine | | | | | | | | | | | | | | | | | | | | | | | | | | | | | | | | | | | | | | | X | | | | | | |
| Red Clover | | X | | | | | | | | | | | | | | | | | | | | | | | | | | | | | | | | | | | | | X | | | | | | |
| Rhodiola | X | | X | | | | | | | | | | | | | | | | | | | | | | | | | | | | | | | | | | | | X | X | | | | | |
| Sage | | | | | | | | X | X | | X | | | | | | | | X | | | X | X | X | X | | X | | X | X | | | | | | X | X | X | X | | | | X | | X |
| Skullcap | | | | X | X | | | | | | | | X | | | | | | X | | | | | | | | | | | | | | | | | X | X | X | X | | | | | | |
| St. John's Wort | | | | | | | | X | | | | | X | | | | | | X | X | | | | | | | | | | | | | | | | X | X | X | X | | | | | | X |
| Tulsi | X | | X | | | | | | | | | | | | | | | | | | | | | | | | | | | | | | | | | | | X | X | | | | | | |
| Valerian | X | | | | | | | | | | | | | | | | | | X | | | | | | | | | | | | | | | | | X | X | X | X | | | | | | |
| Vervain | | | | | | | | | | | | | | | | | | | | | | | | | | | | | | | | | X | | | | X | | X | | | | | | |
| Wood Betony | | | | | | | | | | | | | | | | | | | | | | | | | | | | | | | | | | | | | | X | X | | | | | | |

| Herbs By Classifications | Adaptogens | Alterative | Amphoteric | Analgesic | Anodyne | Antacid & Anti-ulcer | Anthelmintics | Antibiotic | Anticatarrhal | Antiemetics | Antifungal | Antihemorrhagic | Anti-Inflammatory | Antilithics-Gallstone | Antilithics-Urinary | Antiprotozoal | Antipyretic | Antirheumatic | Antispasmodic | Antiviral | Aperient | Astringent | Bitters | Cardiotonic | Carminative | Cathartic | Cholagogue | Demulcent | Diaphoretic | Diuretic | Emmenagogue | Expectorant | Galactogogue | Hematinic | Hepatic | Hypnotic | Hypotensive | Nervine Tonics | Nervine Relaxants | Nervine Stimulants | Oxytocic | Rubefacient | Sialogogue | Vasodilator | Vulnerary |
|---|---|---|---|---|---|---|---|---|---|---|---|---|---|---|---|---|---|---|---|---|---|---|---|---|---|---|---|---|---|---|---|---|---|---|---|---|---|---|---|---|---|---|---|---|---|
| **Nervine** |  |  |  |  |  |  |  |  |  |  |  |  |  |  |  |  |  |  |  |  |  |  |  |  |  |  |  |  |  |  |  |  |  |  |  |  |  |  |  |  |  |  |  |  |  |
| **Nervine Stimulants** |  |  |  |  |  |  |  |  |  |  |  |  |  |  |  |  |  |  |  |  |  |  |  |  |  |  |  |  |  |  |  |  |  |  |  |  |  |  |  |  |  |  |  |  |  |
| American Ginseng | X |  |  |  |  |  |  |  |  |  |  |  |  |  |  |  |  |  |  |  |  |  |  |  |  |  |  |  |  |  |  |  |  |  |  |  |  |  |  | X |  |  |  |  |  |
| Angelica |  |  |  |  |  |  |  |  |  |  |  |  |  |  |  |  | X | X |  |  |  | X |  |  |  |  |  |  |  | X |  |  |  |  |  |  |  |  | X | X |  |  |  |  |
| Ashwagandha | X |  | X |  |  |  |  |  |  |  |  |  |  |  |  |  |  |  |  |  |  |  |  |  |  |  |  |  |  |  |  |  | X |  | X |  | X | X | X |  |  |  |  |  |
| Black Pepper |  |  |  |  |  |  |  |  |  |  |  |  |  |  |  |  |  |  |  |  |  |  |  |  |  |  |  |  |  |  |  |  |  |  |  |  |  |  |  | X |  | X | X |  |  |
| Cardamom |  |  |  |  |  |  |  |  |  | X |  |  |  |  |  |  |  |  |  |  |  |  |  | X |  |  |  |  |  |  |  |  |  |  |  |  |  |  |  | X |  |  | X |  |  |
| Cayenne |  |  | X | X | X |  |  | X | X |  |  | X | X |  |  |  |  | X |  |  |  |  |  | X |  |  |  |  | X |  |  |  |  |  |  |  | X |  |  | X |  | X | X | X | X |
| Cinnamon |  |  |  |  |  |  |  | X |  | X | X |  |  |  |  |  |  |  |  |  |  |  |  |  | X |  |  |  |  |  |  |  |  |  |  |  | X |  |  | X |  |  | X | X |  |
| Cloves |  |  |  | X | X |  | X |  |  | X | X |  |  |  |  |  |  |  |  | X |  |  |  |  | X |  |  |  |  |  |  |  |  |  |  |  |  |  |  | X |  |  |  |  |  |
| Damiana |  |  |  |  |  |  |  |  |  |  |  |  |  |  |  |  |  |  |  |  |  |  |  |  |  |  |  |  |  |  |  |  |  |  |  |  |  |  |  | X |  |  |  |  |  |
| Elecampane |  |  |  |  |  |  | X | X | X |  |  |  |  |  |  |  |  |  |  |  |  |  |  |  |  |  |  |  |  |  |  | X |  |  |  |  |  |  |  | X |  |  |  |  |  |
| Garlic |  | X |  |  |  |  | X | X | X |  | X |  |  |  |  | X |  | X |  | X |  |  |  | X | X |  |  |  |  |  |  | X |  |  |  |  | X |  |  | X |  | X |  | X | X |
| Ginger |  |  |  | X |  |  | X | X | X | X |  |  | X | X |  | X | X | X | X |  | X |  | X |  | X |  |  |  | X | X | X | X |  |  |  |  | X |  |  | X | X | X |  | X |  |
| Ginkgo | X |  |  |  |  |  |  |  |  |  |  |  |  |  |  |  |  |  |  |  |  |  | X |  |  |  |  |  |  |  |  |  |  |  |  |  |  |  |  | X |  |  |  | X |  |
| Ginkgo Biloba | X |  |  |  |  |  |  |  |  |  |  |  |  |  |  |  |  |  |  |  |  |  | X |  |  |  |  |  |  |  |  |  |  |  |  |  |  |  |  | X |  |  |  | X |  |
| Ginseng |  | X |  |  |  |  |  |  |  |  |  |  |  |  |  |  |  |  |  |  |  |  |  |  |  |  |  |  |  |  |  |  |  |  |  |  |  |  |  | X |  |  |  | X |  |
| Gotu Kola | X |  | X |  |  | X |  |  |  |  |  |  |  |  |  | X |  |  |  |  |  |  |  |  |  |  |  |  |  |  |  |  |  |  |  |  |  | X |  | X |  |  |  |  | X |
| Gravel Root |  |  |  |  |  |  |  |  |  |  |  |  |  |  | X |  | X |  |  |  |  |  |  |  |  |  |  |  | X |  |  |  |  |  |  |  |  |  |  | X |  |  |  |  |  |
| Guarana |  |  |  |  |  |  |  |  |  |  |  |  |  |  |  |  |  |  |  |  |  | X |  |  |  |  |  |  |  |  |  |  |  |  |  |  |  |  |  | X |  |  |  |  |  |
| Horseradish |  |  |  |  |  |  |  |  |  |  |  |  |  |  |  |  |  |  |  |  |  |  |  |  |  |  |  |  |  |  |  | X |  |  | X |  |  |  |  | X |  | X |  |  |  |
| Juniper |  |  |  |  |  |  |  | X |  |  |  |  |  |  | X |  |  | X |  |  |  |  |  |  | X |  |  |  |  | X |  |  |  |  |  |  |  |  |  | X | X |  |  |  |  |
| Juniper Berries |  |  |  |  |  |  |  | X |  |  |  |  |  |  | X |  |  | X |  |  |  |  |  |  | X |  |  |  |  | X |  |  |  |  |  |  |  |  |  | X | X |  |  |  |  |
| Kola Nut |  |  |  |  |  |  |  |  |  |  |  |  |  |  |  |  |  |  |  |  |  |  |  |  |  |  |  |  |  |  |  |  |  |  |  |  |  |  |  | X |  |  |  |  |  |
| Rhodiola | X |  | X |  |  |  |  |  |  |  |  |  |  |  |  |  |  |  |  |  |  |  |  |  |  |  |  |  |  |  |  |  |  |  |  |  |  |  | X | X |  |  |  |  |  |
| Rosemary |  |  |  |  |  |  |  |  |  | X |  |  | X |  |  |  |  | X | X |  |  |  | X | X |  |  |  |  |  |  |  |  |  |  |  |  |  |  |  | X |  | X |  | X |  |
| Siberian Ginseng | X |  |  |  |  |  |  |  |  |  |  |  |  |  |  |  |  |  |  |  |  |  |  |  |  |  |  |  |  |  |  |  |  |  |  |  |  | X |  | X |  |  |  |  |  |
| Yarrow |  |  |  | X | X |  |  | X | X |  |  | X | X |  |  |  |  |  | X |  |  | X | X | X |  |  |  |  | X |  |  |  |  |  |  |  | X |  |  | X |  |  |  | X | X |
| Yerba Mate |  |  |  |  |  |  |  |  |  |  |  |  |  |  |  |  |  |  |  |  |  |  |  |  |  |  |  |  |  |  |  |  |  |  |  |  |  |  |  | X |  |  |  |  |  |

| Herbs By Classifications | Adaptogens | Alterative | Amphoteric | Analgesic | Anodyne | Antacid & Anti-ulcer | Anthelmintics | Antibiotic | Anticatarrhal | Antiemetics | Antifungal | Antihemorrhagic | Anti-Inflammatory | Antilithics-Gallstone | Antilithics-Urinary | Antiprotozoal | Antipyretic | Antirheumatic | Antispasmodic | Antiviral | Aperient | Astringent | Bitters | Cardiotonic | Carminative | Cathartic | Cholagogue | Demulcent | Diaphoretic | Diuretic | Emmenagogue | Expectorant | Galactogogue | Hematinic | Hepatic | Hypnotic | Hypotensive | Nervine Tonics | Nervine Relaxants | Nervine Stimulants | Oxytocic | Rubefacient | Sialogogue | Vasodilator | Vulnerary |
|---|---|---|---|---|---|---|---|---|---|---|---|---|---|---|---|---|---|---|---|---|---|---|---|---|---|---|---|---|---|---|---|---|---|---|---|---|---|---|---|---|---|---|---|---|---|
| **Oxytocic** | | | | | | | | | | | | | | | | | | | | | | | | | | | | | | | | | | | | | | | | | | | | | |
| Angelica | | | | | | | | | | | | | | | | | | X | X | | | | X | | | | | | | | X | | | | | | | | | X | X | | | | |
| Black Cohosh | X | | | X | X | | | | | | | | | | | | | | X | | | | | | | | | | | | X | | | | | | | | X | | X | | | | |
| Blue Cohosh | | | | | | | | | | | | | | | | | | | | | | | | | | | | | | | X | | | | | | | | | | X | | | | |
| Cotton Root Bark | | | | | | | | | | | | | | | | | | | | | | | | | | | | | | | | | | | | | | | | | X | | | | |
| Cramp Bark | | | | | | | | | | | | | | | | | | | X | | | | | | | | | | | | X | | | | | X | | | X | | X | | | | |
| Ginger | | | | X | | | X | X | X | X | | | X | X | | X | X | X | X | X | X | | X | X | X | | | | | X | X | X | | | X | | X | | | X | X | X | | X | |
| Juniper | | | | | | | | X | | | | | | | X | | | X | | | | | | | X | | | | | X | | | | | | | | | | X | X | | | | |
| Juniper Berries | | | | | | | | X | | | | | | | X | | | X | | | | | | | X | | | | | X | | | | | | | | | | X | X | | | | |
| Marjoram | | | | X | X | | | X | X | | | | X | | | | | X | X | X | X | X | X | | X | | | | | | | | | | | | | X | X | | X | X | X | X | X |
| Pennyroyal | | | | | | | | | | | | | | | | | | | | | | | | | | | | | | | X | | | | | | | | | | X | | | | |
| Raspberry Leaf | | | | | | | | | | | | X | | | | | X | | | | | X | | | | | | | | | | | | | | | | | | | X | | | | |
| Rue | | | | | | | X | X | | | | | | | | | | | | | | | | | | | | | | | X | | | | | | | | | | X | | | | |
| Shepherd's Purse | | | | | | | | | | | | X | | | | | | | | | | X | | | | | | | | | | | | | | | | | | | X | | | | |
| Squaw Vine | | | | | | | | | | | | | | | | | | | | | | | | | | | | | | | | | | | | | | | | | X | | | | |

| Herbs By Classifications | Adaptogens | Alterative | Amphoteric | Analgesic | Anodyne | Antacid & Anti-ulcer | Anthelmintics | Antibiotic | Anticatarrhal | Antiemetics | Antifungal | Antihemorrhagic | Anti-Inflammatory | Antilithics-Gallstone | Antilithics-Urinary |
|---|---|---|---|---|---|---|---|---|---|---|---|---|---|---|---|
| **Rubefacient** | | | | | | | | | | | | | | | |
| Allspice | | | | | | | | X | | | | | | | |
| Arnica | | | | X | X | | | | | | | | X | | |
| Black Mustard | | | | | | | | | | | | | | | |
| Black Pepper | | | | | | | | | | | | | | | |
| Camphor | | | | | | | | | | | | | | | |
| Cayenne | | | X | X | X | | | X | X | | X | X | | | |
| Eucalyptus | | | | | | | | X | | | | | | | |
| Garden Sage | | | | | | | | X | X | | X | | X | | X |
| Garlic | | X | | | | | X | X | X | | X | | | X | |
| Ginger | | | | X | | | X | X | X | X | | | | | |
| Horseradish | | | | | | | | | | | | | | | |
| Marjoram | | | | X | X | | | X | X | | | | X | | |
| Mustard | | | | | | | | | | | | | | | |
| Onion | | | | | | | | X | | | X | | | | |
| Peppermint | | | | X | | | | X | X | X | | | X | X | |
| Rosemary | | | | X | | | | | X | | X | | | | |

| Herbs By Classifications | Antiprotozoal | Antipyretic | Antirheumatic | Antispasmodic | Antiviral | Aperient | Astringent | Bitters | Cardiotonic | Carminative | Cathartic | Cholagogue | Demulcent | Diaphoretic | Diuretic |
|---|---|---|---|---|---|---|---|---|---|---|---|---|---|---|---|
| **Rubefacient** | | | | | | | | | | | | | | | |
| Allspice | | | | X | X | | | | | X | | | | | |
| Arnica | | | X | | | | | | | | | | | | |
| Black Mustard | | | | | | | | | | | | | | | |
| Black Pepper | | | | | | | | | | | | | | | |
| Camphor | | | | | | | | | | | | | | | |
| Cayenne | | | X | | | | | | X | | | | | X | |
| Eucalyptus | | | | | | | | | | | | | | | |
| Garden Sage | | X | X | X | X | | X | X | | X | | | | X | X |
| Garlic | X | | | | X | | | | X | X | | | | | |
| Ginger | X | X | X | X | X | | X | X | X | X | | | | X | X |
| Horseradish | | | | | | | | | | | | | | | |
| Marjoram | | | X | X | X | X | X | X | | X | | | | | |
| Mustard | | | | | | | | | | | | | | | |
| Onion | | | | X | | | | | | | | | | | |
| Peppermint | | | | X | X | | | | | X | | X | | X | |
| Rosemary | | | X | X | | | | | | X | | | | X | |

| Herbs By Classifications | Emmenagoguc | Expectorant | Galactogogue | Hematinic | Hepatic | Hypnotic | Hypotensive | Nervine Tonics | Nervine Relaxants | Nervine Stimulants | Oxytocic | Rubefacient | Sialogogue | Vasodilator | Vulnerary |
|---|---|---|---|---|---|---|---|---|---|---|---|---|---|---|---|
| **Rubefacient** | | | | | | | | | | | | | | | |
| Allspice | | | | | | | | | | | | X | | X | |
| Arnica | | | | | | | | | | | | X | | | X |
| Black Mustard | | | | | | | | | | | | X | | | |
| Black Pepper | | | | | | | | | | X | | X | X | | |
| Camphor | | | | | | | | | | | | X | | | |
| Cayenne | | | | | | | X | | | | | X | X | X | X |
| Eucalyptus | | | | | | | | | | | | X | | | |
| Garden Sage | X | | | | X | | | X | X | | | X | | | X |
| Garlic | | X | | | X | | X | | | X | | X | | X | X |
| Ginger | | X | | | X | | | | | X | X | X | X | X | |
| Horseradish | | | | | | | | | | X | | X | | | |
| Marjoram | | | | | | | | X | X | | X | X | X | X | X |
| Mustard | | | | | | | | | | | | X | | | |
| Onion | | X | | | | | X | | | | | X | | | |
| Peppermint | X | | | | | | | | | | | X | X | | |
| Rosemary | | | | | | | | | | X | | X | | X | |

## Herbs By Classifications

Category: **Sialogogue**

| Herbs By Classifications | Anise seed | Black Pepper | Cardamom | Cayenne | Cinnamon | Echinacea | Fennel | Fennel Seeds | Licorice | Licorice Root | Lovage | Marjoram | Peppermint | Sage | Yerba Santa |
|---|---|---|---|---|---|---|---|---|---|---|---|---|---|---|---|
| Adaptogens | | | | | | | | | × | × | | | | | |
| Alterative | | | | | | × | | | × | × | × | | | | |
| Amphoteric | | | | × | | | | | × | × | | | | | |
| Analgesic | | | | × | | | | | | | | × | | | |
| Anodyne | | | | × | | | | | | | | × | | | |
| Antacid & Anti-ulcer | | | | | | | | | × | × | | | | | |
| Anthelmintics | | | | | | | | | | | | | | | |
| Antibiotic | | | | × | × | × | | | × | × | × | | | | |
| Anticatarrhal | | | | × | | | | | × | × | × | × | | × | |
| Antiemetics | | | × | × | | | × | × | | × | | × | | | |
| Antifungal | | | | | × | × | | | | | | | | × | |
| Antihemorrhagic | | | | × | | | | | | | | | | | |
| Anti-Inflammatory | | | | × | | × | | | × | × | | × | | × | |
| Antilithics-Gallstone | | | | | | | | | | | | | × | | |
| Antilithics-Urinary | | | | | | | | | | | | | | | |
| Antiprotozoal | | | | | | | | | × | × | | | | | |
| Antipyretic | | | | | | × | | | | | | | × | | |
| Antirheumatic | | | | × | | | | | × | × | | | | | |
| Antispasmodic | | | | | | | × | × | | | | × | × | × | |
| Antiviral | | | | | | × | | | × | × | | × | | × | |
| Aperient | | | | | | | × | × | × | × | × | | | | |
| Astringent | | | | | | | | | | | | × | | × | |
| Bitters | | | | | | | | | × | × | | | | × | |
| Cardiotonic | | | | × | | | | | | | | | | | |
| Carminative | | × | × | | | | × | × | | | | × | × | × | |
| Cathartic | | | | | | | | | × | × | | | | | |
| Cholagogue | | | | | | | | | × | × | | | | | |
| Demulcent | | | | | | | | | × | × | × | | | | |
| Diaphoretic | | | | × | | × | | | | | × | | × | × | |
| Diuretic | | | | | | | | | | | × | | | | |
| Emmenagogue | | | | | | | | | | | | | × | × | |
| Expectorant | | | | | | | | | × | × | × | | | | × |
| Galactogogue | × | | | | | | × | × | | | | | | | |
| Hematinic | | | | | | × | | | | | | | | | |
| Hepatic | | | | | | | | | × | × | × | | | | |
| Hypnotic | | | | | | | | | | | | | | | |
| Hypotensive | | | | × | × | | | | | | | | | | |
| Nervine Tonics | | | | | | | | | | | | × | × | | |
| Nervine Relaxants | | | | | | | | | | | | × | × | | |
| Nervine Stimulants | | × | × | × | × | | | | | | | | | | |
| Oxytocic | | | | | | | | | | | | × | | | |
| Rubefacient | | × | | × | | | | | | | | × | × | | |
| Sialogogue | × | × | × | × | × | × | × | × | × | × | × | × | × | × | × |
| Vasodilator | | | | × | × | | | | | | | × | | | |
| Vulnerary | | | | × | | × | | | | | | × | | × | |

Table columns 1–23:

| Herbs By Classifications | Adaptogens | Alterative | Amphoteric | Analgesic | Anodyne | Antacid & Anti ulcer | Anthelmintics | Antibiotic | Anticatarrhal | Antiemetics | Antifungal | Antihemorrhagic | Anti-Inflammatory | Antilithics-Gallstone | Antilithics-Urinary | Antiprotozoal | Antipyretic | Antirheumatic | Antispasmodic | Antiviral | Aperient | Astringent | Bitters |
|---|---|---|---|---|---|---|---|---|---|---|---|---|---|---|---|---|---|---|---|---|---|---|---|
| **Vasodilator** | | | | | | | | | | | | | | | | | | | | | | | |
| Allspice | | | | | | | | X | | | | | | | | | | | X | X | | | |
| Astragalus | X | | X | | | | | | | | | | | | | | | | | X | | | |
| Butcher's Broom | | | | | | | | | | | | | | | | | | | | | | | |
| Cacao | | | | | | | | | | | | | | | | | | | | | | | |
| Cayenne | | | X | X | X | | | X | X | | | X | X | | | | X | X | | | | | |
| Cinnamon | | | | | | | | X | | X | X | | | | | | | | X | | | X | |
| Garlic | | X | | | | | X | X | X | | X | | | | | X | | | | X | | | |
| Ginger | | | | X | | | X | X | X | X | | X | X | | | X | X | X | X | X | | | X |
| Ginkgo | X | | | | | | | | | | | | | | | | | | | | | | |
| Ginkgo Biloba | X | | | | | | | | | | | | | | | | | | | | | | |
| Ginseng | | | X | | | | | | | | | | | | | | | | | | | | |
| Hawthorn | X | | | | | | | | | | | | | | | | | | | | | | |
| Horse Chestnut | | | | | | | | | | | | | | | | | | | | | | | |
| Linden | | | | | | | | | | | | | | | | | | | | | | | |
| Marjoram | | | | X | X | | | X | X | | | | X | | | | | | X | X | X | X | X |
| Mistletoe | | | | | | | | | | | | | | | X | | | | | | | | |
| Onion | | | | | | | | X | | | X | | X | | | | | | | X | | | |
| Prickly Ash | | X | | | | | | | | | | | | | | | | | | | | | |
| Rosemary | | | X | | | | | | X | | | | X | | | | | X | X | | | | |
| Turmeric | X | | X | X | X | X | X | X | | | | | X | X | | | | X | | | | | |
| Yarrow | | | X | X | | | | X | X | | | X | X | | | | X | | | | | X | |

Table columns 24–45:

| Herbs By Classifications | Cardiotonic | Carminative | Cathartic | Cholagogue | Demulcent | Diaphoretic | Diuretic | Emmenagogue | Expectorant | Galactogogue | Hematinic | Hepatic | Hypnotic | Hypotensive | Nervine Tonics | Nervine Relaxants | Nervine Stimulants | Oxytocic | Rubefacient | Sialogogue | Vasodilator | Vulnerary |
|---|---|---|---|---|---|---|---|---|---|---|---|---|---|---|---|---|---|---|---|---|---|---|
| **Vasodilator** | | | | | | | | | | | | | | | | | | | | | | |
| Allspice | | X | | | | | | | | | | | | | | | | | X | | X | |
| Astragalus | X | | | | | | | | | | X | X | | X | | | | | | | X | |
| Butcher's Broom | | | | | | | | | | | | | | | | | | | | | X | |
| Cacao | | | | | | | | | | | | | | | | | | | | | X | |
| Cayenne | X | | | | | X | | | | | | | | X | | | X | | X | | X | X |
| Cinnamon | X | X | | | X | | | | | | | | | X | | | | | | | X | |
| Garlic | X | X | | | | X | | | X | | | | | X | | | | | | | X | X |
| Ginger | | X | | | | X | X | X | | | | X | | X | | | X | X | X | | X | |
| Ginkgo | X | | | | | | | | | | | | | | | | | | | | X | |
| Ginkgo Biloba | X | | | | | | | | | | | | | | | | | | | | X | |
| Ginseng | | | | | | | | | | | | | | | | | | | | | X | |
| Hawthorn | X | | | | | | X | | | | | | | | | | | | | | X | |
| Horse Chestnut | | | | | | | | | | | | | | | | | | | | | X | |
| Linden | X | | | | | | | | | | | | X | X | X | X | | | | | X | |
| Marjoram | | X | | | | | | | | | | | | | X | X | | X | X | X | X | X |
| Mistletoe | | | | | | | | | | | | | | X | | | | | | | X | |
| Onion | | | | | | | | | X | | | | | X | | | | | | | X | |
| Prickly Ash | | | | | | | | | | | | | | | | | | | | | X | |
| Rosemary | | | | X | | X | | | | | | X | | | | | | | X | | X | |
| Turmeric | | | | X | | | | | | | | X | | | | | | | | | X | |
| Yarrow | X | | | | | X | | | | | | | | X | | | | | | | X | X |

The table lists herbs (column headers) against herbal-action classifications (row labels); an "X" marks that the herb has that action. Because of the page width it is presented here in two column-groups.

| Herbs By Classifications | Aloe Vera | Arnica | Calendula | Cayenne | Chamomile | Comfrey | Echinacea | Elder | Elderberry | Elderflower | Garden Sage | Garlic | Goldenseal | Gotu Kola | Gumweed | Lavender |
|---|---|---|---|---|---|---|---|---|---|---|---|---|---|---|---|---|
| Vulnerary | X | X | X | X | X | X | X | X | X | X | X | X | X | X | X | X |
| Vasodilator |  |  |  | X |  |  |  |  |  |  |  | X |  |  |  |  |
| Sialogogue |  |  |  | X |  |  | X |  |  |  |  |  |  |  |  |  |
| Rubefacient |  | X |  | X |  |  |  |  |  |  |  | X |  |  |  |  |
| Oxytocic |  |  |  |  |  |  |  |  |  |  |  |  |  |  |  |  |
| Nervine Stimulants |  |  |  | X |  |  |  |  |  |  | X |  |  | X |  |  |
| Nervine Relaxants |  |  |  |  | X |  |  |  |  |  | X |  |  |  |  |  |
| Nervine Tonics |  |  |  |  | X |  |  |  |  |  | X |  |  | X |  |  |
| Hypotensive |  |  |  |  | X |  |  |  |  |  | X | X |  |  |  |  |
| Hypnotic |  |  |  |  |  |  |  |  |  |  |  | X |  |  |  |  |
| Hepatic |  |  |  |  |  |  |  |  |  |  | X |  |  |  |  |  |
| Hematinic |  |  |  |  | X |  |  |  |  |  |  |  |  |  |  |  |
| Galactogogue |  |  |  |  |  |  |  |  |  |  |  |  |  |  |  |  |
| Expectorant |  |  |  |  | X |  |  | X | X | X |  | X |  | X |  |  |
| Emmenagogue |  |  | X |  | X |  |  |  |  |  | X |  |  |  |  |  |
| Diuretic |  |  |  |  |  |  |  | X | X | X | X |  |  |  |  |  |
| Diaphoretic |  |  |  | X | X |  |  | X | X | X | X |  |  |  |  |  |
| Demulcent | X |  |  |  | X |  |  |  |  |  |  |  |  |  |  |  |
| Cholagogue |  |  |  |  |  |  |  |  |  |  |  |  |  |  |  |  |
| Cathartic |  |  |  |  |  |  |  |  |  |  |  |  |  |  |  |  |
| Carminative |  |  |  |  | X |  |  |  |  |  | X |  |  | X |  |  |
| Cardiotonic |  |  |  |  |  |  |  |  |  |  | X |  |  |  |  |  |
| Bitters |  |  |  |  | X |  |  |  |  |  | X |  | X |  |  |  |
| Astringent |  |  |  |  |  |  |  |  |  |  | X |  |  |  |  |  |
| Aperient | X |  |  |  |  |  |  |  |  |  |  |  |  |  |  |  |
| Antiviral |  |  |  |  | X | X | X | X | X | X |  |  |  |  |  |  |
| Antispasmodic |  |  |  |  | X |  |  |  |  |  | X |  |  |  |  | X |
| Antirheumatic |  | X |  |  | X | X |  |  |  |  | X |  |  |  |  |  |
| Antipyretic |  |  |  |  | X |  | X | X | X | X |  |  |  | X |  |  |
| Antiprotozoal |  |  |  |  |  |  |  |  |  |  |  | X | X |  |  |  |
| Antilithics-Urinary |  |  |  |  |  |  |  |  |  |  | X |  |  |  |  | X |
| Antilithics-Gallstone |  |  |  |  |  |  |  |  |  |  |  |  |  |  |  |  |
| Anti-inflammatory | X | X | X | X | X | X | X |  |  |  | X |  |  | X |  |  |
| Antihemorrhagic |  |  | X | X |  | X |  |  |  |  | X |  |  |  |  |  |
| Antifungal | X |  | X |  | X |  | X |  |  |  | X | X | X |  |  |  |
| Antiemetics |  |  |  |  | X |  |  |  |  |  |  |  |  | X | X |  |
| Anticatarrhal |  |  |  | X |  |  |  |  | X |  | X | X |  |  |  |  |
| Antibiotic |  |  | X | X | X |  | X |  |  |  | X | X | X |  | X |  |
| Anthelmintics |  |  |  |  |  |  |  |  |  |  |  | X |  |  |  |  |
| Antacid & Anti-ulcer |  |  | X |  | X | X |  |  |  |  |  |  | X |  |  |  |
| Anodyne |  | X |  | X | X |  |  |  |  |  |  |  |  | X |  |  |
| Analgesic |  | X |  | X | X |  |  |  |  |  |  |  |  | X |  |  |
| Amphoteric |  |  |  | X |  |  |  |  |  |  |  | X |  |  |  |  |
| Alterative | X |  | X |  | X | X |  |  |  |  | X |  |  |  |  |  |
| Adaptogens |  |  |  |  |  |  |  |  |  |  |  |  |  | X |  |  |

| Herbs By Classifications | Mallow | Marjoram | Marshmallow | Marshmallow Root | Myrrh | Nasturtium | Onion | Plantain | Purslane | Sage | St. John's Wort | Sweet Cicely | Thyme | Witch Hazel | Yarrow |
|---|---|---|---|---|---|---|---|---|---|---|---|---|---|---|---|
| Vulnerary | X | X | X | X | X | X |  | X | X | X | X | X | X | X | X |
| Vasodilator |  | X |  |  |  |  |  |  |  |  |  |  |  |  | X |
| Sialogogue |  | X |  |  |  |  |  |  |  | X |  |  |  |  |  |
| Rubefacient |  | X |  |  |  |  |  |  |  |  |  |  |  |  |  |
| Oxytocic |  | X |  |  |  |  |  |  |  |  |  |  |  |  |  |
| Nervine Stimulants |  |  |  |  |  |  |  |  |  |  |  |  |  |  | X |
| Nervine Relaxants |  | X |  |  |  |  |  |  |  | X | X |  |  |  |  |
| Nervine Tonics |  | X |  |  |  |  |  |  |  | X | X |  |  |  |  |
| Hypotensive |  | X |  |  |  |  |  | X |  |  |  |  |  |  | X |
| Hypnotic |  |  |  |  |  |  |  |  |  |  |  |  |  |  |  |
| Hepatic |  |  |  |  |  |  |  |  |  |  |  |  |  |  |  |
| Hematinic |  |  |  |  |  |  |  |  |  |  |  |  |  |  |  |
| Galactogogue |  |  |  |  |  |  |  |  |  |  |  |  |  |  |  |
| Expectorant |  |  |  |  |  | X |  |  |  |  |  |  | X |  |  |
| Emmenagogue |  |  |  |  |  |  |  |  |  | X |  |  |  |  |  |
| Diuretic |  |  |  |  | X |  |  | X | X |  |  |  |  |  |  |
| Diaphoretic |  |  |  |  | X | X |  |  |  | X |  |  |  |  | X |
| Demulcent | X |  | X | X |  |  |  | X | X |  |  |  |  |  |  |
| Cholagogue |  |  |  |  |  |  |  |  |  |  |  |  |  |  |  |
| Cathartic |  |  |  |  |  |  |  |  |  |  |  |  |  |  |  |
| Carminative |  | X |  |  |  |  |  |  |  | X |  |  | X |  |  |
| Cardiotonic |  | X |  |  |  |  |  |  |  |  |  |  |  |  | X |
| Bitters |  | X |  |  | X |  |  |  |  | X |  |  |  |  |  |
| Astringent |  | X |  |  | X |  | X | X | X |  |  |  |  | X | X |
| Aperient | X | X | X | X | X |  |  | X |  |  |  |  |  |  |  |
| Antiviral |  | X |  |  | X | X |  |  |  | X | X |  | X |  |  |
| Antispasmodic |  | X |  |  |  |  |  |  |  | X | X |  | X |  |  |
| Antirheumatic |  | X |  |  |  |  |  |  |  |  |  |  |  |  |  |
| Antipyretic |  |  |  |  |  |  |  |  |  | X |  |  | X |  | X |
| Antiprotozoal |  |  |  |  | X |  |  |  |  |  |  |  |  |  |  |
| Antilithics-Urinary |  |  | X | X | X |  |  |  |  |  |  |  |  |  |  |
| Antilithics-Gallstone |  |  |  |  | X |  |  |  |  |  |  |  |  |  |  |
| Anti-inflammatory | X | X | X | X | X | X | X | X | X | X |  |  |  |  | X |
| Antihemorrhagic |  |  | X |  |  |  |  | X | X |  |  |  | X |  | X |
| Antifungal | X | X | X |  | X | X |  | X |  | X |  |  | X | X |  |
| Antiemetics | X | X | X |  | X |  |  | X |  |  |  |  |  |  |  |
| Anticatarrhal | X | X | X | X | X |  |  |  |  | X | X |  |  |  | X |
| Antibiotic |  | X |  | X | X | X |  | X | X | X | X |  | X |  | X |
| Anthelmintics |  |  |  |  | X |  |  |  |  |  |  |  |  |  |  |
| Antacid & Anti-ulcer |  |  |  |  |  |  |  |  |  |  |  |  |  |  |  |
| Anodyne |  | X |  |  |  |  |  |  |  |  |  |  |  |  | X |
| Analgesic |  | X |  |  |  |  |  |  |  | X |  |  |  | X | X |
| Amphoteric |  |  |  |  | X |  |  | X | X |  |  |  |  |  |  |
| Alterative | X |  | X | X |  | X |  | X | X |  |  |  |  |  |  |
| Adaptogens |  |  |  |  |  |  |  |  |  |  |  |  |  |  |  |

# SECTION III

## Alphabetized Herbs With Classifications

| Herbs in Alphabetical Order | Adaptogens | Alterative | Amphoteric | Analgesic | Anodyne | Antacid & Anti-ulcer | Anthelmintics | Antibiotic | Anticatarrhal | Antiemetics | Antifungal | Antihemorrhagic | Anti-Inflammatory | Antilithics-Gallstone | Antilithics-Urinary | Antiprotozoal | Antipyretic | Antirheumatic | Antispasmodic | Antiviral | Aperient | Astringent | Bitters | Cardiotonic | Carminative | Cathartic | Cholagogue | Demulcent | Diaphoretic | Diuretic | Emmenagogue | Expectorant | Galactogogue | Hematinic | Hepatic | Hypnotic | Hypotensive | Nervine Tonics | Nervine Relaxants | Nervine Stimulants | Oxytocic | Rubefacient | Sialogogue | Vasodilator | Vulnerary |
|---|---|---|---|---|---|---|---|---|---|---|---|---|---|---|---|---|---|---|---|---|---|---|---|---|---|---|---|---|---|---|---|---|---|---|---|---|---|---|---|---|---|---|---|---|---|
| Agrimony | | | | | | | | | | | | | X | | | | | | | | | X | X | | | | | | | X | | | | | | | | | | | | | | | |
| Albizia | | | | | | | | | | | | | | | | | | | | | | | | | | | | | | | | | | X | | | | | | | | | | | |
| Alder Buckthorn | | | | | | | | | | | | | | | | | | | | | | | | | | X | | | | | | | | | | | | | | | | | | | |
| Alfalfa | | X | | | | | | | | | | | | | | X | | | | | X | | | | | | | | | X | | | X | X | | | | | | | | | | | |
| Allspice | | | | | | | | X | | | | | | | | | | | X | X | | | | | X | | | | | | | | | | | | | | | | | X | | X | |
| Aloe Vera | | X | | | | | | | | | X | | X | | | | | | | | X | | | | | | | X | | | | | | | | | | | | | | | | | X |
| Aloe Vera Leaf | | | | | | | | | | | | | | | | | | | | | | | | | | X | | | | | | | | | | | | | | | | | | | |
| Alum | | | | | | | | | | | | | | | | | | | | | | X | | | | | | | | | | | | | | | | | | | | | | | |
| American Ginseng | X | | | | | | | | | | | | | | | | | | | | | | | | | | | | | | | | | | | | | | | | | X | | | |
| American Skullcap | X | | | | | | | | | | | | | | | | | | | | | | | | | | | | | | | | | | | | | | | | | | | | |
| Andrographis | | | | | | | | X | | | | | | | | | | | | X | | | | | | | | | | | | | | | | | | | | | | | X | | |
| Angelica | | | | | | | | | | | | | | | | | | X | X | | | | | | X | | | | | | X | | | | | | | | | | X | X | | | |
| Anise seeds | | | | | | | | | X | | X | | | | | | | X | X | | | | | | X | | | | | | | X | X | | | | | | | | | | X | | |
| Arjuna | | | | | | | | | | | | | | | | | | | | | | | | | | | | | | | | | | | | | X | | | | | | | | |
| Arnica | | | | X | X | | | | | | | | X | | | | | X | | | | | | | | | | | | | | | | | | | | | | | | X | | | X |
| Artichoke | | | | | | | | | | | | | | X | | | | | | | | | X | | | | X | | | | | | | | X | | | | | | | | | | |
| Ashitaba | | | X | | | | | | | | | | | | | | | | | | | | | | | | | | | | | | | | | | | | | | | | | | |
| Ashwagandha | X | | X | | | | | | | | | | | | | | | | | | | | | | | | | | | | | | | X | | X | | X | X | X | | | | | |
| Aspen | | | X | | | | | | | | | | X | | | | X | | | | | | | | | | | | | | | | | | | | | | | | | | | | |
| Astragalus | X | X | | | | | | | | | | | | | | | X | | | | | | | | | | | | X | | | | | X | X | | X | | | | | | | X | |
| Baneberry | | X | | | | | | | | | | | | | | | X | | | | | | | | | | | | | | | | | | | | | | | | | | | | |
| Barberry | | | | | | | | X | | | | | | | | | | | | | | | X | | X | | X | | | | | | | | X | | | | | | | | | | |
| Basil | X | | | | | | | X | | X | X | | | | | | X | | | | | | | | X | | | | X | | | X | | | | | | X | | | | | | | |
| Bay Leaves | | | | | | | | X | | | X | | | | | | | | | | | | | | X | X | X | | X | | | | | | | | | | | | | | | | |
| Bearberry | | | | | | | | | | | | | | | X | | | | | | | | | | | | | | | X | | | | | | | | | | | | | | | |
| Bee Balm | | | | | | | | X | | | | | | | | | | | | | | | | | | | | | | | | | | | | | | | | | | | | | |
| Bergamot | | | | | | | | X | | | X | | X | | | | | | | X | | | | | | | | | X | | | | | | | | | | | | | | | | |
| Bilberry | | | | X | | | | | | | | | | | | | | | | X | | | | | | | | | | | | | | | X | | | | | | | | | | |
| Birch | | X | | | | | | | | | | | X | | | | | X | | X | | | | | | | | | | | | | | | | | | | | | | | | | |
| Bitter Leaf | | | | | | | X | | | | | | | | | | | | | | | | | | | | | | | | | | | | | | | | | | | | | | |
| Bitter Melon | | | | | | | | | | | | | | | | | | | | | | | X | | | | | | | | | | | | | | | | | | | | | | |

| Herbs in Alphabetical Order | Adaptogens | Alterative | Amphoteric | Analgesic | Anodyne | Antacid & Anti-ulcer | Anthelmintics | Antibiotic | Anticatarrhal | Antiemetics | Antifungal | Antihemorrhagic | Anti-Inflammatory | Antilithics-Gallstone | Antilithics-Urinary | Antiprotozoal | Antipyretic | Antirheumatic | Antispasmodic | Antiviral | Aperient | Astringent | Bitters | Cardiotonic | Carminative | Cathartic | Cholagogue | Demulcent | Diaphoretic | Diuretic | Emmenagogue | Expectorant | Galactogogue | Hematinic | Hepatic | Hypnotic | Hypotensive | Nervine Tonics | Nervine Relaxants | Nervine Stimulants | Oxytocic | Rubefacient | Sialogogue | Vasodilator | Vulnerary |
|---|---|---|---|---|---|---|---|---|---|---|---|---|---|---|---|---|---|---|---|---|---|---|---|---|---|---|---|---|---|---|---|---|---|---|---|---|---|---|---|---|---|---|---|---|---|
| Black Cohosh | X | | | X | X | | | | | | | | | | | | | | X | | | | | | | | | | | | X | | | | | | | | X | | X | | | | |
| Black Current | | | | | | | | | | | | | | | | | | X | | | | | | | | | | | | | | | | | | | | | | | | | | | |
| Black haw | | | | | | | | | | | | X | | | | | | X | | | | | | | | | | | | | | | | | | | | | | | | | | | |
| Black hellebore | | | | | | | | | | | | | | | | | | | | | | | | | | X | | | | | | | | | | | | | | | | | | | |
| Black Horehound | | | | | | | | | | X | | | | | | | | | | | | | | | | | | | | | | | | | | | | | | | | | | | |
| Black Mustard | | | | | | | | | | | | | | | | | | | | | | | | | | | | | | | | | | | | | | | | | | X | | | |
| Black Pepper | | | | | | | | | | | | | | | | | | | | | | | | | | | | | | | | | | | | | | | | X | | X | X | | |
| Black Seed | | | | | | | | | | | | | | | | | | | | | | | | | | | | | | | | X | | | | | | | | | | | | | |
| Black Walnut Hull | | | | | | | X | | | | X | | | | | X | | | | | | | | | | | | | | | | | | | | | | | | | | | | | |
| Blackberry | | | | | | | | | | | | X | | | | | | | | | | X | | | | | | | | | | | | | | | | | | | | | | | |
| Blackberry Leaf | | | | | | | | | | | | | | | | | | | | | | X | | | | | | | | | | | | | | | | | | | | | | | |
| Blessed Thistle | | | | | | | | | | | | | | | | | | | | | | | | | | | | | X | | | | X | | | | | | | | | | | | |
| Bloodroot | | | | | | | | | | | | X | | | | | | | | | | | | | | | | | | | | | | | | | | | | | | | | | |
| Blue Cohosh | | | | | | | | | | | | | | | | | | | | | | | | | | | | | X | | | | | | | | | | | | X | | | | |
| Blue Flag | | X | | | | | | | | | | | | | | | | | | | | | | | | | | | | | | | | | | | | | | | | | | | |
| Blue Vervain | | | | | | | | | | | | | | | | | | | | | | | | | | | | | | | | | | | | X | | X | X | | | | | | |
| Boldo | | | | | | | X | | | | | | X | | | | | | | | | | | | | | | | | X | | | | | X | | | | | | | | | | |
| Boneset | | | | | | | | | | | | | | | | | X | | | | | | | | | | | | X | | | | | | | | | | | | | | | | |
| Borage | | | | | | | | | | | | | | | | | | X | | | | | | | | | | | | | | | X | | | | | | | | | | | | |
| Boswellia | | | | X | X | | | | | | | | X | | | | | X | | | | | | | | | | | | | | | | | | | | | | | | | | | |
| Buchu | | | | | | | | | | | | | | | | | | | | | | | | | | | | | | X | | | | | | | | | | | | | | | |
| Buckthorn | | | | | | | | | | | | | | | | | | | | | | | | | | X | X | | | | | | | | | | | | | | | | | | |
| Bupleurum | | | | | | | | | | | | | | | | | | | | | | | | | | | X | | | | | | | | X | | | | | | | | | | |
| Burdock | | X | | | | | | | | | | | | | | | | X | | | X | | | | | | | | | X | | | | | X | | | | | | | | | | |
| Burdock Root | | | | | | | | | | | X | | X | X | | | | X | | | | | | | | | X | | | | | | | X | X | | | | | | | | | | |
| Butcher's Broom | | | | | | | | | | | | | | | | | | | | | | | | | | | | | | | | | | | | | | | | | | | | X | |
| Cacao | | | | | | | | | | | | | | | | | | | | | | | | | | | | | | | | | | | | | | | | | | | | X | |
| Calendula | | X | | X | | | X | | | | X | X | X | | | | | | | | | | | | | X | | | | | | | | | | | | | | | | | | | X |
| California Poppy | | | | | | | | | | | | | | | | | | | | | | | | | | | | | | | | | | | | X | | X | X | | | | | | |
| Camphor | | | | | | | | | | | | | | | | | | | | | | | | | | | | | | | | | | | | | | | | | | X | | | |
| Cannabis | | | | | | | | | | X | | | | | | | | | | | | | | | | | | | | | | | | | | | | | | | | | | | |

| Herbs in Alphabetical Order | Adaptogens | Alterative | Amphoteric | Analgesic | Anodyne | Antacid & Anti-ulcer | Anthelmintics | Antibiotic | Anticatarrhal | Antiemetics | Antifungal | Antihemorrhagic | Anti-Inflammatory | Antilithics-Gallstone | Antilithics-Urinary | Antiprotozoal | Antipyretic | Antirheumatic | Antispasmodic | Antiviral | Aperient | Astringent | Bitters | Cardiotonic | Carminative | Cathartic | Cholagogue | Demulcent | Diaphoretic | Diuretic | Emmenagogue | Expectorant | Galactogogue | Hematinic | Hepatic | Hypnotic | Hypotensive | Nervine Tonics | Nervine Relaxants | Nervine Stimulants | Oxytocic | Rubefacient | Sialogogue | Vasodilator | Vulnerary |
|---|---|---|---|---|---|---|---|---|---|---|---|---|---|---|---|---|---|---|---|---|---|---|---|---|---|---|---|---|---|---|---|---|---|---|---|---|---|---|---|---|---|---|---|---|---|
| Caraway |  |  |  |  |  |  |  |  |  |  |  |  |  |  |  |  |  |  | X |  |  |  |  |  | X |  |  |  |  |  |  |  | X |  |  |  |  |  |  |  |  |  |  |  |  |
| Cardamom |  |  |  |  |  |  |  |  |  | X |  |  |  |  |  |  |  |  |  |  |  |  |  |  | X |  |  |  |  |  |  |  |  |  |  |  |  |  |  | X |  |  | X |  |  |
| Cascara amarga |  |  |  |  |  |  |  |  |  |  |  |  |  |  |  |  |  |  |  |  |  |  |  |  |  | X |  |  |  |  |  |  |  |  |  |  |  |  |  |  |  |  |  |  |  |
| Cascara sagrada |  |  |  |  |  |  |  |  |  |  |  |  |  | X |  |  |  |  |  |  | X |  |  |  |  | X |  |  |  |  |  |  |  |  |  |  |  |  |  |  |  |  |  |  |  |
| Cascarilla |  |  |  |  |  |  | X |  |  |  |  |  |  |  |  |  |  |  |  |  |  |  |  |  |  |  |  |  |  |  |  |  |  |  |  |  |  |  |  |  |  |  |  |  |  |
| Cassia |  |  |  |  |  |  |  |  |  |  |  |  |  |  |  |  |  |  |  |  |  |  |  |  |  | X |  |  |  |  |  |  |  |  |  |  |  |  |  |  |  |  |  |  |  |
| Catnip |  |  |  |  |  |  |  |  |  | X |  |  |  |  |  |  | X |  | X |  |  |  |  |  |  |  |  |  | X |  |  |  |  |  |  | X |  | X | X |  |  |  |  |  |  |
| Cat's Claw |  |  |  |  |  |  |  |  |  |  |  |  | X |  |  |  |  | X |  | X |  |  |  |  |  |  |  |  |  |  |  |  |  |  |  |  | X |  |  |  |  |  |  |  |  |
| Cayenne |  |  | X | X | X |  |  | X | X |  |  | X | X |  |  |  |  |  | X |  |  |  |  | X |  |  |  |  | X |  |  |  |  |  |  |  | X |  |  | X |  | X | X | X | X |
| Celery |  |  |  |  |  |  |  |  |  |  |  |  |  |  |  |  |  |  |  |  |  |  |  |  |  |  |  |  |  | X |  |  |  |  |  |  | X |  |  |  |  |  |  |  |  |
| Celery Seed |  |  |  |  |  |  |  |  |  |  |  |  |  |  | X |  |  |  |  |  |  |  |  |  | X |  |  |  |  |  |  |  |  |  |  |  |  |  |  |  |  |  |  |  |  |
| Centaury |  |  |  |  |  |  |  |  |  |  |  |  |  |  |  |  |  |  |  |  |  |  | X |  |  |  |  |  |  |  |  |  |  |  |  |  |  |  |  |  |  |  |  |  |  |
| Chamomile |  |  |  | X | X | X |  | X |  | X | X |  | X |  |  |  | X | X | X |  |  |  | X |  | X |  |  |  | X |  | X |  |  |  |  | X |  | X | X |  |  |  |  |  | X |
| Chanca Piedra |  |  |  |  |  |  |  |  |  |  |  |  |  |  | X |  |  |  |  |  |  |  |  |  |  |  |  |  |  |  |  |  |  |  |  |  |  |  |  |  |  |  |  |  |  |
| Chaparral |  | X |  |  |  |  |  | X |  |  | X |  |  |  |  | X |  |  |  | X |  |  |  |  |  |  |  |  |  |  |  |  |  |  |  |  |  |  |  |  |  |  |  |  |  |
| Chaste Tree |  |  |  |  |  |  |  |  |  |  |  |  |  |  |  |  |  |  |  |  |  |  |  |  |  |  |  |  |  |  | X |  | X |  |  |  |  |  |  |  |  |  |  |  |  |
| Chenopodium Oil |  |  |  |  |  |  | X |  |  |  |  |  |  |  |  |  |  |  |  |  |  |  |  |  |  |  |  |  |  |  |  |  |  |  |  |  |  |  |  |  |  |  |  |  |  |
| Chia Seeds |  |  |  |  |  |  |  |  |  |  |  |  |  |  |  |  |  |  |  |  |  |  |  |  |  |  |  | X |  |  |  |  |  | X |  |  |  |  |  |  |  |  |  |  |  |
| Chickpeas |  |  |  |  |  |  |  |  |  |  |  |  |  |  |  |  |  |  |  |  |  |  |  |  |  |  |  |  |  | X |  |  |  | X |  |  |  |  |  |  |  |  |  |  |  |
| Chickweed |  |  |  |  |  |  |  |  |  |  |  |  | X |  |  |  |  |  |  |  |  |  |  |  |  |  |  |  |  | X |  |  |  | X |  |  |  |  |  |  |  |  |  |  |  |
| Chicory |  |  |  |  |  |  |  |  |  |  |  |  |  |  |  |  |  |  |  |  |  |  | X |  |  |  | X |  |  | X |  |  |  | X |  |  |  |  |  |  |  |  |  |  |  |
| Chicory Root |  |  |  |  |  |  |  |  |  |  |  |  |  |  |  |  |  |  |  |  |  |  | X |  |  |  | X |  |  | X |  |  |  |  |  |  |  |  |  |  |  |  |  |  |  |
| Chlorella |  | X | X |  |  |  |  |  |  |  |  |  |  |  |  |  |  |  |  |  |  |  |  |  |  |  |  |  |  |  |  |  |  |  |  |  |  |  |  |  |  |  |  |  |  |
| Cilantro |  |  |  |  |  |  |  |  |  | X |  |  |  |  |  |  |  |  |  |  |  |  |  |  | X |  |  |  |  |  |  |  |  |  |  |  |  |  |  |  |  |  |  |  |  |
| Cinnamon |  |  |  |  |  |  |  | X |  | X | X |  |  |  |  |  |  |  |  |  |  |  |  |  | X |  |  |  |  |  | X |  |  |  |  |  | X |  |  | X |  |  | X | X |  |
| Cinquefoil |  |  |  |  |  |  |  |  |  | X |  |  |  |  |  |  |  |  |  |  |  |  |  |  |  |  |  |  |  |  |  |  |  |  |  |  |  |  |  |  |  |  |  |  |  |
| Cleavers |  | X |  |  |  |  |  |  |  |  |  |  |  |  | X |  |  |  |  |  |  |  |  |  |  |  |  |  |  | X |  |  |  |  | X |  |  |  |  |  |  |  |  |  |  |
| Clematis |  |  |  | X |  |  |  |  |  |  |  |  |  |  |  |  |  |  |  |  |  |  |  |  |  |  |  |  |  |  |  |  |  |  |  |  |  |  |  |  |  |  |  |  |  |
| Cloves |  |  |  | X | X |  | X | X |  | X | X |  |  |  |  |  |  |  |  |  |  |  |  |  | X |  |  |  |  |  |  |  |  |  |  |  |  |  |  | X |  |  |  |  |  |
| Coleus Forskohlii |  |  |  |  |  |  |  |  |  |  |  |  |  |  |  |  |  |  |  |  |  |  |  | X |  |  |  |  |  |  |  |  |  |  |  |  |  |  |  |  |  |  |  |  |  |
| Coltsfoot |  |  |  |  |  |  |  |  | X |  |  |  |  |  |  |  |  |  |  |  |  |  |  |  |  |  |  | X |  |  |  | X |  |  |  |  |  |  |  |  |  |  |  |  |  |

| Herbs in Alphabetical Order | Adaptogens | Alterative | Amphoteric | Analgesic | Anodyne | Antacid & Anti-ulcer | Anthelmintics | Antibiotic | Anticatarrhal | Antiemetics | Antifungal | Antihemorrhagic | Anti-Inflammatory | Antilithics-Gallstone | Antilithics-Urinary | Antiprotozoal | Antipyretic | Antirheumatic | Antispasmodic | Antiviral | Aperient | Astringent | Bitters | Cardiotonic | Carminative | Cathartic | Cholagogue | Demulcent | Diaphoretic | Diuretic | Emmenagogue | Expectorant | Galactogogue | Hematinic | Hepatic | Hypnotic | Hypotensive | Nervine Tonics | Nervine Relaxants | Nervine Stimulants | Oxytocic | Rubefacient | Sialogogue | Vasodilator | Vulnerary |
|---|---|---|---|---|---|---|---|---|---|---|---|---|---|---|---|---|---|---|---|---|---|---|---|---|---|---|---|---|---|---|---|---|---|---|---|---|---|---|---|---|---|---|---|---|---|
| Comfrey | | X | | | | X | | | | | | X | X | | | | | | | | | | | | | | | X | | | | X | | | | | | | | | | | | | X |
| Cordyceps | X | | X | | | | | | | | | | | | | | | | | | | | | | | | | | | | | | | | | | | | | | | | | | |
| Coriander | | | | | | | | | X | | | | | | | | | | | | X | | | | X | | | | | | | | | | | | | | | | | | | | |
| Corn Silk | | | | | | | | | | | | | | | X | | | | | | | | | | | | | X | | X | | | | | | | | | | | | | | | |
| Cotton Root Bark | | | | | | | | | | | | | | | | | | | | | | | | | | | | | | | | | | | | | | | | | X | | | | |
| Couchgrass | | | | | | | | | | | | | | | X | | | | | | | | | | | | | | | X | | | | | | | | | | | | | | | |
| Cramp Bark | | | | | | | | | | | | | | | | | | | X | | | | | | | | | | | X | | | | | | | X | | X | | X | | | | |
| Cranberry | | | | | | | | X | | | | | | | | | | | | | | | | | | | | | | | | | | | | | | | | | | | | | |
| Cranesbill | | | | | | | | | | | | X | | | | | | | | | | X | | | | | | | | | | | | | | | | | | | | | | | |
| Cumin | | | | | | | | | | | | | | | | | | | | | | | | | X | | | | | | | | X | | | | | | | | | | | | |
| Cypress | | | | | | | | | | | | X | | | | | | | | | | | | | | | | | | | | | | | | | | | | | | | | | |
| Damiana | | | | | | | | | | | | | | | | | | | | | | | | | | | | | | | | | | | | | | | | X | | | | | |
| Dandelion | | X | | | | | | | | | | | | X | X | | | | | | X | | X | | | | X | | | X | | | | X | X | | | | | | | | | | |
| Dandelion Root | | X | | | | | | | | | | | | X | X | | | | | | X | | X | | | | X | | | X | | | | X | X | | | | | | | | | | |
| Danshen | | | | | | | | | | | | | | | | | | | | | | | | X | | | | | | | | | | | | | | | | | | | | | |
| Devil's Claw | | | | X | X | | | | | | | | X | | | | | X | | | | | | | | | | | | | | | | | | | | | | | | | | | |
| Dill | | | | | | | | | | X | | | | | | | | | | | | | | | X | | | | | | | | X | | | | | | | | | | | | |
| Dill Seed | | | | | | | | | | X | | | | | | | | | | | | | | | X | | | | | | | | X | | | | | | | | | | | | |
| Dong Quai | | | | | | | | | | | | | | | | | | | | | | | | | | | | | | | X | | | X | | | | | | | | | | | |
| Echinacea | | X | | | | | | X | | | X | | X | | | | X | | | X | | | | | | | | | X | | | | | | | | | | | | | | X | | X |
| Elder | | | | | | | | | X | | | | | | | | X | | | X | | | | | | | | | X | X | | X | | | | | | | | | | | | | X |
| Elderberry | | | | | | | | | | | | | | | | | X | | | X | | | | | | | | | X | X | | X | | | | | | | | | | | | | X |
| Elderflower | | | | | | | | | | | | | | | | | X | | | X | | | | | | | | | X | X | | X | | | | | | | | | | | | | X |
| Elecampane | | | | | | | X | X | X | | | | | | | | | | | | | | | | | | | | | | | X | | | | | | | | | | | | | |
| Eleuthero | X | | | | | | | | | | | | | | | | | | | | | | | | | | | | | | | | | | | | | | | | | | | | |
| Eucalyptus | | | | | | | | | X | | | | | | | | | | | | | | | | | | | | | | | X | | | | | | | | | | X | | | |
| Fennel | | | | | | | | | | X | | | | | | | | | X | | X | | | | X | | | | | X | | | X | | | | | | | | | | X | X | |
| Fennel Seeds | | | | | | | | | | X | | | | | | | | | X | | X | | | | X | | | | | X | | | X | | | | | | | | | | X | X | |
| Fenugreek seeds | | | | | | | | | | | | | | | | | | | | | X | | | | | | | X | | | | X | X | | | | | | | | | | | | |
| Feverfew | | | | X | | | | | | | | | | | | | | | | | | | | | | | | | | | | | | | | | | | | | | | | | |
| Fireweed | | | | | | | | | | | X | | | | | | | | | | | | | | | | | | | | | | | | | | | | | | | | | | |

**Herbs in Alphabetical Order**

Columns 1–15 (Adaptogens – Antilithics-Urinary):

| Herbs in Alphabetical Order | Adaptogens | Alterative | Amphoteric | Analgesic | Anodyne | Antacid & Anti-ulcer | Anthelmintics | Antibiotic | Anticatarrhal | Antiemetics | Antifungal | Antihemorrhagic | Anti-Inflammatory | Antilithics-Gallstone | Antilithics-Urinary |
|---|---|---|---|---|---|---|---|---|---|---|---|---|---|---|---|
| Flax |  |  |  |  |  |  |  |  |  |  |  |  |  |  |  |
| Fringe Tree |  |  |  |  |  |  |  |  |  |  |  |  | X |  |  |
| Frankincense |  |  |  | X | X |  |  |  |  |  |  |  | X |  |  |
| French Lavendar |  |  |  |  |  |  |  |  |  |  |  |  |  |  |  |
| Garden Sage |  |  |  |  |  |  |  | X | X |  | X |  | X |  | X |
| Garlic |  | X |  |  |  |  | X | X | X |  | X |  |  |  |  |
| Gentian |  |  |  |  |  |  |  | X |  |  |  |  |  |  |  |
| Geranium |  |  |  |  |  |  |  |  |  |  |  |  |  |  |  |
| Germander |  |  |  |  |  |  |  |  |  |  |  | X |  |  |  |
| Ginger |  |  |  | X |  |  |  | X | X | X |  |  |  |  |  |
| Ginkgo | X |  |  |  |  |  |  |  |  |  |  |  |  |  |  |
| Ginkgo Biloba | X |  |  |  |  |  |  |  |  |  |  |  |  |  |  |
| Ginseng |  |  | X |  |  |  |  |  |  |  |  |  |  |  |  |
| Globe Artichoke |  |  |  |  |  |  |  |  |  |  |  |  |  | X |  |
| Goat's Rue |  |  |  |  |  |  |  |  |  |  |  |  |  |  |  |
| Goldenrod |  |  |  |  |  |  |  |  | X |  |  |  |  |  | X |
| Goldenseal |  |  |  |  |  |  |  |  | X |  |  |  |  |  |  |
| Gotu Kola | X |  | X |  |  | X |  |  |  |  |  |  |  |  |  |
| Gravel Root |  |  |  |  |  |  |  |  |  |  |  |  |  |  | X |
| Greater Celandine |  |  |  |  |  |  |  |  |  |  |  |  | X |  |  |
| Green Tea |  |  |  |  |  |  |  |  |  |  |  |  | X |  |  |
| Guarana |  |  |  |  |  |  |  |  |  |  |  |  |  |  |  |
| Gumweed |  |  |  |  |  |  |  |  | X |  |  |  | X |  |  |
| Hawthorn | X |  |  |  |  |  |  |  |  |  |  |  |  |  |  |
| Hibiscus |  |  |  |  |  |  |  |  |  |  |  |  |  |  |  |
| Hollyhock |  |  |  |  |  |  |  |  |  |  |  |  |  |  |  |
| Holy Basil | X |  | X |  |  |  |  |  |  |  |  |  |  |  |  |
| Hops |  |  |  |  |  |  |  |  |  |  |  |  |  |  |  |
| Horehound |  |  |  |  |  |  |  | X |  |  |  |  |  |  |  |
| Horse Chestnut |  |  |  |  |  |  |  |  |  |  |  |  |  |  |  |

Columns 16–30 (Antiprotozoal – Diuretic):

| Herbs in Alphabetical Order | Antiprotozoal | Antipyretic | Antirheumatic | Antispasmodic | Antiviral | Aperient | Astringent | Bitters | Cardiotonic | Carminative | Cathartic | Cholagogue | Demulcent | Diaphoretic | Diuretic |
|---|---|---|---|---|---|---|---|---|---|---|---|---|---|---|---|
| Flax |  |  |  |  |  | X |  |  |  |  |  |  | X |  |  |
| Fringe Tree |  |  |  |  |  |  |  |  |  |  |  | X |  |  |  |
| Frankincense |  |  | X |  |  |  |  |  |  |  |  |  |  |  |  |
| French Lavendar |  |  |  |  |  |  |  |  |  |  |  |  |  |  |  |
| Garden Sage |  | X | X | X | X |  | X | X |  | X |  |  |  | X | X |
| Garlic | X |  |  |  |  |  |  |  | X | X |  |  |  |  |  |
| Gentian |  |  |  |  |  |  |  | X |  |  |  | X |  |  |  |
| Geranium |  |  |  |  |  |  | X |  |  |  |  |  |  |  |  |
| Germander |  |  |  |  |  |  |  |  |  |  |  |  |  |  |  |
| Ginger |  | X | X | X | X |  |  | X | X | X |  |  |  | X | X |
| Ginkgo |  |  |  |  |  |  |  |  | X |  |  |  |  |  |  |
| Ginkgo Biloba |  |  |  |  |  |  |  |  | X |  |  |  |  |  |  |
| Ginseng |  |  |  |  |  |  |  |  |  |  |  |  |  |  |  |
| Globe Artichoke |  |  |  |  |  |  |  |  |  |  |  |  |  |  |  |
| Goat's Rue |  |  |  |  |  |  |  |  |  |  |  |  |  |  |  |
| Goldenrod |  |  |  |  |  |  |  |  |  |  |  |  |  |  | X |
| Goldenseal | X |  | X |  |  |  |  | X |  |  |  | X |  |  |  |
| Gotu Kola |  |  |  |  |  |  |  |  |  |  |  |  |  |  |  |
| Gravel Root |  |  |  |  |  |  |  |  |  |  |  |  |  |  | X |
| Greater Celandine |  |  |  |  |  |  |  |  |  |  |  | X |  |  |  |
| Green Tea |  |  |  |  |  |  |  |  |  |  |  |  |  |  | X |
| Guarana |  |  |  |  |  |  |  |  |  |  |  |  |  |  |  |
| Gumweed |  |  |  |  |  |  |  |  |  |  |  |  |  |  |  |
| Hawthorn |  |  |  |  |  |  |  |  | X |  |  |  |  |  | X |
| Hibiscus |  |  |  |  |  |  |  |  |  |  |  |  |  |  | X |
| Hollyhock |  |  |  |  |  |  |  |  |  |  |  |  | X |  |  |
| Holy Basil |  |  |  |  |  |  |  |  |  |  |  |  |  |  |  |
| Hops |  |  |  |  |  |  |  |  |  |  |  |  |  |  |  |
| Horehound |  |  |  |  |  |  |  |  |  |  |  |  |  |  |  |
| Horse Chestnut |  |  |  |  |  |  |  |  |  |  |  |  |  |  |  |

Columns 31–45 (Emmenagogue – Vulnerary):

| Herbs in Alphabetical Order | Emmenagogue | Expectorant | Galactogogue | Hematinic | Hepatic | Hypnotic | Hypotensive | Nervine Tonics | Nervine Relaxants | Nervine Stimulants | Oxytocic | Rubefacient | Sialogogue | Vasodilator | Vulnerary |
|---|---|---|---|---|---|---|---|---|---|---|---|---|---|---|---|
| Flax |  |  |  |  |  |  |  |  |  |  |  |  |  |  |  |
| Fringe Tree |  |  |  |  |  |  |  |  |  |  |  |  |  |  |  |
| Frankincense |  |  |  |  |  |  |  |  |  |  |  |  |  |  |  |
| French Lavendar |  |  |  |  |  |  | X |  |  |  |  |  |  |  |  |
| Garden Sage | X |  |  |  | X |  | X | X | X |  |  | X |  |  | X |
| Garlic |  | X |  |  |  |  | X |  |  | X |  |  |  | X | X |
| Gentian |  |  |  |  | X |  |  |  |  |  |  |  |  |  |  |
| Geranium |  |  |  |  |  |  |  |  |  |  |  |  |  |  |  |
| Germander |  |  |  |  |  |  |  |  |  |  |  |  |  |  |  |
| Ginger | X | X |  |  | X |  |  |  |  | X | X | X |  | X |  |
| Ginkgo |  |  |  |  |  |  |  |  |  | X |  |  |  | X |  |
| Ginkgo Biloba |  |  |  |  |  |  |  |  |  | X |  |  |  | X |  |
| Ginseng |  |  |  |  |  |  |  |  |  | X |  |  |  | X |  |
| Globe Artichoke |  |  |  |  |  |  |  |  |  |  |  |  |  |  |  |
| Goat's Rue |  |  | X |  |  |  |  |  |  |  |  |  |  |  |  |
| Goldenrod |  |  |  |  |  |  |  |  |  |  |  |  |  |  |  |
| Goldenseal |  |  |  |  |  |  |  |  |  |  |  |  |  |  | X |
| Gotu Kola |  |  |  |  |  |  |  | X | X |  |  |  |  |  | X |
| Gravel Root |  |  |  |  |  |  |  |  |  |  |  |  |  |  |  |
| Greater Celandine |  |  |  |  |  | X |  |  |  |  |  |  |  |  |  |
| Green Tea |  |  |  |  |  |  |  |  |  |  |  |  |  |  |  |
| Guarana |  |  |  |  |  |  |  |  |  | X |  |  |  |  |  |
| Gumweed |  | X |  |  |  |  |  |  |  |  |  |  |  |  | X |
| Hawthorn |  |  |  |  |  |  | X |  |  |  |  |  |  | X |  |
| Hibiscus |  |  |  |  |  |  |  |  |  |  |  |  |  |  |  |
| Hollyhock |  |  |  |  |  |  |  |  |  |  |  |  |  |  |  |
| Holy Basil |  |  |  |  |  |  |  | X | X |  |  |  |  |  |  |
| Hops |  |  |  |  |  | X |  |  | X |  |  |  |  |  |  |
| Horehound |  | X |  |  |  |  |  |  |  |  |  |  |  |  |  |
| Horse Chestnut |  |  |  |  |  |  |  |  |  |  |  |  |  | X |  |

# Quick Guide To Benefits And Tastes Of Herbs

Herbs in Alphabetical Order — Benefits matrix (Horsemint through Lomatium). Split into two column-groups for width; the property (benefit) labels are the rows.

### Herbs: Horsemint – Kola Nut

| Herbs in Alphabetical Order | Horsemint | Horseradish | Horsetail | Hydrangea Root | Hyssop | Indian Gooseberry | Irish Moss | Jamaican Dogwood | Japanese Knotweed | Jiaogulan | Juniper | Juniper Berries | Kava Kava | Kelp | Kola Nut |
|---|---|---|---|---|---|---|---|---|---|---|---|---|---|---|---|
| Vulnerary |  |  |  |  |  |  |  |  |  |  |  |  |  |  |  |
| Vasodilator |  |  |  |  |  |  |  |  |  |  |  |  |  |  |  |
| Sialogogue |  |  |  |  |  |  |  |  |  |  |  |  |  |  |  |
| Rubefacient |  | X |  |  |  |  |  |  |  |  |  |  |  |  |  |
| Oxytocic |  |  |  |  |  |  |  |  |  |  | X | X |  |  |  |
| Nervine Stimulants |  | X |  |  |  |  |  |  |  |  | X | X |  |  | X |
| Nervine Relaxants |  |  |  |  | X |  |  |  |  |  |  |  | X |  |  |
| Nervine Tonics |  |  |  |  |  |  |  |  |  |  |  |  | X |  |  |
| Hypotensive |  |  |  |  |  |  |  |  |  |  |  |  |  |  |  |
| Hypnotic |  |  |  |  |  |  |  | X |  |  |  |  | X |  |  |
| Hepatic |  | X |  |  |  |  |  |  |  |  |  |  |  |  |  |
| Hematinic |  |  |  |  |  |  |  |  |  |  |  |  |  |  |  |
| Galactogogue |  |  |  |  |  |  |  |  |  |  |  |  |  |  |  |
| Expectorant |  |  |  |  | X |  |  |  |  |  |  |  |  |  |  |
| Emmenagogue |  |  |  |  |  |  |  |  |  |  |  |  |  |  |  |
| Diuretic |  |  | X |  |  |  |  |  |  |  | X | X |  |  |  |
| Diaphoretic |  |  |  |  | X |  |  |  |  |  |  |  |  |  |  |
| Demulcent |  |  |  |  |  |  | X |  |  |  |  |  |  |  |  |
| Cholagogue |  |  |  |  |  |  |  |  |  |  |  |  |  |  |  |
| Cathartic |  |  |  |  |  |  |  |  |  |  |  |  |  |  |  |
| Carminative |  |  |  |  |  |  |  |  |  |  | X | X |  |  |  |
| Cardiotonic |  |  |  |  |  |  |  |  |  |  |  |  |  |  |  |
| Bitters |  |  |  |  |  |  |  |  |  |  |  |  |  |  |  |
| Astringent |  | X |  |  |  |  |  |  |  |  |  |  |  |  |  |
| Aperient |  |  |  |  |  |  |  |  |  |  |  |  |  |  |  |
| Antiviral |  |  |  |  |  |  |  |  | X |  |  |  |  |  |  |
| Antispasmodic |  |  |  |  | X |  |  |  |  |  |  |  |  |  |  |
| Antirheumatic |  |  |  |  |  |  |  |  |  |  | X | X |  |  |  |
| Antipyretic |  |  |  |  |  |  |  | X |  |  |  |  |  |  | X |
| Antiprotozoal |  |  |  |  |  |  |  |  |  |  |  |  |  |  |  |
| Antilithic-Urinary |  | X | X |  |  |  |  |  |  |  | X | X |  |  |  |
| Antilithic-Gallstone |  |  |  |  |  |  |  |  |  |  |  |  |  |  |  |
| Anti-Inflammatory |  |  |  |  | X |  |  |  |  |  |  |  |  |  |  |
| Antihemorrhagic | X |  |  |  |  |  |  |  |  |  |  |  |  |  | X |
| Antifungal |  |  |  |  |  |  |  |  |  |  |  |  |  |  |  |
| Antiemetics |  |  |  |  |  |  |  |  |  |  |  |  |  |  |  |
| Anticatarrhal |  |  |  |  | X |  | X |  |  |  |  |  |  |  |  |
| Antibiotic |  |  |  |  |  |  |  |  |  |  | X | X |  |  |  |
| Anthelmintics |  |  |  |  | X |  |  |  |  |  |  |  |  |  |  |
| Antacid & Anti-ulcer |  |  |  |  |  |  |  |  |  |  |  |  |  |  |  |
| Anodyne |  |  |  |  |  |  |  |  |  |  |  |  | X |  |  |
| Analgesic |  |  |  |  |  |  |  |  |  |  |  |  | X |  |  |
| Amphoteric |  |  |  |  |  |  |  |  |  |  |  |  |  |  |  |
| Alterative |  | X |  |  |  |  |  |  |  |  |  |  |  |  |  |
| Adaptogens |  |  |  |  |  | X |  |  |  | X |  |  | X |  |  |

### Herbs: Korean Ginseng – Lomatium

| Herbs in Alphabetical Order | Korean Ginseng | Kratom | Lady's Mantle | Lamb's Ear | Lavendar | Lemon | Lemon Balm | Lemon Grass | Lemon Verbana | Licorice | Licorice Root | Lily of the Valley | Linden | Lobelia | Lomatium |
|---|---|---|---|---|---|---|---|---|---|---|---|---|---|---|---|
| Vulnerary |  |  |  |  | X |  |  |  |  |  |  |  |  |  |  |
| Vasodilator |  |  |  |  |  |  |  |  |  |  |  |  | X |  |  |
| Sialogogue |  |  |  |  |  |  | X | X |  |  |  |  |  |  |  |
| Rubefacient |  |  |  |  |  |  |  |  |  |  |  |  |  |  |  |
| Oxytocic |  |  |  |  |  |  |  |  |  |  |  |  |  |  |  |
| Nervine Stimulants |  |  |  |  |  |  |  |  |  |  |  |  |  |  |  |
| Nervine Relaxants |  |  |  |  | X |  | X |  | X |  |  |  | X | X |  |
| Nervine Tonics |  |  |  |  | X |  | X |  |  |  |  |  | X |  |  |
| Hypotensive |  |  |  |  | X |  | X |  |  |  |  |  | X |  |  |
| Hypnotic | X |  |  |  | X |  | X |  |  |  |  |  | X |  |  |
| Hepatic |  |  |  |  |  |  |  |  |  | X | X |  |  |  |  |
| Hematinic |  |  |  |  |  |  |  |  |  |  |  |  |  |  |  |
| Galactogogue |  |  |  |  |  |  |  |  |  |  |  |  |  |  |  |
| Expectorant |  |  |  |  |  |  |  |  |  | X | X |  | X |  |  |
| Emmenagogue |  |  |  |  |  |  |  |  |  |  |  |  |  |  |  |
| Diuretic |  |  |  |  |  |  |  |  |  |  |  |  |  |  |  |
| Diaphoretic |  |  |  |  |  |  |  |  |  |  |  |  |  |  |  |
| Demulcent |  |  |  |  |  |  |  |  |  | X | X |  |  |  |  |
| Cholagogue |  |  |  |  | X |  |  |  |  | X | X |  |  |  |  |
| Cathartic |  |  |  |  |  |  |  |  |  | X | X |  |  |  |  |
| Carminative |  |  |  |  | X |  | X |  |  |  |  |  |  |  |  |
| Cardiotonic |  |  |  |  |  |  | X |  |  |  |  | X | X |  |  |
| Bitters |  |  |  |  |  |  |  |  | X |  |  |  |  |  |  |
| Astringent |  |  |  |  |  |  |  |  |  |  |  |  |  |  |  |
| Aperient |  |  |  |  |  |  |  |  |  | X | X |  |  |  |  |
| Antiviral |  |  |  |  | X |  |  |  |  | X | X |  |  |  | X |
| Antispasmodic |  |  |  |  | X |  | X |  | X |  |  |  |  | X |  |
| Antirheumatic |  |  |  |  |  |  |  |  |  | X | X |  |  |  |  |
| Antipyretic |  |  |  |  | X |  |  |  |  |  |  |  |  |  |  |
| Antiprotozoal |  |  |  |  |  |  |  |  |  | X | X |  |  |  |  |
| Antilithic-Urinary |  |  |  |  |  |  |  |  |  |  |  |  |  |  |  |
| Antilithic-Gallstone |  |  | X |  |  |  |  |  |  |  |  |  |  |  |  |
| Anti-Inflammatory |  |  |  |  |  |  |  |  |  | X | X |  |  |  |  |
| Antihemorrhagic | X |  |  |  |  |  |  |  |  |  |  |  |  |  |  |
| Antifungal |  | X |  |  |  |  |  |  |  |  |  |  |  |  |  |
| Antiemetics | X |  | X |  |  |  |  |  |  |  |  |  |  |  |  |
| Anticatarrhal |  |  |  |  |  |  |  |  |  | X | X |  |  |  |  |
| Antibiotic |  |  |  |  |  |  |  |  |  |  |  |  |  |  |  |
| Anthelmintics |  |  |  |  |  |  |  |  |  |  |  |  |  |  |  |
| Antacid & Anti-ulcer |  |  |  |  |  |  |  |  |  | X | X |  |  |  |  |
| Anodyne |  |  |  |  | X |  |  |  |  |  |  |  |  |  |  |
| Analgesic |  |  |  |  | X |  |  |  |  |  |  |  |  |  |  |
| Amphoteric |  |  |  |  |  |  |  |  |  | X | X |  |  |  |  |
| Alterative |  |  |  |  |  |  |  |  |  | X | X |  |  |  |  |
| Adaptogens | X |  |  |  |  |  | X |  |  | X | X |  |  |  |  |

| Herbs in Alphabetical Order | Adaptogens | Alterative | Amphoteric | Analgesic | Anodyne | Antacid & Anti-ulcer | Anthelmintics | Antibiotic | Anticatarrhal | Antiemetics | Antifungal | Antihemorrhagic | Anti-Inflammatory | Antilithics-Gallstone | Antilithics-Urinary | Antiprotozoal | Antipyretic | Antirheumatic | Antispasmodic | Antiviral | Aperient | Astringent | Bitters | Cardiotonic | Carminative | Cathartic | Cholagogue | Demulcent | Diaphoretic | Diuretic | Emmenagogue | Expectorant | Galactogogue | Hematinic | Hepatic | Hypnotic | Hypotensive | Nervine Tonics | Nervine Relaxants | Nervine Stimulants | Oxytocic | Rubefacient | Sialogogue | Vasodilator | Vulnerary |
|---|---|---|---|---|---|---|---|---|---|---|---|---|---|---|---|---|---|---|---|---|---|---|---|---|---|---|---|---|---|---|---|---|---|---|---|---|---|---|---|---|---|---|---|---|---|
| Lovage |  | X |  |  |  |  |  | X | X | X |  |  |  |  |  |  |  |  |  |  |  |  | X |  | X |  |  | X | X | X |  | X |  |  | X |  |  |  |  |  |  |  | X |  |  |
| Maca | X |  | X |  |  |  |  |  |  |  |  |  |  |  |  |  |  |  |  |  |  |  |  |  |  |  |  |  |  |  |  |  |  |  |  |  |  |  |  |  |  |  |  |  |  |
| Maca Root | X |  | X |  |  |  |  |  |  |  |  |  |  |  |  |  |  |  |  |  |  |  |  |  |  |  |  |  |  |  |  |  |  |  |  |  |  |  |  |  |  |  |  |  |  |
| Male Fern |  |  |  |  |  |  | X |  |  |  |  |  |  |  |  |  |  |  |  |  |  |  |  |  |  |  |  |  |  |  |  |  |  |  |  |  |  |  |  |  |  |  |  |  |  |
| Mallow |  | X |  |  |  |  |  |  | X | X |  |  | X |  | X |  |  |  |  |  | X |  |  |  |  |  |  | X |  |  |  |  |  |  |  |  |  |  |  |  |  |  |  |  | X |
| Marjoram |  |  |  | X | X |  |  | X | X |  |  |  | X |  |  |  |  |  | X | X | X | X | X |  | X |  |  |  |  |  |  |  |  |  |  |  |  | X | X |  | X | X | X | X | X |
| Marshmallow |  | X |  |  |  |  |  |  | X | X |  |  | X |  | X |  |  |  |  |  | X |  |  |  |  |  |  | X |  |  |  |  |  |  |  |  |  |  |  |  |  |  |  |  | X |
| Marshmallow Root |  | X |  |  |  |  |  |  | X | X |  |  | X |  | X |  |  |  |  |  | X |  |  |  |  |  |  | X |  |  |  |  |  |  |  |  |  |  |  |  |  |  |  |  | X |
| Meadowsweet |  |  |  |  |  | X |  |  |  |  |  |  | X |  |  |  | X | X |  |  |  | X |  |  |  |  |  |  |  |  |  |  |  |  |  |  |  |  |  |  |  |  |  |  |  |
| Milk Thistle | X |  |  |  |  | X |  |  |  |  |  |  |  | X |  | X |  |  |  |  |  |  |  |  |  |  | X |  |  |  |  |  |  |  | X |  |  |  |  |  |  |  |  |  |  |
| Mint |  |  |  |  |  |  |  |  |  | X |  |  |  |  |  |  |  |  |  |  |  |  |  |  |  |  |  |  |  |  |  |  |  |  |  |  |  |  |  |  |  |  |  |  |  |
| Mistletoe |  |  |  |  |  |  |  |  |  |  |  |  |  |  |  |  | X |  |  |  |  |  |  |  |  |  |  |  |  |  |  |  |  |  |  | X | X |  |  |  |  |  |  | X |  |
| Motherwort |  |  |  |  |  |  |  |  |  |  |  |  |  |  |  |  |  |  | X |  |  |  |  | X | X |  |  |  |  |  | X |  |  |  |  |  | X | X | X |  | X |  |  |  |  |
| Mucuna Pruriens | X |  |  |  |  |  |  |  |  |  |  |  |  |  |  |  |  |  |  |  |  |  |  |  |  |  |  |  |  |  |  |  |  |  |  |  |  |  |  |  |  |  |  |  |  |
| Mullein |  |  |  |  |  |  |  |  | X |  |  |  | X |  |  |  |  |  | X |  |  |  |  |  |  |  |  | X |  |  |  | X |  |  |  |  |  |  |  |  |  |  |  |  |  |
| Mustard |  |  |  |  |  |  |  |  |  |  |  |  |  |  |  |  |  |  |  |  |  |  |  |  |  |  |  |  |  |  |  |  |  |  |  |  |  |  |  |  |  | X |  |  |  |
| Myrrh |  |  |  |  |  |  |  | X |  |  | X |  |  |  |  | X |  |  |  |  |  |  |  |  |  |  |  |  |  |  |  |  |  |  |  |  |  |  |  |  |  |  |  |  | X |
| Nasturtium | X | X | X |  |  |  |  | X | X | X | X | X | X | X | X |  | X | X | X | X | X | X | X |  |  |  |  | X |  | X |  |  |  |  |  |  |  |  |  |  |  |  |  |  | X |
| Neem |  |  |  |  |  |  | X | X |  |  | X |  |  |  |  |  |  |  |  |  |  |  |  |  |  |  |  |  |  |  |  |  |  |  |  |  |  |  |  |  |  |  |  |  |  |
| Nettle |  | X |  |  |  |  |  |  | X |  |  | X | X |  |  |  |  |  | X |  |  |  |  |  |  |  |  | X |  | X |  |  | X | X | X |  |  |  |  |  |  |  |  |  |  |
| Oak Bark |  |  |  |  |  |  |  |  |  |  |  |  |  |  |  |  |  |  |  |  |  | X |  |  |  |  |  |  |  |  |  |  |  |  |  |  |  |  |  |  |  |  |  |  |  |
| Oak Moss |  |  |  |  |  |  |  |  |  |  |  | X |  |  |  |  |  |  |  |  |  |  |  |  |  |  |  |  |  |  |  |  |  |  |  |  |  |  |  |  |  |  |  |  |  |
| Oat Straw |  |  |  |  |  |  |  |  |  |  |  |  |  |  |  |  |  |  |  |  |  |  |  |  |  |  |  |  |  |  |  |  |  |  |  |  |  | X |  |  |  |  |  |  |  |
| Oats |  |  |  |  |  |  |  |  |  |  |  |  |  |  |  |  |  |  |  |  |  |  |  |  |  |  |  | X |  |  |  |  |  |  |  |  |  |  |  |  |  |  |  |  |  |
| Okra |  |  |  |  |  |  |  |  |  |  |  |  |  |  |  |  |  |  |  |  |  |  |  |  |  |  |  | X |  |  |  |  |  |  |  |  |  |  |  |  |  |  |  |  |  |
| Olive |  |  |  |  |  |  |  |  |  |  |  |  |  |  |  |  |  |  |  |  |  |  |  |  |  |  |  |  |  |  |  |  |  |  |  |  | X |  |  |  |  |  |  |  |  |
| Olive Leaf |  |  |  |  |  |  |  | X |  |  | X |  |  |  |  |  |  |  |  | X |  |  |  |  |  |  |  |  |  |  |  |  |  |  |  |  | X |  |  |  |  |  |  |  |  |
| Onion |  |  |  |  |  |  |  | X |  |  | X |  | X |  |  |  |  |  |  | X |  |  |  | X |  |  |  |  |  |  |  | X |  |  |  |  | X |  |  |  |  |  |  |  |  |
| Oregano |  |  |  | X |  |  |  | X | X |  |  |  | X |  |  |  | X |  | X | X |  |  |  |  |  |  |  |  | X |  |  | X |  |  |  |  |  |  |  |  |  |  |  |  |  |

| Herbs in Alphabetical Order | Adaptogens | Alterative | Amphoteric | Analgesic | Anodyne | Antiacid & Anti-ulcer | Anthelmintics | Antibiotic | Anticatarrhal | Antiemetics | Antifungal | Antihemorrhagic | Anti-Inflammatory | Antilithics-Gallstone | Antilithics-Urinary |
| --- | --- | --- | --- | --- | --- | --- | --- | --- | --- | --- | --- | --- | --- | --- | --- |
| Oregon Grape | | X | | | | | | X | | | X | | | X | |
| Oregon Grape Root | | X | | | | | | X | | | X | | | X | |
| Panax ginseng | X | | | | | | | | | | | | | | |
| Papaya Seed | | | | | | | X | | | | | | | | |
| Parsley | | | | | | | | | | | | | | | X |
| Parsley Root | | | | | | | | | | | | | | | X |
| Passionflower | X | | | | | | | | | | | | | | |
| Passionvine | | | | | | | | | | | | | | | |
| Pau D'Arco | | | | | | | | X | | | X | | | | |
| Pennyroyal | | | | | | | | | | | | | | | |
| Peppermint | | | | X | | | | X | X | X | | | | X | |
| Pineapple Bromelain | | | | | | | | | | | | | | | |
| Plantain | | X | | | | | | X | | | | X | X | | |
| Pleurisy Root | | | | | | | | | | | | | | | |
| Poke Root | | X | | | | | | | | | | | | | |
| Pomegranate | | | | | | | X | | | | | | | | |
| Poplar | | | | X | | | | | | | | | X | | |
| Prickly Ash | | | | | | | | | | | | | | | |
| Prune | | | | | | | | | | | | | | | |
| Psyllium | | | | | | | | | | | | | | | |
| Pumpkin | | | | | | | | | | | | | | | |
| Pumpkin Seed | | | | | | | X | | | | | | | | |
| Puncture Vine | X | | | | | | | | | | | | | | |
| Purslane | | X | X | | | | | X | X | X | X | X | X | | |
| Raspberry Leaf | | | | | | | | | | | | X | | | |
| Red Clover | | X | | | | | | | | | | | | | |
| Rehmannia | | | | | | | | | | | | | | | |
| Reishi mushrooms | X | X | | | | | | | | | | | | | |
| Rhodiola | X | X | | | | | | | | | | | | | |
| Rhubarb | | | X | | | | | | | | | | | | |

| Herbs in Alphabetical Order | Antiprotozoal | Antipyretic | Antirheumatic | Antispasmodic | Antiviral | Aperient | Astringent | Bitters | Cardiotonic | Carminative | Cathartic | Cholagogue | Demulcent | Diaphoretic | Diuretic |
| --- | --- | --- | --- | --- | --- | --- | --- | --- | --- | --- | --- | --- | --- | --- | --- |
| Oregon Grape | | | | | | | | | | | | X | | | |
| Oregon Grape Root | | | | | | | | | | | | X | | | |
| Panax ginseng | | | | | | | | | | | | | | | |
| Papaya Seed | | | | | | | | | | | | | | | |
| Parsley | | | | | | | | | | X | | | | | X |
| Parsley Root | | | | | | | | | | | | | | | |
| Passionflower | | | | X | | | | | | | | | | | |
| Passionvine | | | | | | | | | | | | | | | |
| Pau D'Arco | | | | | X | | | | | | | | | | |
| Pennyroyal | | | | | | | | | | | | | | | |
| Peppermint | | X | | X | X | | | | | X | | | | X | |
| Pineapple Bromelain | | | X | | | | | | | | | | | | |
| Plantain | | | | | | | X | | | | | | X | | X |
| Pleurisy Root | | | | | | | | | | | | | | | |
| Poke Root | | | | | | | | | | | | | | | |
| Pomegranate | | | | | | | | | | | | | | | |
| Poplar | | X | | | | | | | | | | | | | |
| Prickly Ash | | | | | | | | | | | | | | | |
| Prune | | | | | | | | | | | X | | | | |
| Psyllium | | | | | | X | | | | | | | | | |
| Pumpkin | | | | | | | | | | | | | | | X |
| Pumpkin Seed | | | | | | | | | | | | | | | |
| Puncture Vine | | | | | | | | | | | | | | | |
| Purslane | | X | | | | X | X | | | | | | X | X | X |
| Raspberry Leaf | | | | | | | X | | | | | | | | |
| Red Clover | | | | | | | | | | | | | | | |
| Rehmannia | | | | | | | | | | | | | | | |
| Reishi mushrooms | | | | | | | | | | | | | | | |
| Rhodiola | | | | | | | | | | | | | | | |
| Rhubarb | | | | | | X | | | | | X | | | | |

| Herbs in Alphabetical Order | Emmenagogue | Expectorant | Galactogogue | Hematinic | Hepatic | Hypnotic | Hypotensive | Nervine Tonics | Nervine Relaxants | Nervine Stimulants | Oxytocic | Rubefacient | Sialogogue | Vasodilator | Vulnerary |
| --- | --- | --- | --- | --- | --- | --- | --- | --- | --- | --- | --- | --- | --- | --- | --- |
| Oregon Grape | | | | | X | | | | | | | | | | |
| Oregon Grape Root | | | | | X | | | | | | | | | | |
| Panax ginseng | | | | | | | | X | | | | | | | |
| Papaya Seed | | | | | | | | | | | | | | | |
| Parsley | X | | | X | | | X | | | | | | | | |
| Parsley Root | | | | | | | | | | | | | | | |
| Passionflower | | | | | | X | X | X | X | | | | | | |
| Passionvine | | | | | | | | | X | | | | | | |
| Pau D'Arco | | | | | | | | | | | | | | | |
| Pennyroyal | X | | | | | | | | | | X | | | | |
| Peppermint | X | | | | | | | | | | | X | X | | |
| Pineapple Bromelain | | | | | | | | | | | | | | | |
| Plantain | | | | | | | | | | | | | | | X |
| Pleurisy Root | | X | | | | | | | | | | | | | |
| Poke Root | | | | | | | | | | | | | | | |
| Pomegranate | | | | | | | | | | | | | | | |
| Poplar | | | | | | | | | | | | | | | |
| Prickly Ash | | | | | | | | | | | | | | X | |
| Prune | | | | | | | | | | | | | | | |
| Psyllium | | | | | | | | | | | | | | | |
| Pumpkin | | | | | | | | | | | | | | | |
| Pumpkin Seed | | | | | | | | | | | | | | | |
| Puncture Vine | | | | | | | | | | | | | | | |
| Purslane | | | | | | | | | | | X | | | | X |
| Raspberry Leaf | | | | | | | | | X | | | | | | |
| Red Clover | | | | | | | | | | | | | | | |
| Rehmannia | | | | X | | | | | | | | | | | |
| Reishi mushrooms | | | | | | | | | | | | | | | |
| Rhodiola | | | | | | | | | X | X | | | | | |
| Rhubarb | | | | | | | | | | | | | | | |

| Herbs in Alphabetical Order | Adaptogens | Alterative | Amphoteric | Analgesic | Anodyne | Antacid & Anti-ulcer | Anthelmintics | Antibiotic | Anticatarrhal | Antiemetics | Antifungal | Antihemorrhagic | Anti-Inflammatory | Antilithics-Gallstone | Antilithics-Urinary | Antiprotozoal | Antipyretic | Antirheumatic | Antispasmodic | Antiviral | Aperient | Astringent | Bitters | Cardiotonic | Carminative | Cathartic | Cholagogue | Demulcent | Diaphoretic | Diuretic | Emmenagogue | Expectorant | Galactogogue | Hematinic | Hepatic | Hypnotic | Hypotensive | Nervine Tonics | Nervine Relaxants | Nervine Stimulants | Oxytocic | Rubefacient | Sialogogue | Vasodilator | Vulnerary |
|---|---|---|---|---|---|---|---|---|---|---|---|---|---|---|---|---|---|---|---|---|---|---|---|---|---|---|---|---|---|---|---|---|---|---|---|---|---|---|---|---|---|---|---|---|---|
| Rose |  |  |  |  |  |  |  |  |  |  |  |  |  |  |  |  |  |  |  |  |  | X |  |  |  |  |  |  |  |  |  |  |  |  |  |  |  |  |  |  |  |  |  |  |  |  |
| Rosemary |  |  |  | X |  |  |  | X |  |  | X |  | X |  |  |  |  | X | X | X |  |  |  |  | X |  | X |  | X | X |  |  |  |  |  |  |  |  |  | X |  | X |  | X |  |
| Rue |  |  |  |  |  |  | X | X |  |  |  |  |  |  |  |  |  |  |  |  |  |  |  |  |  |  |  |  |  |  | X |  |  |  |  |  |  |  |  |  | X |  |  |  |  |
| Saffron | X |  |  |  |  |  |  |  |  |  |  |  |  |  |  |  |  |  |  |  |  |  |  |  |  |  |  |  |  |  |  |  |  |  |  |  |  |  |  |  |  |  |  |  |  |
| Sage |  |  |  | X |  |  |  | X | X |  | X |  | X |  |  |  |  | X | X | X |  | X | X |  | X |  |  |  | X |  |  |  |  |  |  |  |  | X | X |  |  |  | X |  | X |
| Sarsaparilla |  | X |  |  |  |  |  |  |  |  |  |  |  |  |  |  |  |  |  |  |  |  |  |  |  |  |  |  |  |  |  |  |  |  |  |  |  |  |  |  |  |  |  |  |  |
| Savory |  |  | X | X | X |  | X | X | X | X | X |  | X |  |  |  |  | X | X | X | X | X | X | X | X | X | X | X | X | X | X | X | X | X | X |  |  |  |  |  |  |  |  |  |  |
| Schisandra | X |  | X |  |  |  |  |  |  |  |  |  |  |  |  |  |  |  |  |  |  |  |  |  |  |  |  |  |  |  |  |  |  |  | X |  |  |  |  |  |  |  |  |  |  |
| Senna |  |  |  |  |  |  |  |  |  |  |  |  |  |  |  |  |  |  |  |  | X |  |  |  |  | X |  |  |  |  |  |  |  |  |  |  |  |  |  |  |  |  |  |  |  |
| Sesame Seeds |  |  |  |  |  |  | X |  |  |  |  |  |  |  |  |  |  |  |  |  |  |  |  |  |  |  |  |  |  |  |  |  |  |  |  |  |  |  |  |  |  |  |  |  |  |
| Savory |  |  | X | X | X |  | X | X | X | X | X |  | X |  |  |  |  | X | X | X | X | X | X | X | X | X | X | X | X | X | X | X | X | X | X |  |  |  |  |  |  |  |  |  |  |
| Shatavari |  |  |  |  |  |  |  |  |  |  |  |  |  |  |  |  |  |  |  |  |  |  |  |  |  |  |  |  |  |  |  |  | X |  |  |  |  |  |  |  |  |  |  |  |  |
| Shepherd's Purse |  |  |  |  |  |  |  |  |  |  |  | X |  |  |  |  |  |  |  |  |  | X |  |  |  |  |  |  |  |  |  |  |  |  |  |  |  |  |  |  |  |  |  |  |  |
| Shiitake Mushroom |  |  |  |  |  |  |  |  |  |  |  |  |  |  |  |  |  |  |  | X |  |  |  |  |  |  |  |  |  |  |  |  |  |  |  |  |  |  |  |  |  |  |  |  |  |
| Shilajit | X |  |  |  |  |  |  |  |  |  |  |  |  |  |  |  |  |  |  |  |  |  |  |  |  |  |  |  |  |  |  |  |  |  |  |  |  |  |  |  |  |  |  |  |  |
| Siberian Ginseng | X |  |  |  |  |  |  |  |  |  |  |  |  |  |  |  |  |  |  |  |  |  |  |  |  |  |  |  |  |  |  |  |  |  |  |  | X |  |  | X |  |  |  |  |  |
| Skullcap |  |  |  | X | X |  |  |  |  |  |  |  | X |  |  |  |  |  | X | X |  |  |  |  |  |  |  |  |  |  |  |  |  |  |  | X | X | X | X |  |  |  |  |  |  |
| Slippery Elm |  |  |  |  |  |  |  |  |  |  |  |  |  |  |  |  |  |  |  |  |  |  |  |  |  |  |  | X |  |  |  | X |  |  |  |  |  |  |  |  |  |  |  |  |  |
| Spearmint |  |  |  |  |  |  |  |  |  | X |  |  |  |  |  |  |  |  |  |  |  |  |  |  |  |  |  |  |  |  |  |  |  |  |  |  |  |  |  |  |  |  |  |  |  |
| Spirulina |  |  | X |  |  |  |  |  |  |  |  |  |  |  |  |  |  |  |  |  |  |  |  |  |  |  |  |  |  |  |  |  |  |  |  |  |  |  |  |  |  |  |  |  |  |
| Squaw Vine |  |  |  |  |  |  |  |  |  |  |  |  |  |  |  |  |  |  |  |  |  |  |  |  |  |  |  |  |  |  |  |  |  |  |  |  |  |  |  |  | X |  |  |  |  |
| St. John's Wort |  |  |  |  |  |  |  | X |  |  |  |  | X |  |  |  |  |  | X | X |  |  |  |  |  |  |  |  |  |  |  |  |  |  |  |  |  | X | X |  |  |  |  |  | X |
| Stinging Nettle |  | X |  |  |  |  |  |  | X |  |  | X | X |  |  |  |  | X |  |  |  |  |  |  |  |  |  |  |  | X |  |  | X | X |  |  |  |  |  |  |  |  |  |  |  |
| Suma | X |  |  |  |  |  |  |  |  |  |  |  |  |  |  |  |  |  |  |  |  |  |  |  |  |  |  |  |  |  |  |  |  |  |  |  |  |  |  |  |  |  |  |  |  |
| Sweet Annie |  |  |  |  |  |  |  |  |  |  |  |  |  |  |  |  | X |  |  |  |  |  |  |  |  |  |  |  |  |  |  |  |  |  |  |  |  |  |  |  |  |  |  |  |  |
| Sweet Cicely |  |  |  |  |  |  |  | X |  |  | X |  |  |  |  |  |  |  |  |  |  |  |  |  |  |  |  |  |  |  |  |  |  |  |  |  |  |  |  |  |  |  |  |  | X |
| Sweet Root |  |  |  |  |  |  |  |  |  |  | X |  |  |  |  |  |  |  |  |  |  |  |  |  |  |  |  |  |  |  |  |  |  |  |  |  |  |  |  |  |  |  |  |  |  |
| Tansy |  |  |  | X |  |  |  |  |  |  |  |  |  |  |  |  |  | X |  |  |  |  |  |  |  |  |  |  |  |  | X |  |  |  |  |  |  |  |  |  |  |  |  |  |  |
| Tea Tree Oil |  |  |  |  |  |  |  |  |  |  | X |  |  |  |  |  |  |  |  | X |  |  |  |  |  |  |  |  |  |  |  |  |  |  |  |  |  |  |  |  |  |  |  |  |  |
| Teasel Root |  |  |  |  |  |  |  |  |  |  |  |  | X |  |  |  |  | X | X | X |  |  |  |  |  |  |  |  | X |  |  |  |  |  |  |  |  |  |  |  |  |  |  |  |  |

| Herbs in Alphabetical Order | Adaptogens | Alterative | Amphoteric | Analgesic | Anodyne | Antacid & Anti-ulcer | Anthelmintics | Antibiotic | Anticatarrhal | Antiemetics | Antifungal | Antihemorrhagic | Anti-Inflammatory | Antilithics-Gallstone | Antilithics-Urinary | Antiprotozoal | Antipyretic | Antirheumatic | Antispasmodic | Antiviral | Aperient | Astringent | Bitters | Cardiotonic | Carminative | Cathartic | Cholagogue | Demulcent | Diaphoretic | Diuretic | Emmenagogue | Expectorant | Galactogogue | Hematinic | Hepatic | Hypnotic | Hypotensive | Nervine Tonics | Nervine Relaxants | Nervine Stimulants | Oxytocic | Rubefacient | Sialogogue | Vasodilator | Vulnerary |
|---|---|---|---|---|---|---|---|---|---|---|---|---|---|---|---|---|---|---|---|---|---|---|---|---|---|---|---|---|---|---|---|---|---|---|---|---|---|---|---|---|---|---|---|---|---|
| Thuja | | | | | | | | | | | | | | | | | | | | X | | | | | | | | | | | | | | | | | | | | | | | | | | X |
| Thyme | | | | | | | X | X | | | X | | | | | | X | X | | X | | X | | | X | | | | X | | | X | | | | | | | | | | | | | |
| Tinospora Cordifolia | | | | | | | | | | | | | | | | | | | | | | | | | | | X | | | | | | | | | | | | | | | | | | |
| Tormentil | | | | | | | | | | | | X | | | | | | | | | | | | | | | | | | | | | | | | | | | | | | | | | |
| Tulsi | X | | X | | | | | | | | | | | | | | | | | | | | | | | | | | | | | | | | | | | X | X | | | | | | |
| Turkey Rhubarb | | | | | | | | | | | | | X | | | | | | | | | X | | | | | | | | | | | | | | | | | | | | | | | |
| Turmeric | X | | X | X | X | X | X | X | | | | X | X | | | | | X | | | | | | X | | | X | | | | | | | | X | | | | | | | | | X | |
| Usnea | | | | | | | | X | | | | | | | | | | | | | | | | | | | | | | | | | | | | | | | | | | | | | |
| Uva Ursi | | X | | | | | | X | X | | X | | | | X | | | X | | | | X | | | | | | | | X | | | | | | | | | | | | | | | |
| Valerian | X | | | | | | | | | | | | | | | | | | X | | | | | | | | | | | | | | | | | X | X | X | X | | | | | | |
| Vervain | | | | | | | | | | | | | | | | | | | | | | | | | | | | | | | | | X | | X | | | X | X | | | | | | |
| Weld | | | | | | | | | | | | X | | | | | | | | | | | | | | | | | | | | | | | | | | | | | | | | | |
| White Oak | | | | | | | | | | | | X | | | | | | | | | | X | | | | | | | | | | | | | | | | | | | | | | | |
| White Oak Bark | | | | | | | | | | | | X | | | | | | | | | | X | | | | | | | | | | | | | | | | | | | | | | | |
| White Willow | | | | X | X | | | | | | | | X | | | | X | X | | | | | | | | | | | | | | | | | | | | | | | | | | | |
| White Willow Bark | | | | X | X | | | | | | | | X | | | | X | X | | | | | | | | | | | | | | | | | | | | | | | | | | | |
| Wild Cherry Bark | | | | | | | | | | | | | X | | | | | | X | | | | | | | | | | | | | X | | | | | | | | | | | | | |
| Wild Indigo | | X | | | | | | | | | | | | | | | | | | | | | | | | | | | | | | | | | | | | | | | | | | | |
| Wild Yam | | | | | | | | | | | | | | | | | | | X | | | | | | | | X | | | | | | | | | | X | | | | | | | | |
| Willow | | | | X | X | | | | | | | | X | | | | X | X | | | | | | | | | | | | | | | | | | | | | | | | | | | |
| Chamomile | | | | X | X | | | | | | | | X | | | | X | X | | | | | | | | | | | | | | | | | | | | | | | | | | | |
| Wintergreen | | | | | | | | | | | | | | | | | | X | | | | | | | | | | | | | | | | | | | | | | | | | | | |
| Witch Hazel | | | | | | | | | | | | X | | | | | | | | | | X | | | | | | | | | | | | | | | | | | | | | | | X |
| Wood Betony | | | | | | | | | | | | | | | | | | | | | | | | | | | | | | | | | | | | | | X | X | | | | | | |
| Wormseed | | | | | | | X | | | | | | | | | | | | | | | | | | | | | | | | | | | | | | | | | | | | | | |
| Wormwood | | | | | | | X | X | | | | | | | | X | | | | | | | X | | | | | | | | X | | | | | | | | | | | | | | |
| Yarrow | | | | X | X | | | X | X | | | X | X | | | | X | | | | | X | | X | | | | | X | | | | | | | | X | | | | | | | X | X |
| Yellow Dock | | X | | | | | | | | | | X | | | | | | | | | | | | | | X | X | | | | | | | X | X | | | | | | | | | | |
| Yerba Mate | | | | | | | | | | | | | | | | | | | | | | | | | | | | | | | | | | | | | | | | X | | | | | |
| Yerba Santa | | | | | | | | | | | | | | | | | | | | | | | | | | | | | | | | X | | | | | | | | | | | X | | |

# SECTION IV

Organized by Taste Profile

| Herbs In Alphabetical Order | Astringent | Bitter | No Taste | Pungent | Salty | Sour | Sweet | Umami | Details |
|---|---|---|---|---|---|---|---|---|---|
| **Astringent** | | | | | | | | | |
| Agrimony | X | X | | | | | | | Slightly bitter and astringent taste, mildly sweet or nutty.  Suitable for teas & infusions. |
| Alum | X | | | | | | | | Not typically consumed as food or spice.  Often used for medicine or a pickling agent. |
| Arjuna | X | X | | | | | | | The astringent taste is described as dry, puckering, or tannic. |
| Bayberry | X | X | | | | | | | Astringent and slightly bitter.  Bayberry leaves have been used in some traditional dishes. |
| Bearberry | X | X | | | | | | | Astringent and slightly bitter.  It is primarily used for health benefits, not culinary taste. |
| Black haw | X | X | | | | | | | Bitter and astringent tastes. |
| Black Walnut Hull | X | X | | | | | | | Bitter and somewhat astringent.  Not typically consumed for their taste. |
| Blackberry Leaf | X | X | | | | | | | Mildly astringent or slightly bitter taste.  Often used in herbal teas or infusions. |
| Boswellia | X | X | | | | | | | Bitter or slightly astringent.  Used to prepare teas for medicinal purposes. |
| Buchu | X | X | | | | | | | Mildly bitter or astringent taste.  Used in traditional herbal medicine. |
| Cat's Claw | X | X | | | | | | | Bitter and astringent tastes. |
| Celery | X | X | | | X | | X | | Astringent, slightly salty, mildly bitter, & mildly sweet taste.  Used in soups, salads, snacks, etc. |
| Celery Seed | X | X | | X | | | | | Astringent, slightly bitter, & pungent taste like concentrated celery.  Used as a spice in recipes. |
| Cramp Bark | X | | | | | | | | Astringent.  Used in herbal formulations, such as teas and tinctures. |
| Germander | X | X | | | | | | | Bitter and astringent.  Not consumed as food.  Potential toxicity. |
| Green Tea | X | X | | | | | X | X | Astringent & bitter.  Can be slightly sweet if high quality & brewed correctly.  Umami notes. |
| Kola Nut | X | X | | | | | X | | Bitterness with slight sweetness and astringency.  Flavoring in beverages like cola sodas. |
| Lady's Mantle | X | | | | | | | | Astringent.  Used in herbal preparations for its potential health benefits. |
| Lavender | X | | | | | | X | | Slight sweet, floral, herbaceous flavor, & mildly astringent.  Use sparingly due to potent flavor. |
| Lovage | X | X | | X | | | | | Mildly astringent, hint of bitterness, slightly pungent or peppery.  Adds depth or complexity. |
| Meadowsweet | X | | | | | | X | | Sweet and slightly astringent. |
| Oak Bark | X | X | | | | | | | Astringent and bitter.  Not consumed as food.  Used in traditional medicine. |
| Olive Leaf | X | X | | | | | | | Mildly bitter and may be slightly astringent.  Used in herbal teas and supplements. |
| Oregon Grape Root | X | X | | | | | | | Bitter and slightly astringent.  Not consumed as food.  Used in herbal preparations. |
| Peppermint | X | | | X | | | X | | Cool, sweetness, subtle bitterness, with a pungency.  Used in various foods and beverages. |
| Prickly Ash | X | X | | X | | | | | Astringent, can be bitter.  Tingling or numbing sensation contributes to pungent, spicy quality. |
| Raspberry Leaf | X | X | | | | | | | Astringent or slightly bitter.  Is often used for herbal teas. |
| Shepherd's Purse | X | X | | | | | | | Slightly bitter and astringent.  The leaves are edible and used in salads or cooked dishes. |
| Tormentil | X | X | | | | | | | Astringent and bitter.  Used in teas and as a flavoring agent. |
| Tulsi | X | X | | X | | | X | | Slightly astringent, mildly bitter, sweet undertones, & subtle pungency.  Wide culinary uses. |
| Turkey Rhubarb | X | X | | | | | | | Astringent and bitter.  Not consumed as food.  Used in traditional medicine. |
| Usnea | X | X | | | | | | | Bitter and astringent.  Not consumed as food.  Used in traditional medicine. |
| Uva Ursi | X | X | | | | | | | Astringent & slightly bitter.  It is primarily used for medicine, not culinary taste.  Can be toxic. |
| White Oak | X | | | | | | | | Astringent.  Not commonly consumed for taste.  Traditionally used medicinally. |
| White Oak Bark | X | | | | | | | | Astringent.  Not commonly consumed for taste.  Traditionally used medicinally. |
| Wild Yam | X | X | | | | | | | Astringent and bitter.  Not used for culinary purposes.  Traditionally used in herbal medicines. |
| Willow | X | X | | | | | | | Astringent and bitter.  Not used for culinary purposes.  Traditionally used in herbal medicines. |
| Willow Bark | X | X | | | | | | | Astringent and bitter.  Not used for culinary purposes.  Traditionally used in herbal medicines. |
| Witch Hazel | X | | | | | | | | Astringent.  Not consumed for taste.  Traditionally used medicinally.  Can be toxic. |
| Yerba Santa | X | X | | | | | | | Bitter & somewhat astringent.  Not used for culinary purposes.  Used in herbal medicines. |

| Herbs In Alphabetical Order | Astringent | Bitter | No Taste | Pungent | Salty | Sour | Sweet | Umami | Details |
|---|---|---|---|---|---|---|---|---|---|
| **Bitter** | | | | | | | | | |
| Agrimony | X | X | | | | | | | Slightly bitter and astringent taste, mildly sweet or nutty.  Suitable for teas & infusions. |
| Albizia | | X | | | | | | | Slightly bitter.  Not typically consumed as food, due to potential toxicity. |
| Alder Buckthorn | | X | | | | | | | Bitter.  Not typically consumed as food, due to potential toxicity. |
| Aloe Vera | | X | | | | | | | Mild, slightly bitter.  Consuming in large amounts may have a laxative effect.  Use caution. |
| Aloe Vera Leaf | | X | | | | | | | Mild, slightly bitter.  Consuming in large amounts may have a laxative effect.  Use caution. |
| American Ginseng | | X | | | | | X | | Mildly bitter and slightly sweet.  May taste slightly earthy or herbal.  Used in teas and tonics. |
| American Skullcap | | X | | | | | | | Slightly bitter.  Often used with other herbs to balance or complement the overall taste. |
| Andrographis | | X | | | | | | | One of the bitterest herbs. |
| Angelica | | X | | X | | | | | A complex flavor that has bitter and sweet notes. |
| Arjuna | X | X | | | | | | | The astringent taste is described as dry, puckering, or tannic. |
| Artichoke | | X | | | | | X | | Bitter and slightly sweet. |
| Ashitaba | | X | | | | | X | | Bitter and somewhat sweet notes. |
| Ashwagandha | | X | | | | | | | Bitterness that is somewhat earthy or reminiscent of the taste of roots. |
| Baneberry | | X | | | | | | | Not consumed as food because it is toxic. |
| Bayberry | X | X | | | | | | | Astringent and slightly bitter.  Bayberry leaves have been used in some traditional dishes. |
| Bay Leaves | | X | | X | | | | | Bitter & pungent in fresh form.  When dried they taste herbal like thyme or oregano. |
| Bearberry | X | X | | | | | | | Astringent and slightly bitter.  It is primarily used for health benefits, not culinary taste. |
| Bergamot | | X | | | | | | | Citrusy and mildly bitter.  Used in culinary applications when a slight citrusy note is desired. |
| Bitter Leaf | | X | | | | | | | Used in cooking, especially African cuisines.  Balanced with other flavors. |
| Bitter Melon | | X | | | | | | | Bitterness with hints of astringency.  Used in Asian cooking: stir-fries, soups, and other dishes. |
| Black Cohosh | | X | | | | | | | Not typically consumed for taste. |
| Black haw | X | X | | | | | | | Bitter and astringent tastes. |
| Black Horehound | | X | | X | | | | | Bitter and pungent or slightly spicy taste. |
| Black Mustard | | X | | X | | | | | Pungent and slightly bitter.  Used in condiments, pickles & spice blends to add heat and flavor. |
| Black Seed | | X | | | | | | | Slightly bitter.  Can be used in culinary dishes and health remedies. |
| Black Walnut Hull | X | X | | | | | | | Bitter and somewhat astringent.  Not typically consumed for their taste. |
| Blackberry Leaf | X | X | | | | | | | Mildly astringent or slightly bitter taste.  Often used in herbal teas or infusions. |
| Blessed Thistle | | X | | | | | | | Not commonly consumed for taste, but used medicinally. |
| Bloodroot | | X | | | | | | | Not used for culinary purposes, because it is extremely toxic.  Medicinal use is controversial. |
| Blue Cohosh | | X | | | | | | | Bitterness is a common taste associated with medicinal herbs. |
| Blue Flag | | X | | X | | | | | Bitter and acrid or sharp, pungent taste.  Not consumed as food, due to toxicity. |
| Blue Vervain | | X | | | | | | | Bitter taste.  Typically used in herbal formulations, teas, or tinctures. |
| Boldo | | X | | | | | | | Bitter.  Often used in herbal medicine and to flavor certain foods and beverages. |
| Boneset | | X | | | | | | | Bitter taste.  Used in traditional medicine. |
| Boswellia | X | X | | | | | | | Bitter or slightly astringent.  Used to prepare teas for medicinal purposes. |
| Buchu | X | X | | | | | | | Mildly bitter or astringent taste.  Used in traditional herbal medicine. |
| Buckthorn | | X | | | | | | | Bitter.  Typically not consumed due to their laxative effects. |
| Bupleurum | | X | | | | | | | Bitter taste.  Often used in traditional Chinese medicine. |
| Burdock | | X | | | | | X | | Slightly bitter with mildly sweet undertones.  Often used in soups, stir-fries, and teas. |
| Burdock Root | | X | | | | | X | | Slightly bitter and mildly sweet and earthy flavor.  Often used in soups, stir-fries, and teas. |
| Butcher's Broom | | X | | | | | | | Bitter.  Typically use in herbal formulations rather than being consumed for taste. |
| Cacao | | X | | | | | X | X | Bitter, can have some sweetness if high quality dark chocolate, & umami (a savory rich taste). |
| Calendula | | X | | | | | | | Mild, slightly bitter or peppery taste.  Used in culinary applications like salads or as garnishes. |
| California Poppy | | X | | | | | | | Mildly bitter.  Not typically used for taste.  Often used in teas or tinctures. |
| Caraway | | X | | X | | | X | | Slightly sweet & warm taste reminiscent of anise or licorice.  Slightly bitter or slightly pungent. |
| Cascara amarga | | X | | | | | | | Bitter.  Used as herbal supplements or teas for a laxative effect.  Not used as food. |
| Cascara sagrada | | X | | | | | | | Bitter.  Used as herbal supplements or teas for a laxative effect.  Not used as food. |
| Cascarilla | | X | | | | | | | Bitter.  Mostly used in certain beverages. |
| Cassia | | X | | | | | | | Slightly bitter and nutty taste.  Uncommon to use in cooking.  Used in teas. |
| Catnip | | X | | | | | | | Mildly bitter and minty.  Not used in culinary.  Used as teas or herbal blends. |
| Cat's Claw | X | X | | | | | | | Bitter and astringent tastes. |
| Celery | X | X | | | X | | X | | Astringent, slightly salty, mildly bitter, & mildly sweet taste.  Used in soups, salads, snacks, etc. |
| Celery Seed | X | X | | X | | | | | Astringent, slightly bitter, & pungent taste like concentrated celery.  Used as a spice in recipes. |
| Centaury | | X | | | | | | | Bitter.  Often used in herbal formulations as medicine, including teas and tinctures. |
| Chamomile | | X | | | | | X | | Mildly sweet, slightly bitter, and herbaceous taste.  Floral or slightly fruity.  Used to make teas. |
| Chanca Piedra | | X | | | | | | | Bitter.  Not typically consumed as food, instead it is used for health benefits. |
| Chaparral | | X | | | | | | | Bitter.  Not typically consumed as food, instead it is used for health benefits. |
| Chaste Tree | | X | | | | | | | Bitterness.  Consumed in the form of extracts, tinctures, or capsules rather than for its taste. |
| Chicory | | X | | | | | | | Bitter taste can be pronounced.  Used in salads, mixed with greens, or a coffee substitute. |
| Chicory Root | | X | | | | | | | Bitter, with a slightly woody and nutty flavor.  Used as a coffee substitute. |

| Herbs In Alphabetical Order | Astringent | Bitter | No Taste | Pungent | Salty | Sour | Sweet | Umami | Details |
|---|---|---|---|---|---|---|---|---|---|
| **Bitter** | | | | | | | | | |
| Coleus Forskohlii | | X | | | | | | | Not typically consumed for taste, and more often used in supplements. |
| Coltsfoot | | X | | | | | | | Bitter taste. Not commonly consumed for taste. Historically used in traditional medicine. |
| Comfrey | | X | | | | | | | Bitter taste. Internal use not recommended, because it can be toxic to the liver. |
| Cotton Root Bark | | X | | | | | | | Bitter. Used for potential medicinal properties in traditional herbal remedies. |
| Cumin | | X | | | | | | | Mild bitterness with a warm, earthy flavor. Added to savory recipes: curries, stews, etc. |
| Damiana | | X | | X | | | | | Bitter and pungent. Not consumed for flavor. Used in herbal teas or supplements. |
| Dandelion | | X | | | | | X | | Older leaves are bitter. Younger leaver are slightly sweet. Culinary uses. Salads & teas. |
| Dandelion Root | | X | | | | | | | Bitter and earthy flavor. Used in culinary and herbal preparations like teas and tinctures. |
| Danshen | | X | | X | | | | | Bitter and slightly pungent. Not consumed for taste. Used it traditional herbal formulas. |
| Devil's Claw | | X | | | | | | | Bitter. Not consumed for taste. Used in herbal formulas like teas and supplements. |
| Dill | | X | | | | | X | | Fresh and herbaceous flavor with mild anise or licorice undertones. Mild bitterness. |
| Dill Seed | | X | | | | | | | Warm & slightly bitter. More concentrated dill flavor. Uses: pickling, baking, & savory dishes. |
| Dong Quai | | X | | X | | | | | Bitter and pungent. Not consumed for flavor. Used in herbal teas or supplements. |
| Echinacea | | X | | | | | | | Bitter. Not consumed for taste. Used in herbal teas and supplements to boost immunity. |
| Elder | | X | | | | | X | | Sweet and somewhat tart taste. My contain some bitterness. Parts can be toxic. |
| Elecampane | | X | | X | | | | | Bitter and pungent taste. Not consumed as food. Used in herbal formulas: teas and tinctures. |
| Eleuthero | | X | | | | | | | Bitter. Not consumed for taste. Used in herbal formulas like teas and supplements. |
| Fenugreek | | X | | | | | X | | Bitter with underlying sweet notes. Used in Indian, Middle Eastern, & North African cuisines. |
| Feverfew | | X | | | | | | | Bitter. Not consumed for taste. Used in herbal formulas like teas and supplements. |
| Fo Ti Root | | X | | | | | X | | Slightly bitter and sweet. Used in traditional Chinese medicine. |
| Frankincense | | X | | | | | | | Bitter with a resinous woody flavor. Not a culinary ingredient. Used medicinally. |
| Garden Sage | | X | | | | | | | Bitter taste with earthy undertones. Used to season meats, stews, and savory dishes. |
| Gentian | | X | | | | | | | Highly bitter. Used to produce certain aperitifs and herbal bitters. |
| Germander | X | X | | | | | | | Bitter and astringent. Not consumed as food. Potential toxicity. |
| Ginkgo | | X | | | | | | | Bitter. Not consumed for taste. Used in supplements. |
| Ginkgo Biloba | | X | | | | | | | Bitter. Not consumed for taste. Used in supplements. |
| Ginseng | | X | | | | | X | | Slightly bitter & subtle sweetness. Used in teas, extracts, or as an ingredient in certain foods. |
| Globe Artichoke | | X | | | | | | | Mildly bitter. Used in salads, dips, and other culinary applications. |
| Goldenseal | | X | | | | | | | Bitter. Historically used in traditional medicine. |
| Gotu Kola | | X | | | | | X | | Bitter and slightly sweet. Used as an herbal tea, included in salads, or other dishes. |
| Greater Celandine | | X | | | | | | | Bitter. Contains toxic compounds, approach with caution. |
| Green Tea | X | X | | | | | X | X | Astringent & bitter. Can be slightly sweet if high quality & brewed correctly. Umami notes. |
| Guarana | | X | | | | | | | Bitter. Often used in energy drinks and supplements due to its caffeine content. |
| Holy Basil | | X | | X | | | | | Mild bitterness and pungent taste. Used in various dishes and teas. |
| Hops | | X | | | | | | | Bitter. Used in beer to balance the sweetness of malt. |
| Horehound | | X | | | | | | | Bitter. Used medicinally in herbal teas, lozenges, or candies. |
| Horse Chestnut | | X | | | | | | | Bitter. Can be toxic in large quantities. Raw seeds are not safe due to their toxicity. |
| Hyssop | | X | | | X | | | | Bitter and slightly pungent or peppery. Used to flavor dishes or in teas. |
| Jamaican Dogwood | | X | | | | | | | Not consumed as food. Often used in tinctures or extracts for medicinal purposes. |
| Jiaogulan | | X | | | | | X | | Sweet and slightly bitter. Often used as a herbal tea. |
| Juniper | | X | | X | | | X | | Slightly sweet and pungent piney flavor with some bitterness. Can be used sparingly in dishes. |
| Juniper Berries | | X | | X | | | X | | Slightly sweet and pungent piney flavor with some bitterness. Can be used sparingly in dishes. |
| Kava Kava | | X | | | | | | | Bitter. Preparation method can influence the taste. Capsules & extracts help avoid the taste. |
| Kola Nut | X | X | | | | | X | | Bitterness with slight sweetness and astringency. Flavoring in beverages like cola sodas. |
| Korean Ginseng | | X | | | | | X | | Bitter with slight sweetness. Used in traditional medicine in teas or herbal preparations. |
| Kratom | | X | | | | | | | Strong bitter taste. Often used in sweet beverages or foods to mask the taste. |
| Lamb's Ear | | X | X | | | | | | No taste. Not consumed as food. Used in teas. |
| Lily of the Valley | | X | | | | | | | Highly toxic. Not consumed as food. |
| Lobelia | | X | | X | | | | | Intensely bitter. It can be pungent and acrid. Not consumed as food. Can be toxic. |
| Lovage | X | X | | X | | | | | Mildly astringent, hint of bitterness, slightly pungent or peppery. Adds depth or complexity. |
| Male Fern | | X | | | | | | | Not consumed as it contains toxic compounds. |
| Milk Thistle | | X | | | | | | | Bitter. |
| Motherwort | | X | | | | | | | Bitter. Used in traditional herbal medicine. |
| Mucuna Pruriens | | X | | | | | | | Bitter. Used in traditional medicine and supplements. |
| Mugwort | | X | | | | | | | Slightly bitter. Used in traditional medicine and occasionally in some culinary practices. |
| Mullein | | X | | | | | | | Mildly bitter an mucilagninous (slightly slimy). Used in herbal teas or other preparations. |
| Mustard | | X | | X | | | X | | Pungent and slightly bitter. Can have a slightly sweet taste when prepared as a condiment. |
| Myrrh | | X | | | | | | | Bitter. Traditionally used for medicinal qualities. |
| Nasturtium | | X | | X | | | | | Peppery and pungent. Reminiscent of watercress. Taste can be mildly spicy and slightly bitter. |
| Neem | | X | | | | | | | Extremely bitter. Used in traditional Ayurvedic medicine. |

| Herbs In Alphabetical Order | Astringent | Bitter | No Taste | Pungent | Salty | Sour | Sweet | Umami | Details |
|---|---|---|---|---|---|---|---|---|---|
| **Bitter** | | | | | | | | | |
| Nettle | | X | | | | | | | Slightly bitter. May have an earthy or grassy flavor. Used in culinary preparations and teas. |
| Oak Bark | X | X | | | | | | | Astringent and bitter. Not consumed as food. Used in traditional medicine. |
| Olive | | X | | | X | | | | Salty & sometimes bitter. Savory. Taste can vary due to variety and ripeness. |
| Olive Leaf | X | X | | | | | | | Mildly bitter and may be slightly astringent. Used in herbal teas and supplements. |
| Oregano | | X | | X | | | | | Pungency and slight bitterness contributes to its savory flavor profile. Used in many cuisines. |
| Oregon Grape | | X | | | | X | | | Bitter and sour. Berries are tart and acidic. Berries are used in jams and jellies. |
| Oregon Grape Root | X | X | | | | | | | Bitter and slightly astringent. Not consumed as food. Used in herbal preparations. |
| Panax ginseng | | X | | | | | X | | Slightly bitter. Can have a slightly sweet or earthy undertone. Used in traditional medicine. |
| Papaya Seed | | X | | X | | | | | Peppery and slightly bitter. Pungent taste. Used as a spice of condiment. |
| Parsley | | X | | X | | | | | Fresh, slightly bitter, mild peppery, and herbaceous taste. Pungent. Adds flavor to dishes. |
| Parsley Root | | X | | X | | | | | Fresh, slightly bitter, and mild peppery. Pungent. Used in soups, stews, & vegetable dishes. |
| Passionflower | | X | | | | | | | Not consumed for taste. Traditionally used in herbal medicine. |
| Pau D'Arco | | X | | | | | | | Bitter. Not consumed as food. Prepared as herbal infusions or teas. |
| Pennyroyal | | X | | X | | | | | Strong minty flavor with a tinge of bitterness. It can be toxic, especially in large doses. |
| Pleurisy Root | | X | | | | | | | Bitter. Not consumed as food. Used in traditional medicine. |
| Poke Root | | X | | | | | | | Extreme bitterness. Not consumed as food, due to potential toxicity. |
| Prickly Ash | X | X | | X | | | | | Astringent, can be bitter. Tingling or numbing sensation contributes to pungent, spicy quality. |
| Puncture Vine | | X | | | | | | | Bitter. Not consumed as food. Used in traditional medicine. |
| Raspberry Leaf | X | X | | | | | | | Astringent or slightly bitter. Is often used for herbal teas. |
| Rehmannia | | X | | | | | X | | Sweet and slightly bitter. Commonly used in traditional Chinese medicine. |
| Reishi mushrooms | | X | | | | | | | Strong bitterness. Not consumed as food. Used in traditional Chinese medicine. |
| Rhodiola | | X | | | | | | | Bitter. Usually in traditional medicine and consumed as a supplement. |
| Rosemary | | X | | X | | | | | Pungent, resinous flavor, with slight bitterness. Adds depth to a variety of dishes. |
| Rue | | X | | X | | | | | Bitter & pungent. A strong sharp flavor. Can be toxic. |
| Sage | | X | | X | | | | | Pungent with a strong, slightly bitter & earthy flavor. Used in cooking, especially savory dishes. |
| Sarsaparilla | | X | | | | | X | | Sweet, slightly bitter, and a mild root beer-like taste. Commonly uses in beverages. |
| Schisandra | | X | | X | X | X | X | | Bitter, pungent, salty, sour, & sweet flavors. Used in teas, infusions, tinctures, & extracts. |
| Senna | | X | | | | | | | Bitter. Not consumed as food. Often used as for laxative properties. |
| Shatavari | | X | | | | | X | | Sweet and bitter, with a cooling effect. Commonly used in Ayurvedic medicine. |
| Shepherd's Purse | X | X | | | | | | | Slightly bitter and astringent. The leaves are edible and used in salads or cooked dishes. |
| Shilajit | | X | | | | | | | Bitter and earthy flavor. Used in traditional Ayurvedic medicine. |
| Siberian Ginseng | | X | | | | | | | Not used for culinary purposes. Traditionally used in herbal medicine. |
| Skullcap | | X | | | | | | | Bitter. Used in traditional herbal remedies or teas. |
| Spirulina | | X | | | | | | | Slightly bitter or seaweed-like. Used in smoothies, juices, or recipes that blend other tastes. |
| St. John's Wort | | X | | | | | | | Bitter. Not used for culinary purposes. Traditionally used in herbal medicines. |
| Stinging Nettle | | X | | | | | | | Slightly bitter. Used in culinary applications. Leaves used in teas and infusions. |
| Sweet Annie | | X | | | | | | | Slightly bitter. Used for medicinal purposes. Also known as sweet wormwood. |
| Tansy | | X | | | | | | | Bitter. Historically used in culinary applications. Can be toxic in large quantities. |
| Tinospora Cordifolia | | X | | | | | | | Bitter. Used in traditional medicine. Especially Ayurveda medicine. |
| Tormentil | X | X | | | | | | | Astringent and bitter. Used in teas and as a flavoring agent. |
| Tulsi | X | X | | X | | | X | | Slightly astringent, mildly bitter, sweet undertones, & subtle pungency. Wide culinary uses. |
| Turkey Rhubarb | X | X | | | | | | | Astringent and bitter. Not consumed as food. Used in traditional medicine. |
| Turmeric | | X | | X | | | | | Mildly bitter, earthy undertones, pungent, and peppery. Used in savory & sweet dishes. |
| Usnea | X | X | | | | | | | Bitter and astringent. Not consumed as food. Used in traditional medicine. |
| Uva Ursi | X | X | | | | | | | Astringent & slightly bitter. It is primarily used for medicine, not culinary taste. Can be toxic. |
| Valerian | | X | | | | | | | Strong, earthy, and somewhat bitter. Not consumed for taste. Used in teas & supplements. |
| Vervain | | X | | | | | | | Bitter. Not used for culinary purposes. Traditionally used in herbal medicines. |
| White Willow Bark | | X | | | | | | | Bitter. Not used for culinary purposes. Traditionally used in herbal medicines. |
| Wild Cherry Bark | | X | | | | | | | Bitter. Not used for culinary purposes. Traditionally used in herbal medicines. |
| Wild Indigo | | X | | | | | | | Bitter. Not used for culinary purposes. Traditionally used in herbal medicines. |
| Wild Yam | X | X | | | | | | | Astringent and bitter. Not used for culinary purposes. Traditionally used in herbal medicines. |
| Willow | X | X | | | | | | | Astringent and bitter. Not used for culinary purposes. Traditionally used in herbal medicines. |
| Willow Bark | X | X | | | | | | | Astringent and bitter. Not used for culinary purposes. Traditionally used in herbal medicines. |
| Wood Betony | | X | | | | | | | Mildly bitter. Used for potential medicinal properties rather than its culinary uses. |
| Wormseed | | X | | X | | | | | Pungent. Strong, herbal, & slightly bitter. Used in Mexican and Central American cuisines. |
| Wormwood | | X | | | | | | | Intensely bitter. Often used to produce the alcoholic beverage absinthe. |
| Yarrow | | X | | | | | | | Bitter. Used in herbal teas or infusions. Small amounts add flavor to certain dishes. |
| Yellow Dock | | X | | | | | | | Bitter. Not used for culinary purposes. Traditionally used in herbal medicines. |
| Yerba Mate | | X | | | | | | | Bitter, with earthy & vegetal undertones. Used as a tea. Sweeteners added to balance taste. |
| Yerba Santa | X | X | | | | | | | Bitter & somewhat astringent. Not used for culinary purposes. Used in herbal medicines. |

| Herbs In Alphabetical Order | Astringent | Bitter | No Taste | Pungent | Salty | Sour | Sweet | Umami | Details |
|---|---|---|---|---|---|---|---|---|---|
| **No Taste** | | | | | | | | | |
| Chia Seeds | | | X | | | | | | Neutral or slightly nutty taste.  Blends without altering flavor.  Used in a wide range of recipes. |
| Chickpeas | | | X | | | | | | Mild nutty taste.  Versatile legumes used in various cuisines & dishes.  Salads, stews, hummus. |
| Chlorella | | | X | | | | | | Neutral to mildly earthy.  Mainly consumed as capsules or mixed in smoothies or juices. |
| Cinquefoil | | | X | | | | | | Not consumed for their taste.  Known for its historical uses in traditional medicine. |
| Cleavers | | | X | | | | | | Not consumed for their taste.  Sometimes used in herbal teas. |
| Clematis | | | X | | | | | | Considered toxic and not consumed. |
| Cordyceps | | | X | | | | | | No taste.  Taste is influenced by the overall dish, rather than having a distinct taste of its own. |
| Couchgrass | | | X | | | | | | Bland taste.  Used medicinally. |
| Cranesbill | | | X | | | | | | No taste.  Not used as food.  Historically used as medicine. |
| Cypress | | | X | | | | | | Not typically consumed as food.  May have toxic compounds. |
| Flax | | | X | | | | X | | Mildly, slightly nutty taste with a neutral or slightly sweet flavor.  Used in cooking or baking. |
| Fringe Tree | | | X | | | | | | No taste.  Not used as food.  Historically used as medicine. |
| French Lavender | | | X | | | | | | Floral and herbaceous flavor.  Not used for taste.  Used for fragrance in teas, and cooking. |
| Geranium | | | X | | | | | | Not all geraniums are edible.  Edible ones have a floral and slightly citrusy taste. |
| Goat's Rue | | | X | | | | | | Not consumed for taste.  Historically used in traditional medicine. |
| Goldenrod | | | X | | | | | | Not consumed for food.  Not all species are edible, and proper identification is crucial. |
| Gravel Root | | | X | | | | | | Not consumed for taste.  Traditionally used in herbal medicine. |
| Gumweed | | | X | | | | | | Not consumed for taste.  Not all species are edible, and proper identification is crucial. |
| Hollyhock | | | X | | | | | | Not consumed for taste.  Not all parts of the plant are edible, proper identification is crucial. |
| Horsemint | | | X | | | | | | Not consumed for taste.  Used in traditional medicine like herbal teas. |
| Horsetail | | | X | | | | | | Not consumed for taste.  Some species may be toxic in large amounts. |
| Hydrangea Root | | | X | | | | | | Not consumed for taste.  Used in traditional medicine. |
| Lamb's Ear | | | X | | | | | | No taste.  Not consumed as food.  Used in teas. |
| Mistletoe | | | X | | | | | | Not consumed as food.  It contains compounds that can be harmful, & lead to health issues. |
| Oak Moss | | | X | | | | | | Not typically consumed as food. |
| Oat Straw | | | X | | | | | | Not typically consumed as food.  Used in herbal teas and supplements. |
| Passionvine | | | X | | | | | | No taste.  Not used as food.  Historically used as medicine. |
| Pineapple Bromelain | | | X | | | | | | Breaks down protein, and works as a meat tenderizer. |
| Plantain | | | X | | | | X | | Unripe: no taste.  Ripe: starchy and slightly sweet.  Used in various cuisines. |
| Poplar | | | X | | | | | | No taste.  Not consumed as food.  Used for potential medicinal properties. |
| Psyllium | | | X | | | | | | No taste.  Used as a dietary fiber supplement.  Mixed with water or other liquids. |
| Pumpkin Seed | | | X | | | | | | Neutral, slightly nutty taste.  Can be influenced by how they are prepared. |
| Squaw Vine | | | X | | | | | | No taste.  Historically used in Native American and folk medicine. |
| Tea Tree Oil | | | X | | | | | | Not ingested.  Used for topical applications and aromatherapy.  Can be toxic. |
| Teasel Root | | | X | | | | | | No taste.  Not used for culinary purposes.  Traditionally used in herbal medicines. |
| Thuja | | | X | | | | | | Not consumed as food.  Can be toxic when ingested.  Used for medicinal purposes. |
| Weld | | | X | | | | | | Not commonly consumed for taste, can be used medicinally. |

| Herbs In Alphabetical Order | Astringent | Bitter | No Taste | Pungent | Salty | Sour | Sweet | Umami | Details |
|---|---|---|---|---|---|---|---|---|---|
| **Pungent** | | | | | | | | | |
| Angelica | | X | | X | | | | | A complex flavor that has bitter and sweet notes. |
| Bay Leaves | | X | | X | | | | | Bitter & pungent in fresh form.  When dried they taste herbal like thyme or oregano. |
| Basil | | | | X | | | X | | Sweet and slightly savory or pungent notes.  Used in pesto, salads, and pasta. |
| Bee Balm | | | | X | | | | | Slightly pungent with minty and citrusy notes.  Used in herbal teas and for culinary purposes. |
| Black Horehound | | X | | X | | | | | Bitter and pungent or slightly spicy taste. |
| Black Mustard | | X | | X | | | | | Pungent and slightly bitter.  Used in condiments, pickles & spice blends to add heat and flavor. |
| Black Pepper | | | | X | | | | | Pungent with heat or spiciness.  Enhances the perception of other tastes in a recipe. |
| Blue Flag | | X | | X | | | | | Bitter and acrid or sharp, pungent taste.  Not consumed as food, due to toxicity. |
| Camphor | | | | X | | | | | Pungent/Medicinal or somewhat menthol-like.  Potentially toxic, and not for consumption. |
| Cannabis | | | | X | | | X | | The taste can vary and be earthy, herbal, skunky, sweet or fruity, or spicy or pungent. |
| Caraway | | X | | X | | | X | | Slightly sweet & warm taste reminiscent of anise or licorice.  Slightly bitter or slightly pungent. |
| Cardamom | | | | X | | | X | | Sweet 7 slightly floral.  Spicy or pungent.  Citrusy undertones.  Used in sweet & savory dishes. |
| Cayenne | | | | X | | | | | Pungent due to spiciness.  A key element in various cuisines worldwide. |
| Celery Seed | X | X | | X | | | | | Astringent, slightly bitter, & pungent taste like concentrated celery.  Used as a spice in recipes. |
| Chenopodium Oil | | | | X | | | | | A pungent taste.  It can be toxic in large quantities. |
| Cilantro | | | | X | | | X | | Citrusy, slightly sweet, and pungent.  It is a common ingredient in many cuisines. |
| Cinnamon | | | | X | | | X | | Sweet and pungent (slightly spicy).  Used in sweet and savory dishes.  Versatile spice. |
| Cloves | | | | X | | | X | | Pungent and a sweetness with a rich, slightly bitter undertone.  Used in sweet & savory dishes. |
| Coriander | | | | X | | | X | | Complex taste: citrusy & slightly sweet, with mildly pungent undertones. |
| Damiana | | X | | X | | | | | Bitter and pungent.  Not consumed for flavor.  Used in herbal teas or supplements. |
| Danshen | | X | | X | | | | | Bitter and slightly pungent.  Not consumed for taste.  Used it traditional herbal formulas. |
| Dong Quai | | X | | X | | | | | Bitter and pungent.  Not consumed for flavor.  Used in herbal teas or supplements. |
| Elecampane | | X | | X | | | | | Bitter and pungent taste.  Not consumed as food.  Used in herbal formulas: teas and tinctures. |
| Eucalyptus | | | | X | | | | | Pungent and menthol-like.  Used in cough drops, throat lozenges, teas, and essential oils. |
| Garlic | | | | X | | | | | Pungent and strong flavor.  Used in savory dishes. |
| Ginger | | | | X | | | | | Pungent and spicy.  Used in herbal teas, sweets, and savory dishes. |
| Holy Basil | | X | | X | | | | | Mild bitterness and pungent taste.  Used in various dishes and teas. |
| Horseradish | | | | X | | | | | Strong and pungent, with a spicy kick.  Commonly used as a condiment. |
| Juniper | | X | | X | | | X | | Slightly sweet and pungent piney flavor with some bitterness.  Can be used sparingly in dishes. |
| Juniper Berries | | X | | X | | | X | | Slightly sweet and pungent piney flavor with some bitterness.  Can be used sparingly in dishes. |
| Lobelia | | X | | X | | | | | Intensely bitter.  It can be pungent and acrid.  Not consumed as food.  Can be toxic. |
| Lomatium | | | | X | | | | | Pungent and sometimes resinous taste.  Used in traditional herbal medicine. |
| Lovage | X | X | | X | | | | | Mildly astringent, hint of bitterness, slightly pungent or peppery.  Adds depth or complexity. |
| Chamomile | | | | X | | | X | | Sweet and slightly pungent.  Used in culinary dishes and beverages. |
| Mustard | | X | | X | | | X | | Pungent and slightly bitter.  Can have a slightly sweet taste when prepared as a condiment. |
| Nasturtium | | X | | X | | | | | Peppery and pungent.  Reminiscent of watercress.  Taste can be mildly spicy and slightly bitter. |
| Onion | | | | X | | | X | | Pungent & savory.  Can have a subtle sweetness.  Used in many cuisines. |
| Oregano | | X | | X | | | | | Pungency and slight bitterness contributes to its savory flavor profile.  Used in many cuisines. |
| Papaya Seed | | X | | X | | | | | Peppery and slightly bitter.  Pungent taste.  Used as a spice of condiment. |
| Parsley | | X | | X | | | | | Fresh, slightly bitter, mild peppery, and herbaceous taste.  Pungent.  Adds flavor to dishes. |
| Parsley Root | | X | | X | | | | | Fresh, slightly bitter, and mild peppery.  Pungent.  Used in soups, stews, & vegetable dishes. |
| Pennyroyal | | X | | X | | | | | Strong minty flavor with a tinge of bitterness.  It can be toxic, especially in large doses. |
| Peppermint | X | | | X | | | X | | Cool, sweetness, subtle bitterness, with a pungency.  Used in various foods and beverages. |
| Prickly Ash | X | X | | X | | | | | Astringent, can be bitter.  Tingling or numbing sensation contributes to pungent, spicy quality. |
| Rosemary | | X | | X | | | | | Pungent, resinous flavor, with slight bitterness.  Adds depth to a variety of dishes. |
| Rue | | X | | X | | | | | Bitter & pungent.  A strong sharp flavor.  Can be toxic. |
| Sage | | X | | X | | | | | Pungent with a strong, slightly bitter & earthy flavor.  Used in cooking, especially savory dishes. |
| Savory | | | | X | | | | | Pungent with earthy, minty, and peppery notes.  Used in culinary applications. |
| Schisandra | | X | | X | X | X | X | | Bitter, pungent, salty, sour, & sweet flavors.  Used in teas, infusions, tinctures, & extracts. |
| Spearmint | | | | X | | | X | | Sweet and slightly pungent.  Milder than peppermint.  Used in teas, beverages, and dishes. |
| Thyme | | | | X | | | X | | Pungent and savory, may have sweet undertones.  Used in culinary applications. |
| Tulsi | X | X | | X | | | X | | Slightly astringent, mildly bitter, sweet undertones, & subtle pungency.  Wide culinary uses. |
| Turmeric | | X | | X | | | | | Mildly bitter, earthy undertones, pungent, and peppery.  Used in savory & sweet dishes. |
| Wormseed | | X | | X | | | | | Pungent.  Strong, herbal, & slightly bitter.  Used in Mexican and Central American cuisines. |

| Herbs In Alphabetical Order | Astringent | Bitter | No Taste | Pungent | Salty | Sour | Sweet | Umami | Details |
|---|---|---|---|---|---|---|---|---|---|
| **Salty** | | | | | | | | | |
| Celery | X | X | | | X | | X | | Astringent, slightly salty, mildly bitter, & mildly sweet taste.  Used in soups, salads, snacks, etc. |
| Hyssop | | X | | | X | | | | Bitter and slightly pungent or peppery.  Used to flavor dishes or in teas. |
| Irish Moss | | | | | X | | | | Hint of sea-like brininess.  Gelling agent for jellies, desserts, and plant-based recipes. |
| Kelp | | | | | X | | X | X | Salty and savory profile with a subtle sweetness.  Imparts Umami to dishes. |
| Olive | | X | | | X | | | | Salty & sometimes bitter.  Savory.  Taste can vary due to variety and ripeness. |
| Schisandra | | X | | X | X | X | X | | Bitter, pungent, salty, sour, & sweet flavors.  Used in teas, infusions, tinctures, & extracts. |

| Herbs In Alphabetical Order | Astringent | Bitter | No Taste | Pungent | Salty | Sour | Sweet | Umami | Details |
|---|---|---|---|---|---|---|---|---|---|
| **Sour** | | | | | | | | | |
| Barberry | | | | | | X | | | A sour taste that can be tangy.  Used in jams, jellies, and certain Middle Eastern dishes. |
| Bilberry | | | | | | X | X | | Sweet and slightly tart or sour taste.  Used in jams, desserts, and baked goods. |
| Black Current | | | | | | X | X | | Sweet and slightly tart taste.  Suitable for culinary applications: jams, desserts, and beverages. |
| Blackberry | | | | | | X | X | | Sweet and slightly tart taste.  Culinary uses: desserts, jams, and sauces. |
| Cranberry | | | | | | X | | | Tart and sour.  Culinary uses: juices, sauces, and baked goods. |
| Hibiscus | | | | | | X | | | A tart and tangy flavor.  Used in tea. |
| Indian Gooseberry | | | | | | X | | | Sour or tangy.  Used in pickles, jams, or as fresh fruit. |
| Japanese Knotweed | | | | | | X | | | Sour or tart taste.  Used in jams or pies. |
| Lemon | | | | | | X | X | | Strong sourness, with slight sweetness.  Used in savory and sweet dishes. |
| Lemon Balm | | | | | | X | X | | Mildly sweet and citrusy, reminiscent of lemon.  Used in salads, beverages, and desserts. |
| Lemon Grass | | | | | | X | | | A strong lemon flavor with a hint of earthiness.  Used in soups, curries, and savory dishes. |
| Lemon Verbana | | | | | | X | | | Strong lemon flavor.  Used in teas, desserts, and other dishes. |
| Oregon Grape | | X | | | | X | | | Bitter and sour.  Berries are tart and acidic.  Berries are used in jams and jellies. |
| Pomegranate | | | | | | X | X | | Sweet with a hint of tartness.  Used in dishes and beverages. |
| Purslane | | | | | | X | | | Mildly slightly sour or tangy flavor.  Subtle citrus like taste.  Used in salads. |
| Rhubarb | | | | | | X | | | Sour.  Sugar is often added to balance out the tartness.  Commonly used in cooking & baking. |
| Schisandra | | X | | X | X | X | X | | Bitter, pungent, salty, sour, & sweet flavors.  Used in teas, infusions, tinctures, & extracts. |

| Herbs In Alphabetical Order | Astringent | Bitter | No Taste | Pungent | Salty | Sour | Sweet | Umami | Details |
|---|---|---|---|---|---|---|---|---|---|
| **Sweet** | | | | | | | | | |
| Alfalfa | | | | | | | X | | Mildly sweet & somewhat grassy or earthy flavor. Used in salads, sandwiches or smoothies. |
| Allspice | | | | | | | X | | Sweet & warm, with a hint of pepper. Combined spice flavors: cinnamon, cloves, & nutmeg. |
| American Ginseng | | X | | | | | X | | Mildly bitter and slightly sweet. May taste slightly earthy or herbal. Used in teas and tonics. |
| Anise | | | | | | | X | | Sweet and licorice like taste. Commonly used in cooking, baking, & beverages. |
| Anise seeds | | | | | | | X | | Sweet and licorice like taste. Commonly used in cooking, baking, & beverages. |
| Artichoke | | X | | | | | X | | Bitter and slightly sweet. |
| Ashitaba | | X | | | | | X | | Bitter and somewhat sweet notes. |
| Astragalus | | | | | | | X | | Slightly sweet and earthy flavor. Commonly used in herbal formulations and teas. |
| Basil | | | | X | | | X | | Sweet and slightly savory or pungent notes. Used in pesto, salads, and pasta. |
| Bilberry | | | | | | X | X | | Sweet and slightly tart or sour taste. Used in jams, desserts, and baked goods. |
| Black Current | | | | | | X | X | | Sweet and slightly tart taste. Suitable for culinary applications: jams, desserts, and beverages. |
| Blackberry | | | | | | X | X | | Sweet and slightly tart taste. Culinary uses: desserts, jams, and sauces. |
| Borage | | | | | | | X | | Mild, cucumber-like taste. Slightly sweet &refreshing. Used in salads, beverages, & garnishes. |
| Burdock | | X | | | | | X | | Slightly bitter with mildly sweet undertones. Often used in soups, stir-fries, and teas. |
| Burdock Root | | X | | | | | X | | Slightly bitter and mildly sweet and earthy flavor. Often used in soups, stir-fries, and teas. |
| Cacao | | X | | | | | X | X | Bitter, can have some sweetness if high quality dark chocolate, & umami (a savory rich taste). |
| Cannabis | | | | X | | | X | | The taste can vary and be earthy, herbal, skunky, sweet or fruity, or spicy or pungent. |
| Caraway | | X | | X | | | X | | Slightly sweet & warm taste reminiscent of anise or licorice. Slightly bitter or slightly pungent. |
| Cardamom | | | | X | | | X | | Sweet 7 slightly floral. Spicy or pungent. Citrusy undertones. Used in sweet & savory dishes. |
| Celery | X | X | | | X | | X | | Astringent, slightly salty, mildly bitter, & mildly sweet taste. Used in soups, salads, snacks, etc. |
| Chamomile | | X | | | | | X | | Mildly sweet, slightly bitter, and herbaceous taste. Floral or slightly fruity. Used to make teas. |
| Chickweed | | | | | | | X | | Slightly sweet, and may have a subtle earthy flavor. Often used in salads, sandwiches, etc. |
| Cilantro | | | | X | | | X | | Citrusy, slightly sweet, and pungent. It is a common ingredient in many cuisines. |
| Cinnamon | | | | X | | | X | | Sweet and pungent (slightly spicy). Used in sweet and savory dishes. Versatile spice. |
| Chamomile | | | | X | | | X | | Pungent and a sweetness with a rich, slightly bitter undertone. Used in sweet & savory dishes. |
| Coriander | | | | X | | | X | | Complex taste: citrusy & slightly sweet, with mildly pungent undertones. |
| Corn Silk | | | | | | | X | | Mildly sweet. Used in herbal teas and supplements for potential health benefits. |
| Dandelion | | X | | | | | X | | Older leaves are bitter. Younger leaver are slightly sweet. Culinary uses. Salads & teas. |
| Dill | | X | | | | | X | | Fresh and herbaceous flavor with mild anise or licorice undertones. Mild bitterness. |
| Elder | | X | | | | | X | | Sweet and somewhat tart taste. My contain some bitterness. Parts can be toxic. |
| Elderberry | | | | | | | X | | Sweet and somewhat tart taste. Used in jams, syrups, and beverages. |
| Elderflower | | | | | | | X | | Sweet and slightly floral taste. Culinary uses in syrups, cordials, and desserts. |
| Fennel | | | | | | | X | | Sweet and mildly licorice or anise-like. Used in salads, soups, and other recipes. |
| Fennel Seeds | | | | | | | X | | Sweet and mildly licorice or anise-like. Used in spice blends, sausages, and baked goods. |
| Fenugreek | | X | | | | | X | | Bitter with underlying sweet notes. Used in Indian, Middle Eastern, & North African cuisines. |
| Fireweed | | | | | | | X | | Mildly sweet. Used in salads, teas, and other culinary preparations. |
| Flax | | | X | | | | X | | Mildly, slightly nutty taste with a neutral or slightly sweet flavor. Used in cooking or baking. |
| Fo Ti Root | | X | | | | | X | | Slightly bitter and sweet. Used in traditional Chinese medicine. |
| Ginseng | | X | | | | | X | | Slightly bitter & subtle sweetness. Used in teas, extracts, or as an ingredient in certain foods. |
| Gotu Kola | | X | | | | | X | | Bitter and slightly sweet. Used as an herbal tea, included in salads, or other dishes. |
| Green Tea | X | X | | | | | X | X | Astringent & bitter. Can be slightly sweet if high quality & brewed correctly. Umami notes. |
| Hawthorn | | | | | | | X | | Slightly sweet with a tart undertone. Used in teas, jams, and syrups. |
| Jiaogulan | | X | | | | | X | | Sweet and slightly bitter. Often used as a herbal tea. |
| Juniper | | X | | X | | | X | | Slightly sweet and pungent piney flavor with some bitterness. Can be used sparingly in dishes. |
| Juniper Berries | | X | | X | | | X | | Slightly sweet and pungent piney flavor with some bitterness. Can be used sparingly in dishes. |
| Kelp | | | | | X | | X | X | Salty and savory profile with a subtle sweetness. Imparts Umami to dishes. |
| Kola Nut | X | X | | | | | X | | Bitterness with slight sweetness and astringency. Flavoring in beverages like cola sodas. |
| Korean Ginseng | | X | | | | | X | | Bitter with slight sweetness. Used in traditional medicine in teas or herbal preparations. |
| Lavender | X | | | | | | X | | Slight sweet, floral, herbaceous flavor, & mildly astringent. Use sparingly due to potent flavor. |
| Lemon | | | | | | X | X | | Strong sourness, with slight sweetness. Used in savory and sweet dishes. |
| Lemon Balm | | | | | | X | X | | Mildly sweet and citrusy, reminiscent of lemon. Used in salads, beverages, and desserts. |
| Licorice | | | | | | | X | | Pronounced sweetness. Used in candies, teas, or various culinary & medicinal preparations. |
| Licorice Root | | | | | | | X | | Sweet with subtle earthy & woody undertones. Used in teas, candies, & traditional medicines. |
| Linden | | | | | | | X | | Sweet and mildly floral. Used in herbal teas and infusions. |
| Maca | | | | | | | X | | Sweet & malt-like flavor. May have earthy or nutty undertones. A natural sweetener. |
| Maca Root | | | | | | | X | | Sweet and nutty flavor. Used in smoothies, desserts & other dishes needing a sweet flavor. |
| Mallow | | | | | | | X | | Slightly sweet. Similar to spinach or lettuce. Used in salads and other dishes. |
| Marjoram | | | | | | | X | | Mild & sweet, slightly similar to oregano but milder. Used for soups, stews, sauces, & meats. |
| Marshmallow | | | | | | | X | | Sweet. Adds subtle sweetness to herbal teas and infusions. |
| Marshmallow Root | | | | | | | X | | Sweet. Adds subtle sweetness to herbal teas and infusions. |

| Herbs In Alphabetical Order | Astringent | Bitter | No Taste | Pungent | Salty | Sour | Sweet | Umami | Details |
|---|---|---|---|---|---|---|---|---|---|
| **Sweet** | | | | | | | | | |
| Meadowsweet | X | | | | | | X | | Sweet and slightly astringent. |
| Mint | | | | X | | | X | | Sweet and slightly pungent. Used in culinary dishes and beverages. |
| Mustard | | X | | X | | | X | | Pungent and slightly bitter. Can have a slightly sweet taste when prepared as a condiment. |
| Oats | | | | | | | X | | Mildly sweet. Oats can take on flavors of other ingredients. |
| Okra | | | | | | | X | X | Mildly sweet & slightly umami. Taste is influenced by the way it is cooked & ingredients used. |
| Onion | | | | X | | | X | | Pungent & savory. Can have a subtle sweetness. Used in many cuisines. |
| Panax ginseng | | X | | | | | X | | Slightly bitter. Can have a slightly sweet or earthy undertone. Used in traditional medicine. |
| Peppermint | X | | | X | | | X | | Cool, sweetness, subtle bitterness, with a pungency. Used in various foods and beverages. |
| Plantain | | | X | | | | X | | Unripe: no taste. Ripe: starchy and slightly sweet. Used in various cuisines. |
| Pomegranate | | | | | | X | X | | Sweet with a hint of tartness. Used in dishes and beverages. |
| Prune | | | | | | | X | | Sweet and slightly tangy. Used in culinary applications. |
| Pumpkin | | | | | | | X | | Mildly sweet. Used in sweet dishes and desserts. |
| Red Clover | | | | | | | X | | Slightly sweet. Used in herbal teas. |
| Rehmannia | | X | | | | | X | | Sweet and slightly bitter. Commonly used in traditional Chinese medicine. |
| Rose | | | | | | | X | | Sweet and floral. Used to add delicate sweetness to various dishes and beverages. |
| Saffron | | | | | | | X | | Subtle sweetness with floral and earthy notes. It imparts a unique flavor to dishes. |
| Sarsaparilla | | X | | | | | X | | Sweet, slightly bitter, and a mild root beer-like taste. Commonly uses in beverages. |
| Schisandra | | X | | X | X | X | X | | Bitter, pungent, salty, sour, & sweet flavors. Used in teas, infusions, tinctures, & extracts. |
| Sesame Seeds | | | | | | | X | | Slightly sweet and nutty. Used in baking, cooking, and garnishing various dishes. |
| Shatavari | | X | | | | | X | | Sweet and bitter, with a cooling effect. Commonly used in Ayurvedic medicine. |
| Slippery Elm | | | | | | | X | | Mucilaginous and slightly sweet. Primarily used medicinally in teas and formulations. |
| Spearmint | | | | X | | | X | | Sweet and slightly pungent. Milder than peppermint. Used in teas, beverages, and dishes. |
| Suma | | | | | | | X | | Slightly sweet & earthy flavor. Used in traditional medicine, not used in culinary applications. |
| Sweet Cicely | | | | | | | X | | Sweet and anise-like flavor. Used to sweeten dishes: desserts, salads, and beverages. |
| Sweet Root | | | | | | | X | | Licorice root that is sweet. Used in herbal teas, candies, and various dishes. |
| Thyme | | | | X | | | X | | Pungent and savory, may have sweet undertones. Used in culinary applications. |
| Tulsi | X | X | | X | | | X | | Slightly astringent, mildly bitter, sweet undertones, & subtle pungency. Wide culinary uses. |
| Wintergreen | | | | | | | X | | Sweet and minty. Used in food and beverages to provide a minty and refreshing taste. |

| Herbs In Alphabetical Order | Astringent | Bitter | No Taste | Pungent | Salty | Sour | Sweet | Umami | Details |
|---|---|---|---|---|---|---|---|---|---|
| **Umami** | | | | | | | | | |
| Cacao | | X | | | | | X | X | Bitter, can have some sweetness if high quality dark chocolate, & umami (a savory rich taste). |
| Green Tea | X | X | | | | | X | X | Astringent & bitter.  Can be slightly sweet if high quality & brewed correctly.  Umami notes. |
| Kelp | | | | | X | | X | X | Salty and savory profile with a subtle sweetness.  Imparts Umami to dishes. |
| Okra | | | | | | | X | X | Mildly sweet & slightly umami.  Taste is influenced by the way it is cooked & ingredients used. |
| Shiitake Mushroom | | | | | | | | X | Rich umami flavor.  Savory and meaty.  Used in traditional and modern dishes. |

# SECTION V

Alphabetized Herbs with Taste Profiles

| Herbs In Alphabetical Order | Astringent | Bitter | No Taste | Pungent | Salty | Sour | Sweet | Umami | Details |
|---|---|---|---|---|---|---|---|---|---|
| Agrimony | X | X | | | | | | | Slightly bitter and astringent taste, mildly sweet or nutty. Suitable for teas & infusions. |
| Albizia | | X | | | | | | | Slightly bitter. Not typically consumed as food, due to potential toxicity. |
| Alder Buckthorn | | X | | | | | | | Bitter. Not typically consumed as food, due to potential toxicity. |
| Alfalfa | | | | | | | X | | Mildly sweet & somewhat grassy or earthy flavor. Used in salads, sandwiches or smoothies. |
| Allspice | | | | | | | X | | Sweet & warm, with a hint of pepper. Combined spice flavors: cinnamon, cloves, & nutmeg. |
| Aloe Vera | | X | | | | | | | Mild, slightly bitter. Consuming in large amounts may have a laxative effect. Use caution. |
| Aloe Vera Leaf | | X | | | | | | | Mild, slightly bitter. Consuming in large amounts may have a laxative effect. Use caution. |
| Alum | X | | | | | | | | Not typically consumed as food or spice. Often used for medicine or a pickling agent. |
| American Ginseng | | X | | | | | X | | Mildly bitter and slightly sweet. May taste slightly earthy or herbal. Used in teas and tonics. |
| American Skullcap | | X | | | | | | | Slightly bitter. Often used with other herbs to balance or complement the overall taste. |
| Andrographis | | X | | | | | | | One of the bitterest herbs. |
| Angelica | | X | | X | | | | | A complex flavor that has bitter and sweet notes. |
| Anise seeds | | | | | | | X | | Sweet and licorice like taste. Commonly used in cooking, baking, & beverages. |
| Arjuna | X | X | | | | | | | The astringent taste is described as dry, puckering, or tannic. |
| Arnica | | | X | | | | | | Not consumed orally due to its potential toxicity. Used topically as creams, ointments, or gels. |
| Artichoke | | X | | | | | X | | Bitter and slightly sweet. |
| Ashitaba | | X | | | | | X | | Bitter and somewhat sweet notes. |
| Ashwagandha | | X | | | | | | | Bitterness that is somewhat earthy or reminiscent of the taste of roots. |
| Aspen | | | X | | | | | | Not typically consumed as food or spice, due to potential toxicity. Often used for medicine. |
| Astragalus | | | | | | | X | | Slightly sweet and earthy flavor. Commonly used in herbal formulations and teas. |
| Baneberry | | X | | | | | | | Not consumed as food because it is toxic. |
| Barberry | | | | | | X | | | A sour taste that can be tangy. Used in jams, jellies, and certain Middle Eastern dishes. |
| Basil | | | | X | | | X | | Sweet and slightly savory or pungent notes. Used in pesto, salads, and pasta. |
| Bayberry | X | X | | | | | | | Astringent and slightly bitter. Bayberry leaves have been used in some traditional dishes. |
| Bay Leaves | | X | | X | | | | | Bitter & pungent in fresh form. When dried they taste herbal like thyme or oregano. |
| Bearberry | X | X | | | | | | | Astringent and slightly bitter. It is primarily used for health benefits, not culinary taste. |
| Bee Balm | | | | X | | | | | Slightly pungent with minty and citrusy notes. Used in herbal teas and for culinary purposes. |
| Bergamot | | X | | | | | | | Citrusy and mildly bitter. Used in culinary applications when a slight citrusy note is desired. |
| Bilberry | | | | | | X | X | | Sweet and slightly tart or sour taste. Used in jams, desserts, and baked goods. |
| Birch | | X | | | | | | | Not commonly used for food, it can be toxic. |
| Bitter Leaf | | X | | | | | | | Used in cooking, especially African cuisines. Balanced with other flavors. |
| Bitter Melon | | X | | | | | | | Bitterness with hints of astringency. Used in Asian cooking: stir-fries, soups, and other dishes. |
| Black Cohosh | | X | | | | | | | Not typically consumed for taste. |
| Black Current | | | | | | X | X | | Sweet and slightly tart taste. Suitable for culinary applications: jams, desserts, and beverages. |
| Black-eyed Susan | | | X | | | | | | No taste. Not used as food. Historically used as medicine. |
| Black haw | X | X | | | | | | | Bitter and astringent tastes. |
| Black hellebore | | | X | | | | | | Not consumed as food, it is toxic and considered dangerous. |
| Black Horehound | | X | | X | | | | | Bitter and pungent or slightly spicy taste. |
| Black Mustard | | X | | X | | | | | Pungent and slightly bitter. Used in condiments, pickles & spice blends to add heat and flavor. |
| Black Pepper | | | | X | | | | | Pungent with heat or spiciness. Enhances the perception of other tastes in a recipe. |
| Black Seed | | X | | | | | | | Slightly bitter. Can be used in culinary dishes and health remedies. |
| Black Walnut Hull | X | X | | | | | | | Bitter and somewhat astringent. Not typically consumed for their taste. |
| Blackberry | | | | | | X | X | | Sweet and slightly tart taste. Culinary uses: desserts, jams, and sauces. |
| Blackberry Leaf | X | X | | | | | | | Mildly astringent or slightly bitter taste. Often used in herbal teas or infusions. |
| Blessed Thistle | | X | | | | | | | Not commonly consumed for taste, but used medicinally. |
| Bloodroot | | X | | | | | | | Not used for culinary purposes, because it is extremely toxic. Medicinal use is controversial. |
| Blue Cohosh | | X | | | | | | | Bitterness is a common taste associated with medicinal herbs. |
| Blue Flag | | X | | X | | | | | Bitter and acrid or sharp, pungent taste. Not consumed as food, due to toxicity. |
| Blue Vervain | | X | | | | | | | Bitter taste. Typically used in herbal formulations, teas, or tinctures. |
| Boldo | | X | | | | | | | Bitter. Often used in herbal medicine and to flavor certain foods and beverages. |
| Boneset | | X | | | | | | | Bitter taste. Used in traditional medicine. |
| Borage | | | | | | | X | | Mild, cucumber-like taste. Slightly sweet &refreshing. Used in salads, beverages, & garnishes. |
| Boswellia | X | X | | | | | | | Bitter or slightly astringent. Used to prepare teas for medicinal purposes. |
| Buchu | X | X | | | | | | | Mildly bitter or astringent taste. Used in traditional herbal medicine. |
| Buckthorn | | X | | | | | | | Bitter. Typically not consumed due to their laxative effects. |
| Bupleurum | | X | | | | | | | Bitter taste. Often used in traditional Chinese medicine. |
| Burdock | | X | | | | | | X | | Slightly bitter with mildly sweet undertones. Often used in soups, stir-fries, and teas. |
| Burdock Root | | X | | | | | X | | Slightly bitter and mildly sweet and earthy flavor. Often used in soups, stir-fries, and teas. |
| Butcher's Broom | | X | | | | | | | Bitter. Typically use in herbal formulations rather than being consumed for taste. |
| Cacao | | X | | | | | X | X | Bitter, can have some sweetness if high quality dark chocolate, & umami (a savory rich taste). |
| Calendula | | X | | | | | | | Mild, slightly bitter or peppery taste. Used in culinary applications like salads or as garnishes. |

| Herbs In Alphabetical Order | Astringent | Bitter | No Taste | Pungent | Salty | Sour | Sweet | Umami | Details |
|---|---|---|---|---|---|---|---|---|---|
| California Poppy | | X | | | | | | | Mildly bitter. Not typically used for taste. Often used in teas or tinctures. |
| Camphor | | | | X | | | | | Pungent/Medicinal or somewhat menthol-like. Potentially toxic, and not for consumption. |
| Cannabis | | | | X | | | X | | The taste can vary and be earthy, herbal, skunky, sweet or fruity, or spicy or pungent. |
| Caraway | | X | | X | | | X | | Slightly sweet & warm taste reminiscent of anise or licorice. Slightly bitter or slightly pungent. |
| Cardamom | | | | X | | | X | | Sweet 7 slightly floral. Spicy or pungent. Citrusy undertones. Used in sweet & savory dishes. |
| Cascara amarga | | X | | | | | | | Bitter. Used as herbal supplements or teas for a laxative effect. Not used as food. |
| Cascara sagrada | | X | | | | | | | Bitter. Used as herbal supplements or teas for a laxative effect. Not used as food. |
| Cascarilla | | X | | | | | | | Bitter. Mostly used in certain beverages. |
| Cassia | | X | | | | | | | Slightly bitter and nutty taste. Uncommon to use in cooking. Used in teas. |
| Catnip | | X | | | | | | | Mildly bitter and minty. Not used in culinary. Used as teas or herbal blends. |
| Cat's Claw | X | X | | | | | | | Bitter and astringent tastes. |
| Cayenne | | | | X | | | | | Pungent due to spiciness. A key element in various cuisines worldwide. |
| Celery | X | X | | | X | | X | | Astringent, slightly salty, mildly bitter, & mildly sweet taste. Used in soups, salads, snacks, etc. |
| Celery Seed | X | X | | X | | | | | Astringent, slightly bitter, & pungent taste like concentrated celery. Used as a spice in recipes. |
| Centaury | | X | | | | | | | Bitter. Often used in herbal formulations as medicine, including teas and tinctures. |
| Chamomile | | X | | | | | X | | Mildly sweet, slightly bitter, and herbaceous taste. Floral or slightly fruity. Used to make teas. |
| Chanca Piedra | | X | | | | | | | Bitter. Not typically consumed as food, instead it is used for health benefits. |
| Chaparral | | X | | | | | | | Bitter. Not typically consumed as food, instead it is used in traditional medicines. |
| Chaste Tree | | X | | | | | | | Bitterness. Consumed in the form of extracts, tinctures, or capsules rather than for its taste. |
| Chenopodium Oil | | | | X | | | | | A pungent taste. It can be toxic in large quantities. |
| Chia Seeds | | | X | | | | | | Neutral or slightly nutty taste. Blends without altering flavor. Used in a wide range of recipes. |
| Chickpeas | | | X | | | | | | Mild nutty taste. Versatile legumes used in various cuisines & dishes. Salads, stews, hummus. |
| Chickweed | | | | | | | X | | Slightly sweet, and may have a subtle earthy flavor. Often used in salads, sandwiches, etc. |
| Chicory | | X | | | | | | | Bitter taste can be pronounced. Used in salads, mixed with greens, or a coffee substitute. |
| Chicory Root | | X | | | | | | | Bitter, with a slightly woody and nutty flavor. Used as a coffee substitute. |
| Chlorella | | X | | | | | | | Neutral to mildly earthy. Mainly consumed as capsules or mixed in smoothies or juices. |
| Cilantro | | | | X | | | X | | Citrusy, slightly sweet, and pungent. It is a common ingredient in many cuisines. |
| Cinnamon | | | | X | | | X | | Sweet and pungent (slightly spicy). Used in sweet and savory dishes. Versatile spice. |
| Cinquefoil | | X | | | | | | | Not consumed for their taste. Known for its historical uses in traditional medicine. |
| Cleavers | | X | | | | | | | Not consumed for their taste. Sometimes used in herbal teas. |
| Clematis | | X | | | | | | | Considered toxic and not consumed. |
| Cloves | | | | X | | | X | | Pungent and a sweetness with a rich, slightly bitter undertone. Used in sweet & savory dishes. |
| Coleus Forskohlii | | X | | | | | | | Not typically consumed for taste, and more often used in supplements. |
| Coltsfoot | | X | | | | | | | Bitter taste. Not commonly consumed for taste. Historically used in traditional medicine. |
| Comfrey | | X | | | | | | | Bitter taste. Internal use not recommended, because it can be toxic to the liver. |
| Cordyceps | | X | | | | | | | No taste. Taste is influenced by the overall dish, rather than having a distinct taste of its own. |
| Coriander | | | | X | | | X | | Complex taste: citrusy & slightly sweet, with mildly pungent undertones. |
| Corn Silk | | | | | | | X | | Mildly sweet. Used in herbal teas and supplements for potential health benefits. |
| Cotton Root Bark | | X | | | | | | | Bitter. Used for potential medicinal properties in traditional herbal remedies. |
| Couchgrass | | | X | | | | | | Bland taste. Used medicinally. |
| Cramp Bark | X | | | | | | | | Astringent. Used in herbal formulations, such as teas and tinctures. |
| Cranberry | | | | | | X | | | Tart and sour. Culinary uses: juices, sauces, and baked goods. |
| Cranesbill | | X | | | | | | | No taste. Not used as food. Historically used as medicine. |
| Cumin | | X | | | | | | | Mild bitterness with a warm, earthy flavor. Added to savory recipes: curries, stews, etc. |
| Cypress | | X | | | | | | | Not typically consumed as food. May have toxic compounds. |
| Damiana | | X | | X | | | | | Bitter and pungent. Not consumed for flavor. Used in herbal teas or supplements. |
| Dandelion | | X | | | | | X | | Older leaves are bitter. Younger leaver are slightly sweet. Culinary uses. Salads & teas. |
| Dandelion Root | | X | | | | | | | Bitter and earthy flavor. Used in culinary and herbal preparations like teas and tinctures. |
| Danshen | | X | | X | | | | | Bitter and slightly pungent. Not consumed for taste. Used it traditional herbal formulas. |
| Devil's Claw | | X | | | | | | | Bitter. Not consumed for taste. Used in herbal formulas like teas and supplements. |
| Dill | | X | | | | | X | | Fresh and herbaceous flavor with mild anise or licorice undertones. Mild bitterness. |
| Dill Seed | | X | | | | | | | Warm & slightly bitter. More concentrated dill flavor. Uses: pickling, baking, & savory dishes. |
| Dong Quai | | X | | X | | | | | Bitter and pungent. Not consumed for flavor. Used in herbal teas or supplements. |
| Echinacea | | X | | | | | | | Bitter. Not consumed for taste. Used in herbal teas and supplements to boost immunity. |
| Elder | | X | | | | | X | | Sweet and somewhat tart taste. My contain some bitterness. Parts can be toxic. |
| Elderberry | | | | | | | X | | Sweet and somewhat tart taste. Used in jams, syrups, and beverages. |
| Elderflower | | | | | | | X | | Sweet and slightly floral taste. Culinary uses in syrups, cordials, and desserts. |
| Elecampane | | X | | X | | | | | Bitter and pungent taste. Not consumed as food. Used in herbal formulas: teas and tinctures. |
| Eleuthero | | X | | | | | | | Bitter. Not consumed for taste. Used in herbal formulas like teas and supplements. |
| Eucalyptus | | | | X | | | | | Pungent and menthol-like. Used in cough drops, throat lozenges, teas, and essential oils. |
| Fennel | | | | | | | X | | Sweet and mildly licorice or anise-like. Used in salads, soups, and other recipes. |

| Herbs In Alphabetical Order | Astringent | Bitter | No Taste | Pungent | Salty | Sour | Sweet | Umami | Details |
|---|---|---|---|---|---|---|---|---|---|
| Fennel Seeds | | | | | | | X | | Sweet and mildly licorice or anise-like. Used in spice blends, sausages, and baked goods. |
| Fenugreek | | X | | | | | X | | Bitter with underlying sweet notes. Used in Indian, Middle Eastern, & North African cuisines. |
| Feverfew | | X | | | | | | | Bitter. Not consumed for taste. Used in herbal formulas like teas and supplements. |
| Fireweed | | | | | | | X | | Mildly sweet. Used in salads, teas, and other culinary preparations. |
| Flax | | | X | | | | X | | Mildly, slightly nutty taste with a neutral or slightly sweet flavor. Used in cooking or baking. |
| Fo Ti Root | | X | | | | | X | | Slightly bitter and sweet. Used in traditional Chinese medicine. |
| Fringe Tree | | | X | | | | | | No taste. Not used as food. Historically used as medicine. |
| Frankincense | | X | | | | | | | Bitter with a resinous woody flavor. Not a culinary ingredient. Used medicinally. |
| French Lavender | | | X | | | | | | Floral and herbaceous flavor. Not used for taste. Used for fragrance in teas, and cooking. |
| Garden Sage | | X | | | | | | | Bitter taste with earthy undertones. Used to season meats, stews, and savory dishes. |
| Garlic | | | | X | | | | | Pungent and strong flavor. Used in savory dishes. |
| Gentian | | X | | | | | | | Highly bitter. Used to produce certain aperitifs and herbal bitters. |
| Geranium | | | X | | | | | | Not all geraniums are edible. Edible ones have a floral and slightly citrusy taste. |
| Germander | X | X | | | | | | | Bitter and astringent. Not consumed as food. Potential toxicity. |
| Ginger | | | | X | | | | | Pungent and spicy. Used in herbal teas, sweets, and savory dishes. |
| Ginkgo | | X | | | | | | | Bitter. Not consumed for taste. Used in supplements. |
| Ginkgo Biloba | | X | | | | | | | Bitter. Not consumed for taste. Used in supplements. |
| Ginseng | | X | | | | | X | | Slightly bitter & subtle sweetness. Used in teas, extracts, or as an ingredient in certain foods. |
| Globe Artichoke | | X | | | | | | | Mildly bitter. Used in salads, dips, and other culinary applications. |
| Goat's Rue | | | X | | | | | | Not consumed for taste. Historically used in traditional medicine. |
| Goldenrod | | | X | | | | | | Not consumed for food. Not all species are edible, and proper identification is crucial. |
| Goldenseal | | X | | | | | | | Bitter. Historically used in traditional medicine. |
| Gotu Kola | | X | | | | | X | | Bitter and slightly sweet. Used as an herbal tea, included in salads, or other dishes. |
| Gravel Root | | | X | | | | | | Not consumed for taste. Traditionally used in herbal medicine. |
| Greater Celandine | | X | | | | | | | Bitter. Contains toxic compounds, approach with caution. |
| Green Tea | X | X | | | | | X | X | Astringent & bitter. Can be slightly sweet if high quality & brewed correctly. Umami notes. |
| Guarana | | X | | | | | | | Bitter. Often used in energy drinks and supplements due to its caffeine content. |
| Gumweed | | | X | | | | | | Not consumed for taste. Not all species are edible, and proper identification is crucial. |
| Hawthorn | | | | | | | X | | Slightly sweet with a tart undertone. Used in teas, jams, and syrups. |
| Hibiscus | | | | | | X | | | A tart and tangy flavor. Used in tea. |
| Hollyhock | | | X | | | | | | Not consumed for taste. Not all parts of the plant are edible, proper identification is crucial. |
| Holy Basil | | X | | X | | | | | Mild bitterness and pungent taste. Used in various dishes and teas. |
| Hops | | X | | | | | | | Bitter. Used in beer to balance the sweetness of malt. |
| Horehound | | X | | | | | | | Bitter. Used medicinally in herbal teas, lozenges, or candies. |
| Horse Chestnut | | X | | | | | | | Bitter. Can be toxic in large quantities. Raw seeds are not safe due to their toxicity. |
| Horsemint | | | X | | | | | | Not consumed for taste. Used in traditional medicine like herbal teas. |
| Horseradish | | | | X | | | | | Strong and pungent, with a spicy kick. Commonly used as a condiment. |
| Horsetail | | | X | | | | | | Not consumed for taste. Some species may be toxic in large amounts. |
| Hydrangea Root | | | X | | | | | | Not consumed for taste. Used in traditional medicine. |
| Hyssop | | X | | | X | | | | Bitter and slightly pungent or peppery. Used to flavor dishes or in teas. |
| Indian Gooseberry | | | | | | X | | | Sour or tangy. Used in pickles, jams, or as fresh fruit. |
| Irish Moss | | | | | X | | | | Hint of sea-like brininess. Gelling agent for jellies, desserts, and plant-based recipes. |
| Jamaican Dogwood | | X | | | | | | | Not consumed as food. Often used in tinctures or extracts for medicinal purposes. |
| Japanese Knotweed | | | | | | X | | | Sour or tart taste. Used in jams or pies. |
| Jiaogulan | | X | | | | | X | | Sweet and slightly bitter. Often used as a herbal tea. |
| Juniper | | X | | X | | | X | | Slightly sweet and pungent piney flavor with some bitterness. Can be used sparingly in dishes. |
| Juniper Berries | | X | | X | | | X | | Slightly sweet and pungent piney flavor with some bitterness. Can be used sparingly in dishes. |
| Kava Kava | | X | | | | | | | Bitter. Preparation method can influence the taste. Capsules & extracts help avoid the taste. |
| Kelp | | | | | X | | X | X | Salty and savory profile with a subtle sweetness. Imparts Umami to dishes. |
| Kola Nut | X | X | | | | | X | | Bitterness with slight sweetness and astringency. Flavoring in beverages like cola sodas. |
| Korean Ginseng | | X | | | | | X | | Bitter with slight sweetness. Used in traditional medicine in teas or herbal preparations. |
| Kratom | | X | | | | | | | Strong bitter taste. Often used in sweet beverages or foods to mask the taste. |
| Lady's Mantle | X | | | | | | | | Astringent. Used in herbal preparations for its potential health benefits. |
| Lamb's Ear | | X | X | | | | | | No taste. Not consumed as food. Used in teas. |
| Lavender | X | | | | | | X | | Slight sweet, floral, herbaceous flavor, & mildly astringent. Use sparingly due to potent flavor. |
| Lemon | | | | | | X | X | | Strong sourness, with slight sweetness. Used in savory and sweet dishes. |
| Lemon Balm | | | | | | X | X | | Mildly sweet and citrusy, reminiscent of lemon. Used in salads, beverages, and desserts. |
| Lemon Grass | | | | | | X | | | A strong lemon flavor with a hint of earthiness. Used in soups, curries, and savory dishes. |
| Lemon Verbana | | | | | | X | | | Strong lemon flavor. Used in teas, desserts, and other dishes. |
| Licorice | | | | | | | X | | Pronounced sweetness. Used in candies, teas, or various culinary & medicinal preparations. |
| Licorice Root | | | | | | | X | | Sweet with subtle earthy & woody undertones. Used in teas, candies, & traditional medicines. |

| Herbs In Alphabetical Order | Astringent | Bitter | No Taste | Pungent | Salty | Sour | Sweet | Umami | Details |
|---|---|---|---|---|---|---|---|---|---|
| Lily of the Valley | | X | | | | | | | Highly toxic. Not consumed as food. |
| Linden | | | | | | | X | | Sweet and mildly floral. Used in herbal teas and infusions. |
| Lobelia | | X | | X | | | | | Intensely bitter. It can be pungent and acrid. Not consumed as food. Can be toxic. |
| Lomatium | | | | X | | | | | Pungent and sometimes resinous taste. Used in traditional herbal medicine. |
| Lovage | X | X | | X | | | | | Mildly astringent, hint of bitterness, slightly pungent or peppery. Adds depth or complexity. |
| Maca | | | | | | | X | | Sweet & malt-like flavor. May have earthy or nutty undertones. A natural sweetener. |
| Maca Root | | | | | | | X | | Sweet and nutty flavor. Used in smoothies, desserts & other dishes needing a sweet flavor. |
| Male Fern | | X | | | | | | | Not consumed as it contains toxic compounds. |
| Mallow | | | | | | | X | | Slightly sweet. Similar to spinach or lettuce. Used in salads and other dishes. |
| Marjoram | | | | | | | X | | Mild & sweet, slightly similar to oregano but milder. Used for soups, stews, sauces, & meats. |
| Marshmallow | | | | | | | X | | Sweet. Adds subtle sweetness to herbal teas and infusions. |
| Marshmallow Root | | | | | | | X | | Sweet. Adds subtle sweetness to herbal teas and infusions. |
| Meadowsweet | X | | | | | | X | | Sweet and slightly astringent. |
| Milk Thistle | | X | | | | | | | Bitter. |
| Mint | | | | X | | | X | | Sweet and slightly pungent. Used in culinary dishes and beverages. |
| Mistletoe | | | X | | | | | | Not consumed as food. It contains compounds that can be harmful, & lead to health issues. |
| Motherwort | | X | | | | | | | Bitter. Used in traditional herbal medicine. |
| Mucuna Pruriens | | X | | | | | | | Bitter. Used in traditional medicine and supplements. |
| Mugwort | | X | | | | | | | Slightly bitter. Used in traditional medicine and occasionally in some culinary practices. |
| Mullein | | X | | | | | | | Mildly bitter an mucilagninous (slightly slimy). Used in herbal teas or other preparations. |
| Mustard | | X | | X | | | X | | Pungent and slightly bitter. Can have a slightly sweet taste when prepared as a condiment. |
| Myrrh | | X | | | | | | | Bitter. Traditionally used for medicinal qualities. |
| Nasturtium | | X | | X | | | | | Peppery and pungent. Reminiscent of watercress. Taste can be mildly spicy and slightly bitter. |
| Neem | | X | | | | | | | Extremely bitter. Used in traditional Ayurvedic medicine. |
| Nettle | | X | | | | | | | Slightly bitter. May have an earthy or grassy flavor. Used in culinary preparations and teas. |
| Oak Bark | X | X | | | | | | | Astringent and bitter. Not consumed as food. Used in traditional medicine. |
| Oak Moss | | | X | | | | | | Not typically consumed as food. |
| Oat Straw | | | X | | | | | | Not typically consumed as food. Used in herbal teas and supplements. |
| Oats | | | | | | | X | | Mildly sweet. Oats can take on flavors of other ingredients. |
| Okra | | | | | | | X | X | Mildly sweet & slightly umami. Taste is influenced by the way it is cooked & ingredients used. |
| Olive | | X | | | X | | | | Salty & sometimes bitter. Savory. Taste can vary due to variety and ripeness. |
| Olive Leaf | X | X | | | | | | | Mildly bitter and may be slightly astringent. Used in herbal teas and supplements. |
| Onion | | | | X | | | X | | Pungent & savory. Can have a subtle sweetness. Used in many cuisines. |
| Oregano | | X | | X | | | | | Pungency and slight bitterness contributes to its savory flavor profile. Used in many cuisines. |
| Oregon Grape | | X | | | | X | | | Bitter and sour. Berries are tart and acidic. Berries are used in jams and jellies. |
| Oregon Grape Root | X | X | | | | | | | Bitter and slightly astringent. Not consumed as food. Used in herbal preparations. |
| Panax ginseng | | X | | | | | X | | Slightly bitter. Can have a slightly sweet or earthy undertone. Used in traditional medicine. |
| Papaya Seed | | X | | X | | | | | Peppery and slightly bitter. Pungent taste. Used as a spice of condiment. |
| Parsley | | X | | X | | | | | Fresh, slightly bitter, mild peppery, and herbaceous taste. Pungent. Adds flavor to dishes. |
| Parsley Root | | X | | X | | | | | Fresh, slightly bitter, and mild peppery. Pungent. Used in soups, stews, & vegetable dishes. |
| Passionflower | | X | | | | | | | Not consumed for taste. Traditionally used in herbal medicine. |
| Passionvine | | | X | | | | | | No taste. Not used as food. Historically used as medicine. |
| Pau D'Arco | | X | | | | | | | Bitter. Not consumed as food. Prepared as herbal infusions or teas. |
| Pennyroyal | | X | | X | | | | | Strong minty flavor with a tinge of bitterness. It can be toxic, especially in large doses. |
| Peppermint | X | | | X | | | X | | Cool, sweetness, subtle bitterness, with a pungency. Used in various foods and beverages. |
| Pineapple Bromelain | | | X | | | | | | Breaks down protein, and works as a meat tenderizer. |
| Plantain | | | X | | | | X | | Unripe: no taste. Ripe: starchy and slightly sweet. Used in various cuisines. |
| Pleurisy Root | | X | | | | | | | Bitter. Not consumed as food. Used in traditional medicine. |
| Poke Root | | X | | | | | | | Extreme bitterness. Not consumed as food, due to potential toxicity. |
| Pomegranate | | | | | | X | X | | Sweet with a hint of tartness. Used in dishes and beverages. |
| Poplar | | | X | | | | | | No taste. Not consumed as food. Used for potential medicinal properties. |
| Prickly Ash | X | X | | X | | | | | Astringent, can be bitter. Tingling or numbing sensation contributes to pungent, spicy quality. |
| Prune | | | | | | | X | | Sweet and slightly tangy. Used in culinary applications. |
| Psyllium | | | X | | | | | | No taste. Used as a dietary fiber supplement. Mixed with water or other liquids. |
| Pumpkin | | | | | | | X | | Mildly sweet. Used in sweet dishes and desserts. |
| Pumpkin Seed | | | X | | | | | | Neutral, slightly nutty taste. Can be influenced by how they are prepared. |
| Puncture Vine | | X | | | | | | | Bitter. Not consumed as food. Used in traditional medicine. |
| Purslane | | | | | | X | | | Mildly slightly sour or tangy flavor. Subtle citrus like taste. Used in salads. |
| Raspberry Leaf | X | X | | | | | | | Astringent or slightly bitter. Is often used for herbal teas. |
| Red Clover | | | | | | | X | | Slightly sweet. Used in herbal teas. |
| Rehmannia | | X | | | | | X | | Sweet and slightly bitter. Commonly used in traditional Chinese medicine. |

| Herbs In Alphabetical Order | Astringent | Bitter | No Taste | Pungent | Salty | Sour | Sweet | Umami | Details |
|---|---|---|---|---|---|---|---|---|---|
| Reishi mushrooms | | X | | | | | | | Strong bitterness. Not consumed as food. Used in traditional Chinese medicine. |
| Rhodiola | | X | | | | | | | Bitter. Usually in traditional medicine and consumed as a supplement. |
| Rhubarb | | | | | | X | | | Sour. Sugar is often added to balance out the tartness. Commonly used in cooking & baking. |
| Rose | | | | | | | X | | Sweet and floral. Used to add delicate sweetness to various dishes and beverages. |
| Rosemary | | X | | X | | | | | Pungent, resinous flavor, with slight bitterness. Adds depth to a variety of dishes. |
| Rue | | X | | X | | | | | Bitter & pungent. A strong sharp flavor. Can be toxic. |
| Saffron | | | | | | | X | | Subtle sweetness with floral and earthy notes. It imparts a unique flavor to dishes. |
| Sage | | X | | X | | | | | Pungent with a strong, slightly bitter & earthy flavor. Used in cooking, especially savory dishes. |
| Sarsaparilla | | X | | | | | X | | Sweet, slightly bitter, and a mild root beer-like taste. Commonly uses in beverages. |
| Savory | | | | X | | | | | Pungent with earthy, minty, and peppery notes. Used in culinary applications. |
| Schisandra | | X | | X | X | X | X | | Bitter, pungent, salty, sour, & sweet flavors. Used in teas, infusions, tinctures, & extracts. |
| Senna | | X | | | | | | | Bitter. Not consumed as food. Often used as for laxative properties. |
| Sesame Seeds | | | | | | | X | | Slightly sweet and nutty. Used in baking, cooking, and garnishing various dishes. |
| Shatavari | | X | | | | | X | | Sweet and bitter, with a cooling effect. Commonly used in Ayurvedic medicine. |
| Shepherd's Purse | X | X | | | | | | | Slightly bitter and astringent. The leaves are edible and used in salads or cooked dishes. |
| Shiitake Mushroom | | | | | | | | X | Rich umami flavor. Savory and meaty. Used in traditional and modern dishes. |
| Shilajit | | X | | | | | | | Bitter and earthy flavor. Used in traditional Ayurvedic medicine. |
| Siberian Ginseng | | X | | | | | | | Not used for culinary purposes. Traditionally used in herbal medicine. |
| Skullcap | | X | | | | | | | Bitter. Used in traditional herbal remedies or teas. |
| Slippery Elm | | | | | | | X | | Mucilaginous and slightly sweet. Primarily used medicinally in teas and formulations. |
| Spearmint | | | | X | | | X | | Sweet and slightly pungent. Milder than peppermint. Used in teas, beverages, and dishes. |
| Spirulina | | X | | | | | | | Slightly bitter or seaweed-like. Used in smoothies, juices, or recipes that blend other tastes. |
| Squaw Vine | | | X | | | | | | No taste. Historically used in Native American and folk medicine. |
| St. John's Wort | | X | | | | | | | Bitter. Not used for culinary purposes. Traditionally used in herbal medicines. |
| Stinging Nettle | | X | | | | | | | Slightly bitter. Used in culinary applications. Leaves used in teas and infusions. |
| Suma | | | | | | | X | | Slightly sweet & earthy flavor. Used in traditional medicine, not used in culinary applications. |
| Sweet Annie | | X | | | | | | | Slightly bitter. Used for medicinal purposes. Also known as sweet wormwood. |
| Sweet Cicely | | | | | | | X | | Sweet and anise-like flavor. Used to sweeten dishes: desserts, salads, and beverages. |
| Sweet Root | | | | | | | X | | Licorice root that is sweet. Used in herbal teas, candies, and various dishes. |
| Tansy | | X | | | | | | | Bitter. Historically used in culinary applications. Can be toxic in large quantities. |
| Tea Tree Oil | | | X | | | | | | Not ingested. Used for topical applications and aromatherapy. Can be toxic. |
| Teasel Root | | | X | | | | | | No taste. Not used for culinary purposes. Traditionally used in herbal medicines. |
| Thuja | | | X | | | | | | Not consumed as food. Can be toxic when ingested. Used for medicinal purposes. |
| Thyme | | | | X | | | X | | Pungent and savory, may have sweet undertones. Used in culinary applications. |
| Tinospora Cordifolia | | X | | | | | | | Bitter. Used in traditional medicine. Especially Ayurveda medicine. |
| Tormentil | X | X | | | | | | | Astringent and bitter. Used in teas and as a flavoring agent. |
| Tulsi | X | X | | X | | | X | | Slightly astringent, mildly bitter, sweet undertones, & subtle pungency. Wide culinary uses. |
| Turkey Rhubarb | X | X | | | | | | | Astringent and bitter. Not consumed as food. Used in traditional medicine. |
| Turmeric | | X | | X | | | | | Mildly bitter, earthy undertones, pungent, and peppery. Used in savory & sweet dishes. |
| Usnea | X | X | | | | | | | Bitter and astringent. Not consumed as food. Used in traditional medicine. |
| Uva Ursi | X | X | | | | | | | Astringent & slightly bitter. It is primarily used for medicine, not culinary taste. Can be toxic. |
| Valerian | | X | | | | | | | Strong, earthy, and somewhat bitter. Not consumed for taste. Used in teas & supplements. |
| Vervain | | X | | | | | | | Bitter. Not used for culinary purposes. Traditionally used in herbal medicines. |
| Weld | | | X | | | | | | Not commonly consumed for taste, can be used medicinally. |
| White Oak | X | | | | | | | | Astringent. Not commonly consumed for taste. Traditionally used medicinally. |
| White Oak Bark | X | | | | | | | | Astringent. Not commonly consumed for taste. Traditionally used medicinally. |
| White Willow | | X | | | | | | | Bitter. Not used for culinary purposes. Traditionally used in herbal medicines. |
| White Willow Bark | | X | | | | | | | Bitter. Not used for culinary purposes. Traditionally used in herbal medicines. |
| Wild Cherry Bark | | X | | | | | | | Bitter. Not used for culinary purposes. Traditionally used in herbal medicines. |
| Chamomile | | X | | | | | | | Bitter. Not used for culinary purposes. Traditionally used in herbal medicines. |
| Wild Yam | X | X | | | | | | | Astringent and bitter. Not used for culinary purposes. Traditionally used in herbal medicines. |
| Willow | X | X | | | | | | | Astringent and bitter. Not used for culinary purposes. Traditionally used in herbal medicines. |
| Willow Bark | X | X | | | | | | | Astringent and bitter. Not used for culinary purposes. Traditionally used in herbal medicines. |
| Wintergreen | | | | | | | X | | Sweet and minty. Used in food and beverages to provide a minty and refreshing taste. |
| Witch Hazel | X | | | | | | | | Astringent. Not consumed for taste. Traditionally used medicinally. Can be toxic. |
| Wood Betony | | X | | | | | | | Mildly bitter. Used for potential medicinal properties rather than its culinary uses. |
| Wormseed | | X | | X | | | | | Pungent. Strong, herbal, & slightly bitter. Used in Mexican and Central American cuisines. |
| Wormwood | | X | | | | | | | Intensely bitter. Often used to produce the alcoholic beverage absinthe. |
| Yarrow | | X | | | | | | | Bitter. Used in herbal teas or infusions. Small amounts add flavor to certain dishes. |
| Yellow Dock | | X | | | | | | | Bitter. Not used for culinary purposes. Traditionally used in herbal medicines. |
| Yerba Mate | | X | | | | | | | Bitter, with earthy & vegetal undertones. Used as a tea. Sweeteners added to balance taste. |
| Yerba Santa | X | X | | | | | | | Bitter & somewhat astringent. Not used for culinary purposes. Used in herbal medicines. |

# SECTION VI

Alphabetized Herbs with Safety Profiles

REMINDER: Consult your medical care provider before using herbs.  Especially if you have an existing medical condition, take prescription medications, or are pregnant or nursing.

People can react differently to a variety of herbs, including allergic reactions.  The use of herbs may interfere with the effectiveness of other medications.  Some herbs may be confused with harmful substances, and can have adverse or deadly consequences.

Considering the issues mentioned you should consult with your medical professional before using herbs.  Your medical professional can discuss diagnosis and treatment options with you.

| Herbs in Alphabetical Order | Toxic | Safe While Pregnant or Lactating |
|---|---|---|
| Agrimony | No | Yes |
| Albizia | No | No |
| Alder Buckthorn | Yes | No |
| Alfalfa | No | Yes-No high doses when pregnant |
| Allspice | No | Yes |
| Aloe Vera | Yes-In large quantities | No-Internally  Yes-Externally |
| Aloe Vera Leaf | Yes-In large quantities | No-Internally  Yes-Externally |
| Alum | Yes-In large quantities | No |
| American Ginseng | No | No |
| American Skullcap | No | No |
| Andrographis | No | No |
| Angelica | No | No |
| Anise seeds | No | Yes |
| Arjuna | No | No |
| Arnica | Yes-internally | No |
| Artichoke | No | Yes |
| Ashitaba | No | No |
| Ashwagandha | No | No |
| Aspen | No | Yes-Pregnancy No-lactating |
| Astragalus | No | Yes-Pregnancy No-lactating |
| Baneberry | Yes | No |
| Barberry | No | No |
| Basil | No | No |
| Bayberry | No | No |
| Bay Leaves | No | No |
| Bearberry | Yes-In large quantities | No |
| Bee Balm | No | No |
| Bergamot | No | No |
| Bilberry | No | Yes |
| Birch | No | Yes |
| Bitter Leaf | No | No |
| Bitter Melon | No | No |
| Black Cohosh | No | No |
| Black Current | No | Yes |
| Black-eyed Susan | No | No |
| Black haw | No | Yes-Pregnancy No-lactating |
| Black hellebore | Yes | No |
| Black Horehound | No | No |
| Black Mustard | No | Yes |
| Black Pepper | No | Yes-except large doses when pregnant |
| Black Seed | No | No |
| Black Walnut Hull | Yes | No |
| Blackberry | No | Yes-Pregnancy No-lactating |
| Blackberry Leaf | No | No |
| Blessed Thistle | Yes | No |
| Bloodroot | Yes | No |
| Blue Cohosh | Yes | No |
| Blue Flag | Yes | No |
| Blue Vervain | No | No |
| Boldo | Yes | No |
| Boneset | Yes-In large quantities | No |
| Borage | No | No |
| Boswellia | No | No |
| Brigham tea | No | Yes |
| Buchu | Yes | No |
| Buckthorn | Yes | No |
| Bugleweed | No | No |
| Bupleurum | No | No |
| Burdock | No | Yes |
| Burdock Root | No | Yes |
| Butcher's Broom | No | No |

| Herbs in Alphabetical Order | Toxic | Safe While Pregnant or Lactating |
| --- | --- | --- |
| Cacao | No | Yes |
| Calendula | No | No-pregnancy Yes-lactating |
| California Poppy | No | No |
| Camphor | Yes | No |
| Cannabis | No | No |
| Caraway | No | No-pregnancy Yes-lactating |
| Cardamom | No | Yes |
| Cascara amarga | Yes | No |
| Cascara sagrada | Yes | No |
| Cascarilla | No | No |
| Cassia | Yes-In large quantities | No |
| Catnip | No | Yes |
| Cat's Claw | No | Yes |
| Cayenne | No | No-large amount while pregnant  Yes-lactation |
| Celery | No | No |
| Celery Seed | No | No |
| Centaury | No | No |
| Chamomile (german) | No | Yes |
| Chanca Piedra | No | No |
| Chaparral | Yes | No |
| Chaste Tree | No | No |
| Chenopodium Oil | Yes | No |
| Chia Seeds | No | Yes |
| Chickpeas | No | Yes |
| Chickweed | No | Yes-Pregnancy No-lactating |
| Chicory | No | Yes |
| Chicory Root | No | Yes |
| Chlorella | No | Yes |
| Cilantro | No | Yes |
| Cinnamon | No | No-In large amounts |
| Cinquefoil | No | No |
| Cleavers | No | No |
| Clematis | Yes | No |
| Cloves | No | No |
| Coleus Forskohlii | No | No |
| Coltsfoot | Yes | No |
| Comfrey | Yes | No |
| Cordyceps | No | No |
| Coriander | No | Yes |
| Corn Silk | No | No |
| Cotton Root Bark | Yes | No |
| Couchgrass | No | No |
| Cramp Bark | No | Yes |
| Cranberry | No | Yes |
| Cranesbill | No | No |
| Cumin | No | No |
| Cypress | Yes | No |
| Damiana | No | No |
| Dandelion | No | Yes |
| Dandelion Root | No | Yes |
| Danshen | No | No |
| Devil's Claw | No | No |
| Dill | No | No |
| Dill Seed | No | No |
| Dong Quai | No | No |
| Echinacea | No | Yes |
| Elder | Yes | No |
| Elderberry | Yes-when raw/unripe | No |
| Elderflower | No | No |
| Elecampane | No | No |
| Eleuthero | No | No |

| Herbs in Alphabetical Order | Toxic | Safe While Pregnant or Lactating |
| --- | --- | --- |
| Eucalyptus | Yes | No |
| Fennel | No | No |
| Fennel Seeds | No | No |
| Fenugreek | No | No |
| Feverfew | No | No |
| Fireweed | No | No |
| Flax | No | No |
| Fo Ti Root | Yes | No |
| Fringe Tree | No | No |
| Frankincense | No | No |
| French Lavendar | No | No |
| Garden Sage | No | No |
| Garlic | No | No-In large amounts |
| Gentian | No | No |
| Geranium | No | No |
| Germander | Yes | No |
| Ginger | No | No |
| Ginkgo | No | No |
| Ginkgo Biloba | No | No |
| Ginseng | No | No |
| Globe Artichoke | No | No |
| Goat's Rue | Yes | No |
| Goldenrod | No | No |
| Goldenseal | No | No |
| Gotu Kola | No | No |
| Gravel Root | No | No |
| Greater Celandine | Yes | No |
| Green Tea | No | No-In large amounts |
| Guarana | No | No |
| Gumweed | No | Yes |
| Hawthorn | No | No |
| Hibiscus | No | No |
| Hollyhock | No | No |
| Holy Basil | No | No |
| Hops | No | No |
| Horehound | No | No |
| Horse Chestnut | Yes | No |
| Horsemint | No | No |
| Horseradish | No | No |
| Horsetail | No | No |
| Hydrangea Root | No | No |
| Hyssop | No | No |
| Indian Gooseberry | No | Yes |
| Irish Moss | No | No |
| Jamaican Dogwood | Yes | No |
| Japanese Knotweed | No | No |
| Jiaogulan | No | No |
| Juniper | Yes | No |
| Juniper Berries | Yes | No |
| Kava Kava | Yes | No |
| Kelp | No | No |
| Kola Nut | No | No |
| Korean Ginseng | No | No |
| Kratom | Yes | No |
| Lady's Mantle | No | No |
| Lamb's Ear | No | No |
| Lavendar | No | Yes |
| Lemon | No | Yes |
| Lemon Balm | No | Yes |
| Lemon Grass | No | No |
| Lemon Verbana | No | No |

| Herbs in Alphabetical Order | Toxic | Safe While Pregnant or Lactating |
|---|---|---|
| Licorice | Yes | No |
| Licorice Root | Yes | No |
| Lily of the Valley | Yes | No |
| Linden | No | No |
| Lobelia | Yes | No |
| Lomatium | Yes | No |
| Lovage | No | No |
| Maca | No | No |
| Maca Root | No | No |
| Male Fern | Yes | No |
| Mallow | No | No |
| Marjoram | No | No |
| Marshmallow | No | Yes |
| Marshmallow Root | No | Yes |
| Meadowsweet | No | No |
| Milk Thistle | No | Yes |
| Mint | No | No-In large amounts |
| Mistletoe | Yes | No |
| Motherwort | No | No |
| Mucuna Pruriens | No | No |
| Mugwort | Yes-In large quantities | No |
| Mullein | No | No |
| Mustard | No | Yes |
| Myrrh | No | No |
| Nasturtium | No | No |
| Neem | Yes | No |
| Nettles | No | Yes-leaves |
| Oak Bark | Yes | No |
| Oak Moss | Yes | No |
| Oat Straw | No | Yes |
| Oats | No | Yes |
| Okra | No | Yes |
| Olive | No | Yes |
| Olive Leaf | No | No |
| Onion | No | Yes |
| Oregano | No | No |
| Oregon Grape | Yes | No |
| Oregon Grape Root | Yes | No |
| Panax ginseng | No | No |
| Papaya Seed | Yes | No |
| Parsley | No | No |
| Parsley Root | No | No |
| Passionflower | No | No |
| Passionvine | No | No |
| Pau D'Arco | No | No |
| Pennyroyal | Yes | No |
| Peppermint | No | Yes |
| Pineapple Bromelain | No | No |
| Plantain | No | Yes |
| Pleurisy Root | No | No |
| Poke Root | Yes | No |
| Pomegranate | No | No |
| Poplar | No | No |
| Prickly Ash | No | No |
| Prune | No | No |
| Psyllium | No | Yes |
| Pumpkin | No | Yes |
| Pumpkin Seed | No | Yes |
| Puncture Vine | No | No |
| Purselane | No | No |
| Raspberry Leaf | No | Yes |

| Herbs in Alphabetical Order | Toxic | Safe While Pregnant or Lactating |
|---|---|---|
| Red Clover | No | No |
| Rehmannia | No | No |
| Reishi mushrooms | No | No |
| Rhodiola | No | No |
| Rhubarb | Yes | No |
| Rose | No | No |
| Rosemary | No | No-pregnancy Yes-lactating |
| Rue | Yes | No |
| Saffron | Yes | No |
| Sage | No | No |
| Sarsaparilla | No | No |
| Savory | No | No |
| Schisandra | No | No |
| Senna | Yes | No |
| Sesame Seeds | No | Yes |
| Shatavari | No | Yes |
| Shepherd's Purse | No | No |
| Shiitake Mushroom | No | Yes |
| Shilajit | No | No |
| Siberian Ginseng | No | No |
| Skullcap | No | Yes |
| Slippery Elm | No | Yes |
| Spearmint | No | No-In large amounts |
| Spirulina | No | No |
| Squaw Vine | No | No |
| St. John's Wort | Yes | No |
| Stinging Nettle | No | No |
| Suma | No | No |
| Sweet Annie | Yes | No |
| Sweet Cicely | No | No |
| Sweet Root | Yes | No |
| Tansy | Yes | No |
| Tea Tree Oil | Yes-if ingested | No |
| Teasel Root | No | No |
| Thuja | Yes | No |
| Thyme | No | No |
| Tinospora Cordifolia | No | No |
| Tormentil | No | No |
| Tulsi | No | No |
| Turkey Rhubarb | Yes | No |
| Turmeric | No | Yes |
| Usnea | Yes-internal use | No |
| Uva Ursi | Yes | No |
| Valerian | No | Yes-Pregnancy No-lactating |
| Vervain | No | No |
| Weld | No | No |
| White Oak | Yes | No |
| White Oak Bark | Yes | No |
| White Willow | Yes | No |
| White Willow Bark | Yes | No |
| Wild Cherry Bark | Yes | No |
| Wild Indigo | Yes | No |
| Wild Yam | No | No |
| Willow | Yes | No |
| Willow Bark | Yes | No |
| Wintergreen | Yes | No |
| Witch Hazel | No | No |
| Wood Betony | No | No |
| Wormseed | Yes | No |
| Wormwood | Yes | No |
| Yarrow | No | No |

| Herbs in Alphabetical Order | Toxic | Safe While Pregnant or Lactating |
| --- | --- | --- |
| Yellow Dock | Yes | No |
| Yerba Mate | No | No |
| Yerba Santa | No | No |

www.ingramcontent.com/pod-product-compliance
Lightning Source LLC
Chambersburg PA
CBHW081604270726
48661CB00020B/3662